WE HAVE NO MICROBES HERE

Carolina Academic Press
Ethnographic Studies in Medical Anthropology Series

Pamela J. Stewart *and* Andrew Strathern
Series Editors

Curing and Healing
Medical Anthropology in Global Perspective
Andrew Strathern *and* Pamela Stewart

Elusive Fragments
Making Power, Propriety and Health in Samoa
Douglass D. Drozdow-St. Christian

Endangered Species
Health, Illness, and Death Among Madagascar's People of the Forest
Janice Harper

Physicians at Work, Patients in Pain
Biomedical Practice and Patient Response in Mexico
Kaja Finkler

Healing the Modern in a Central Javanese City
Steve Ferzacca

The Practice of Concern
Ritual, Well-Being, and Aging in Rural Japan
John W. Traphagan

The Gene and the Genie
Tradition, Medicalization and Genetic Counseling
in a Bedouin Community in Israel
Aviad E. Raz

Social Discord and Bodily Disorders
Healing Among the Yupno of Papua New Guinea
Verena Keck

Indigenous Peoples and Diabetes
Community Empowerment and Wellness
Mariana Leal Ferreira *and* Gretchen Chesley Lang

We Have No Microbes Here
Healing Practices in a Turkish Black Sea Village
Sylvia Wing Önder

WE HAVE NO MICROBES HERE

Healing Practices in a Turkish Black Sea Village

Sylvia Wing Önder
GEORGETOWN UNIVERSITY

CAROLINA ACADEMIC PRESS
Durham, North Carolina

Library of Congress Cataloging-in-Publication Data

Önder, Sylvia Wing.
We have no microbes here : healing practices in a Turkish Black Sea village /
by Sylvia Wing Önder.
    p. cm. -- (Ethnographic studies in medical anthropology)
    Includes bibliographical references.
    ISBN-13: 978-0-89089-573-3
    ISBN-10: 0-89089-573-2
    1. Medical anthropology--Turkey--Medreseönü.
    2. Traditional medicine--Turkey--Medreseönü.
    3. Healing--Turkey--Medreseönü. 4. Women--Medical care--
    Turkey--Medreseönü. 5. Medreseönü (Turkey)--Social life and customs.
    I. Title. II. Series: Carolina Academic Press ethnographic studies in
    medical anthropology series.

GN296.5.T9O53 2005
306.4'61'09561--dc22   2005012970

CAROLINA ACADEMIC PRESS
700 Kent Street
Durham, NC 27701
Telephone (919)489-7486
Fax (919)493-5668
www.cap-press.com

Printed in the United States of America
2019 Printing

Dedicated to Our Mothers

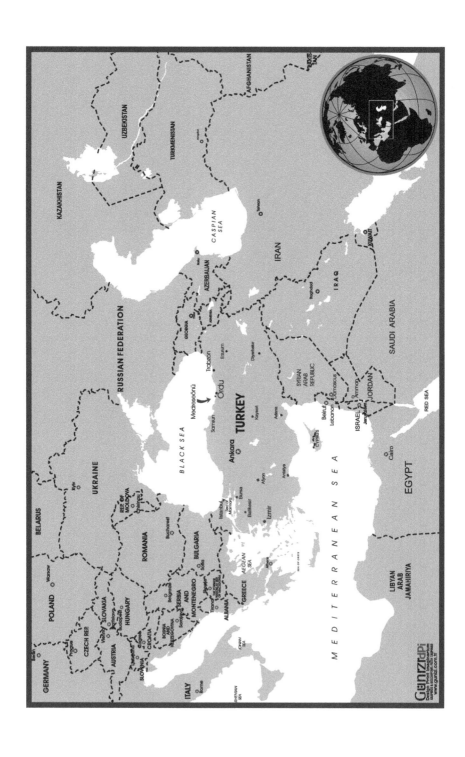

CONTENTS

Acknowledgments

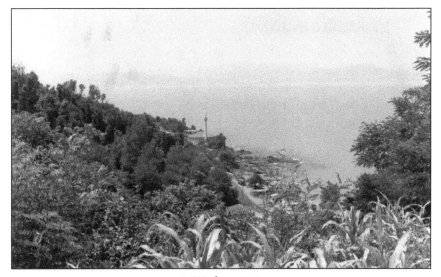

1. Medreseönü

The research and writing of this book would have been impossible without Muammer Önder, whose help with cultural translation and tape transcriptions was invaluable for me and trying for him. His nurturing care for family and friends keeps alive the spirit of Black Sea health care traditions. I thank him for his help with our son, Timur, whose birth was a blessing and whose sunny presence furthered my fieldwork in countless ways.

My mother-in-law, Hamide Önder, inspired me to study traditional healing practices, helped me establish contacts for research, and always exemplified the dynamic combination of inspired innovation and wisdom based on long experience. My father-in-law, İsmail Önder, indulged me with his patience and good-humor.

My parents, Robert and Ingrid Wing, supported my extended academic term and my international adventures. Losing my mother, my great aunt

Sylvia, and my paternal grandmother brought into sharp focus the valuable contributions of female elders. I miss them more than I can express. My grandmother, Gudrun McCowen continues to inspire me from afar with her love and healing circle efforts. I am grateful for all members of my growing family in England, the U.S., Turkey, and beyond—thank you all.

From the Black Sea region, I wish to thank Ayşe and Seyfi Doğan and their daughters Ümran, Nurcan, Gurcan, and Gülsen; Gulşen and Aytun Şahin and their children Canan, Ercan, and Erkan; Nurşen Önder and her children Banu and Baran; Hatice and Hüsamettin Kaya and their children Nihal, Yavuz, and Büşra; and Sezin and Sultan Önder and their newly arrived Afra. Also helpful from gürbet were Sezer and Güller Önder and their sons İsmail, Ünal, and Vedat, as well as their daughters-in-law. I thank Nurten Önder, her mother, her sons Erhan, Tevrat, Tefik, her daughters Rahime and Hayriye, and her daughters-in-law, particularly Emine.

I would like to thank Zekiya Çelebi, Hava and Ahmet Önder, Yeter and Tuncay Doğan, Seyhan and Berhan Önder, Leyla Doğan, Emine Doğan, the Hacigiller, Doctor Halil İbrahim Akbulut, Nurse Rabiye Şahin, Nurse Günnaz Can, Clinic Manager Yusuf Genç, Midwife Nurten Şahin, Midwife Serpil Yavus, Midwife Necla Yardım, her grandmother Zeynep Yıldız, Midwife Nebahat Akkaya, and Secretary Ersin Yılmaz. Medreseönü Mayor Şahin and his successors have graciously allowed me to conduct research in the local villages. Mine and Işın Önder gave me insights into the lives of career nurses.

This study would have been impossible without the assistance and sparkling insights of my graduate school advisers at The Ohio State University, Drs. Pat Mullen, Amy Shuman, and Sabra Webber. As for Dr. Victoria Holbrook, "her ocean encircles both East and West in waves of immersion and discernment." Dr. Richard Davis deserves special thanks for his willingness to substitute on my examination committee.

I wish to acknowledge Dr. Alam Payind, Director of The Ohio State University Middle East Center, not only for his assistance in acquiring funding which helped support this research, through U. S. Title VI Grants, but also for running down a purse-snatcher in Istanbul and thereby saving my passport.

The development of the ideas expressed in this study was encouraged and shaped over the years by Drs. Ahmet Evin, Talat Halman, Walter Feldman, Henry Glassie, Margaret Mills, David Hufford, Marina Roseman, Alma Kunanbaeva, Nan Johnson, Margarita Mazo, Erika Bourguignon, Walter Andrews, Asım Karaömerlioğlu, Erika Gilson, Uli Schamiloglu, and from Georgetown University, Karin Ryding, Scott Redford, Walter Armbrust, Susan

Ossman, and many students and colleagues from the Arabic Department and the Division of Eastern Mediterranean Languages, the College, and the School of Foreign Service. I have been assisted at Georgetown by Middle East Librarian Brenda Bickett, by the staff in the Language Laboratory, especially Peter Janssens, and by Mary Ruof of the Kennedy Institute of Ethics.

While undertaking the writing of this study, I received teaching support from the Institute of Turkish Studies, under the direction of Dr. Sabri Sayarı. Federal support was made available to me through Title VI funding through two Georgetown centers: The National Resource Center on the Middle East and the Center for Eurasian, Russian, and East European Studies, as well as from the National Middle East Language Resource Center.

I wish to thank the Georgetown University Anthropology Reading Group for advice on earlier versions of this work, the American Association of Teachers of Turkic Languages for moral support, and Roger Wing and Laura Cutler for editing help—the remaining faults are mine alone.

There are many more friends and colleagues who helped me along the way, in Turkey (particularly in Istanbul, Ankara, Alanya, and Medreseönü), and in the U.S. (particularly in Philadelphia, Columbus, Annapolis, and Washington). I beg indulgence for not listing names—your contributions enrich my work and my life.

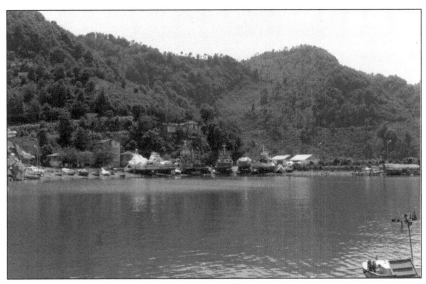

2. A Black Sea Village Port

Important in the final stages of writing this book was the guidance and careful text editing of series editors Dr. Pamela J. Stewart and Dr. Andrew Strathern from the Anthropology Department at the University of Pittsburgh. Greatly appreciated is the help of Carolina Academic Press Acquisitions Editor Bob Conrow, Senior Editor Linda Lacy, Publisher Keith Sipe, Marketing Manager Jennifer Whaley, and Production Managers Erin Ehman and Reuben Ayres (who have had to become experts in the Turkish alphabet), and Tim Colton, who created the cover design.

For the map used in this book, thanks go to Fatih and Türkan Taşpınar of Günizi in Alanya, Turkey.

SERIES EDITORS' PREFACE

Pamela J. Stewart and Andrew Strathern

We Have No Microbes Here: Healing Practices in a Turkish Black Sea Village is a rich ethnographic work that is a delight to read. The work fits neatly into the Ethnographic Studies in Medical Anthropology Series, highlighting a range of topics that are important in many contexts inside of and outside of Turkey.

From our own areas of expertise and regions where we have conducted research, including the Pacific, Asia, and Europe, we will explore a few of these topical themes here.

"Evil Eye"

Önder discusses the beliefs in *nazar* ("Evil Eye") in her study area and the wider belief in this phenomenon amongst Muslims. As a comparative point we note here that historically throughout Europe links between witchcraft and the use of the Evil Eye have been noted.

The church in Medieval Europe played a strong role in associating witchcraft with the Devil. Thus, the acts of those said to be witches were labeled as both dangerous and sinful. This, among many complex factors, then, influenced the infamous witch-hunts in Europe (see Stewart and Strathern 2004 for discussions of witchcraft and the role of rumor and gossip in the persecution of individuals). An escalation in witchcraft fears occurred in post-Reformation times during the sixteenth and seventeenth centuries as waves of hysteria led to witch trials in England, Scotland, Switzerland, Germany and France. During this time as many as 100,000 people may have been prosecuted as witches. Those afraid of being accused were eager to point a finger at others so as to divert accusing eyes from themselves. At least 75% of those accused of being witches were women who were either single or widowed and were propertyless. Those accused were vigorously interrogated and physically pressurized so as to obtain confessions of witchcraft deeds (Duiker and Spielvogel 1998: 547–549). And anti-witchcraft legislation was enacted in European countries that was used to accuse, arrest, torture, legally find guilty, and burn to death those said to be witches (Sidky 1997: 23).

As various political and religious upheavals subsided by the mid-seventeenth century in Europe so did the hysteria over witchcraft. But the fundamental belief in powers to induce misfortune in the affairs of others persisted. An intriguing example of this is evidenced by R.C. Maclagan's study on the Evil Eye that was conducted among the Gaelic-speaking people of the Western Highlands and the Islands off the coast of Scotland during the nineteenth century (1902). As for European witchcraft in general, much has been written about the topic of the Evil Eye in Europe. A subject search on the Internet produces a wealth of information on the topic and references to the literature. The effects of Evil Eye are said to center on the "natural covetousness of the greedy person" using this "diabolical" power which can cause sickness and death in people and livestock. The main outcome of the use of Evil Eye is to diminish what another person possesses, whether that be good health, wealth, or luck. Maclagan quotes an Argyllshire islander as saying: "Witchcraft is all gone now, and it is well it is, for it was a bad thing. But if that is gone, there is another thing that has not gone yet, and that is *Cronachadh* [the misfortunes produced by the use of Evil Eye]. I saw a breeding sow in my own house, and one day a neighbour came in, and she said that that was a splendid sow.... Well, the woman went out, and she was no time away when the sow gave such a scream, and going round about she fell on the floor" (p. 12). This is a typical example of the sorts of stories that Maclagan was told. They involve a person who possesses something that is negatively impacted by the jealous gaze of another. In this particular story the sow did not die but recovered.

Unlike the narrative of the Argyllshire man, other people did not believe that witchcraft had disappeared and maintained that it and the Evil Eye worked in concert to produce misfortunes. An Islay man defined the functioning of the Evil Eye : "Those who have this eye will do injury to beast or person, though they do nothing but look on them" (p. 18). Many of the farmers and those working in fishing in the area that Maclagan studied narrated stories of Evil Eye, and often particular persons were identified as known possessors of these powers. A minister told Maclagan that "The possession was more frequently ascribed to females than to males, and for the most part to elderly women" (p. 24). Another minister said, "They were chiefly women that were suspected, and were generally much disliked in the communities" (ibid.).

Various sorts of devices were described as working to keep the Evil Eye from functioning to cause damage. One of the preventive measures used to protect cows from the Evil Eye, as well as protecting butter and milk from being stolen by witches, was to tie a sprig of a rowan tree to the tail of the cow or in the case of the product of the animal to the butter churn or milk container (Maclagan, pp. 119–120). Another measure was to spit onto the object that the Evil Eye fell upon. An example of this was given by a Ross-shire minister: "A woman there had a child of about nine months old. Another woman came in, and looking at the child on its mother's arm, remarked,... 'You have a pretty, dear boy there.' Without more ado the mother turned the child's face to her and began to spit in it as hard as she could to prevent any bad effect from the other woman's Evil Eye" (p. 126). Maclagan suggests that this practice may be considered to quench the heat (fire) of the Evil Eye, extinguishing its potentially damaging effects.

Another item used in curing the Evil Eye was an *a' chlach nathrach* (the serpent's stone). These were said to be usually round with one hole through them or in some instances two holes through them. The popular account of these given to Maclagan was that "A number of serpents congregating at certain times form themselves into a knot and move around and round on the stone until a hole is worn. They then pass and repass after each other through the hole, leaving a coating of slime round the hole, which by-and-by becomes hard" (p. 170). This congealed slime is said to give the stone healing properties when used to counter Evil Eye effects. The stone would be used along with water which was poured onto the stone and over the person or animal affected. Maclagan states that he tried to obtain one of these eyed healing stones but was told that they were too valuable in curing to relinquish (p. 171).

Of course, the idea of the Evil Eye is spread much more widely throughout the world. It passed with Hispanic traditions from the Mediterranean into the New World; and it is a basic notion underpinning fears of witchcraft in parts of the Pacific region, for example among the Duna people of Papua New Guinea, where it is thought to fall especially from jealous bystanders on fine cuts of pork received in feasts.

From Turkey itself, the medical anthropologist Byron Good has noted that the Evil Eye may be given as a explanation for the onset of illnesses in people (Good 1994: 148–58). Either the Evil Eye or attacks by *jinn* spirits may be cited. In one case a child had tonic-clonic seizures (epilepsy), and the researchers were told: "In essence it happened to him because of an evil eye. There is a woman in the village, if she looks at you she destroys you. That woman looked at him when he was eight months old, the next morning he couldn't speak. His mouth foamed" (p. 150). In this instance the explanation was clear. Evil Eye used against infants is a very common cross-cultural theme. Mothers in the Mount Hagen area of Papua New Guinea in the 1960s would hide their infants' faces from passers-by, particularly from strangers or from other women suspected of being witches, in case their hostile gaze might cause the child to fall sick and die. In circumstances where infant morbidity and mortality rates are high, or are remembered to have been high in the recent past, such fears are strongly reinforced by experiencing the actual deaths of children. Since reproduction of children is so important for local agriculturally based communities, it is obvious that the fear of others' envy also expresses the high value accorded to having healthy children. By a kind of social pact, people do not praise or refer to the healthy appearance of infants. To do so might bring on the envious attentions not only of those said to be witches but also of spirits of the dead who had died in unfavorable circumstances or without descendants, and therefore felt malevolent towards mothers with healthy, handsome children.

Reproductive Health and Practices

Önder provides us with a detailed and interesting set of observations on reproduction and fertility issues within her study area. Some of these are particularly intriguing and poignant observations about the impact of change on the practices of the community and the retention of older ways of dealing with gendered health care. Önder mentions briefly (chapter 7) the practice of burying the placenta and its meanings. We provide a few comparative points here from the Pacific (see Stewart and Strathern 2001: 84–97 for further details).

In the Highlands of Papua New Guinea many practices were followed to help to seek proper growth and fertility (see Strathern and Stewart 2000a: 72–3 for examples from the Hagen, Pangia, and Duna areas). Burial of the placenta formed a part of this cultural complex.

Among the Anganen of the Southern Highlands of Papua New Guinea (Merrett-Balkos 1998): "The umbilical cord is…known as the 'road'…between mother and child. Vital substance, *ip* [grease], flows from the mother to the unborn child along this path and the cord is the source of life for an infant. The *ip* which flows from mother to child comprises the food a woman eats, but it also conveys aspects of identity to the unborn". The connection of the fetus to the mother is referred to as *ronga*, to bind/fasten. *Ronga* and nurturance are sustained after birth through the breast feeding of milk , and through the use of the netbag (a symbolic extension of the womb that is used as a crib and carrier to transport infants, see MacKenzie 1991, and Stewart and Strathern 1997), which has special kinds of leaves placed in it to cushion the child, prevent its spirit from wandering during sleep, and to promote its growth (this practice was also found in Hagen and Pangia in the past). The Anganen mothers "consider themselves the archetypical nourishers and growers of children", (Merrett-Balkos, p. 222) partly because small children consume breast milk which the mother creates from the food that she grows and consumes on the father's land.

The placenta, *nu*, and its attached umbilical cord are either buried or placed high up in the crook of a tree. The *nu* has to be planted in the clan soil of the child's father, thereby fixing the child to the group of his father while at the same time, through the planting of the umbilical cord, strengthening the tie of the mother's connection to her husband's land. The umbilical cord is known as the 'road' and represents relatedness, thus the planting of the cord also affirms the mother's connection to her natal group through the connection that she establishes between affinally related men.

Merrett-Balkos explains further that women nowadays give birth to children in mission health care centers, where they are also fed from mission supplies and gardens. Each mother receives a section of her child's umbilical cord after the delivery, and she tends to keep this with her until she returns home and hides it near to her residence. The mothers themselves negotiate this arrangement in order to preserve the essentials of their previous cultural practices (Merrett-Balkos, p. 221).

The placenta and its associated umbilical cord are considered to be the child's 'base-place'. Merrett-Balkos writes that "the significance of the bond... between a child and its physiological, uterine source is infused with the meaning of the bond between clan members...Tree or ground burial of the placenta is the action which effects this fusion of meaning" (p. 225). In other words there is a metathesis or analogy made between the child's initial 'rootedness' in the mother and its subsequent 'rootedness' in its paternal clan territory. The analogy is given force by the metonymical action of taking and replanting the navel string in the clan ground of the father. But although this reveals a need to transform one kind of connection into another, in fact the tie with the mother and her group is permanent.

In the Hagen (Western Highlands Province, Papua New Guinea) area a comparable set of practics held in the past. The place where the placenta and part of the umbilical cord was buried or planted would be prepared by the child's father, who would make a fence of stakes around it and plant a cordyline sprig in it to mark the spot. Both the cordyline and the child were, from this time on, rooted in the child's paternal ground; yet they also represented the increment of substance brought to that ground by the mother.

"Tradition" and "Modernity"

Önder's study reveals the dynamic interactions between what we label as tradition and modernity in the networks of health care she studied. Particularly revealing are her discussions in chapters 5 and 6 of traditional curing practices held by women of the grandparental generation compared to the practices of clinicians. People expect to use the clinics; but they are also tied by kinship to local communal sources of knowledge, and they try pragmatically to use both resources. They try also to localize introduced practices, bringing them more into line with their own understandings and experience. Interesting here are Önder's accounts of front-stage and back-stage behavior in the clinics (chapter 8); and technical discussions between a doctor and a bone-setter (chapter 6).

While in practical terms people try to use both modern and traditional means of handling illness, Önder also portrays the conflicts between the urban and the rural, the young and the old, and the doctrinal "Islamists" from the cities, usually young males, who criticize the ways of older rural females. Given the emerging significance in the Islamic world of contrasts between Islamist movements of this kind and the diversities of folk cultural practices which have their roots far back in the Islamic past, Önder's discussion is diagnostic of a situation that goes much more widely than her immediate field area (see the essays in Stewart and Strathern 2005a on the multiplicity of Islamic practices in historical and contemporary instances).

In her chapter 1 Önder carefully points out how she is using the term "traditional". It is not a static, but a processual term, marking an ongoing dialectic between past and present: "a negotiation between what people know and what they learn as circumstances change," she writes. We have ourselves explored this dialectic extensively in our studies of the Hagen and Duna people in Papua New Guinea (Strathern and Stewart 2000b, 2004).

"Expressive Genres"

The presentation of poems and songs by Önder enriches the ethnographic presentation of her materials and provides an insight into the aesthetic component in the lives of the people discussed. It is important to present expressive genre materials since they are such an integral aspect of life and they hold much interpretative and philosophical meaning.

Time and again we find that the people themselves are the most adept at summing up their attitudes, problems, experiences, and feelings about their lives or their ideals. We have worked to give space for such voices of people in a number of our publications on Papua New Guinea, concentrating on songs, epics, and ballads (see Stewart and Strathern 2002, 2005b). Önder's inclusion of such materials in her study indicates both her commitment to a contemporary domain of folklore scholarship and her close appreciation of and understanding of people's lives.

As issues surrounding the potential or prospective entry of Turkey into the European Union grow in significance, this book can stand as a sympathetic but objective account of many of the social themes that are important in rural Turkish society, and so can help in the vital process of rendering the lives of people within an expanded vision of Europe intelligible to one another.

Önder's study will be of interest to those in Medical Anthropology, Gender Studies, Islamic Studies, General Anthropology of the wider Mediterranean region, European Studies, and Ritual Studies. Both students and established scholars will no doubt enjoy the narrative style that the author employs to present her research findings.

24 April 2005
University of Pittsburgh
Pittsburgh, PA, USA

REFERENCES

Duiker, William J. and Jackson J. Spielvogel 1998. *World History. Volume II: Since 1500*. 2ⁿᵈ edition. Belmont, CA: Wadsworth publishing.

Good, Byron J. 1994. *Medicine, Rationality, and Experience. An Anthropological Perspective*. Cambridge: Cambridge University Press.

Maclagan, R.C. 1902. *Evil Eye in the Western Highlands. London: David Nutt.*

Mackenzie, Maureen 1991. *Androgynous Objects, String Bags and Gender in Central New Guinea*. Philadelphia: Harwood Academic Publishers.

Merrett-Balkos, Leanne 1998. Just add water: remaking women through childbirth, Anganen, Southern Highlands, Papua New Guinea. In, *Maternities and Modernities. Colonial and Postcolonial Experiences in Asia and the Pacific*, Kalpana Ram and Margaret Jolly (eds.), pp 213–238. Cambridge: Cambridge University Press.

Sidky H. 1997. *Witchcraft, Lycanthropy, Drugs, and Disease. An Anthropological Study of the European Witch-Hunts*. New York: Peter Lang.

Stewart, Pamela J. and Andrew Strathern 1997. Netbags revisited: Cultural narratives from Papua New Gunea. *Pacific Studies* 20(2): 1–30.

Stewart, Pamela J. and Andrew Strathern 2001. *Humors and Substances: Ideas of the Body in New Guinea*. Westport, Conn. and London: Bergin and Garvey, Greenwood Publishing Group.

Stewart, Pamela J. and Andrew Strathern 2002. *Gender, Song, and Sensibility: Folktales and Folksongs in the Highlands of New Guinea*. Westport, Conn. and London: Praeger Publishers, Greenwood Publishing Group.

Stewart Pamela J. and Andrew Strathern 2004. *Witchcraft, Sorcery, Rumors, and Gossip*. For, New Departures in Anthropology Series, Cambridge: Cambridge University Press.

Stewart, Pamela J. and Andrew Strathern eds. 2005a. *Contesting Rituals: Islam and Practices of Identity-Making*. For, Ritual Studies Monograph Series, Durham: N.C.: Carolina Academic Press.

Stewart, Pamela J. and Andrew Strathern eds. 2005b. *Expressive Genres and Historical Change: Indonesia, Papua New Guinea, and Taiwan*. For, Anthropology and Cultural History in Asia and the Indo-Pacific Series, London: Ashgate Publishing.

Strathern and Stewart 2000a. *The Python's Back: Pathways of Comparison between Indonesia and Melanesia*. Westport, Conn. and London: Bergin and Garvey, Greenwood Publishing Group.

Strathern, Andrew and Pamela J. Stewart 2000b. *Arrow Talk: Transaction, Transition, and Contradiction in New Guinea Highlands History.* Kent, Ohio and London: Kent State University Press.

Strathern, Andrew and Pamela J. Stewart 2004. *Empowering the Past, Confronting the Future. The Duna People of Papua New Guinea.* For, Contemporary Anthropology of Religion Series, New York: Palgrave Macmillan.

WE HAVE NO MICROBES HERE

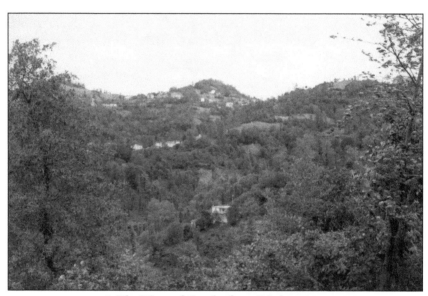

3. The View of Çandır from Medreseönü

CHAPTER 1

APPROACHES

The smooth-riding night bus from Istanbul descends from the high Anatolian plains to follow the twisting Black Sea coast road, rumbling through the gray and sleeping town of Samsun. The trip to Medreseönü takes about 12 hours, with frequent stop along the coast to discharge bleary-eyed and rumpled passengers at small bus depots on the side of the road. By the time it passes Fatsa, the sun is up to illuminate the tortured turns of the road as the bus roars up and around the peninsula which divides Fatsa from Ordu. Encroaching upon the road from above and falling away to the sea below, the verdant tangle of plant life is what Turks from elsewhere think of when they imagine the Black Sea—it is *yemyeşil*, very green. Although the steep hills look wild, they are intensely cultivated, producing a mixed crop of beans, corn, hazelnuts and walnuts, collard greens, many kinds of fruit, cucumbers, tomatoes, eggplant, mushrooms, and many types of herbs and edible greens. As the rising sun burns of the fog, women and children walk their family cows

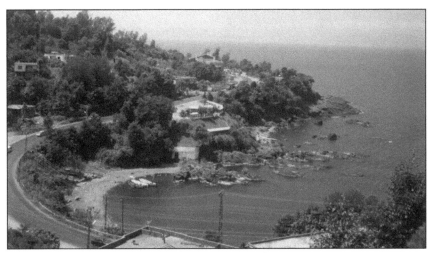

4. The Coast Road

to hazelnut groves to graze in the shaded grass. Men are sweeping the cement sidewalks in front of their businesses—coffeehouses, bus depots, barber shops, gas stations, grocery stores, appliance repair shops, restaurants, bakeries, and dry goods stores. If it is market day, vendors are arranging their colorful wares on push carts—hanging up ready-made shirts and dresses, building pyramids of tomatoes or melons, spreading out bright plastic tubs and buckets, or constructing towers of olive oil cans and detergent boxes.

This is the journey I have made periodically since the summer of 1990, approaching the villages above Medreseönü to visit relatives of my husband and to conduct ethnographic research on health care practices. As the bus rounds the corner past a restaurant perched on a cliff overlooking the rocky shoreline, the large mosque comes into view. This building, along with the municipal government building, the school, two grocery stores, the pharmacy, the wedding salon, four bus company offices, and four coffeehouses, constitutes the center of Medreseönü. The town is nestled in a small bay which shelters a few fishing boats. Behind the buildings along the coastal road the hills rise up so steeply that some cars, especially those driven by inexperienced drivers, cannot make the initial run up the cobbled section of the road leading to the villages, and must coast down backward into the main roads traffic to try again. As large construction trucks and intra-city buses charge around the sharp turns, the local drivers who take passengers up to their village homes deftly dodge, swerving into the oncoming lane to get enough speed and grip to make the ascent. When I arrive with large suitcases and pack into a car with my welcoming party, I join in the whispered prayer for auspicious beginnings *Bismillahirrahmanirrahim* ("In the name of God, the Compassionate, the Merciful") as we charge the hill. Cresting the first slope, we all exhale, joking as we reach the rutted dirt road which, although steep, is out of the reach of the speeding traffic.

Leaving the main road, the car carries along the sounds of traffic until its heated engine is shut off in the open space in front of the house of Aunty Emine and Uncle Ferit. As the bustle of greeting and unloading baggage subsides, a new auditory landscape unfurls in all directions. As different to the stranger as the local language, tastes, and habits, sounds must be recognized and interpreted before they can make sense. Sounds carry meanings which seem obvious to the local inhabitants, meanings integrated into a way of life. To an outsider, the sounds may be indistinguishable, meaningless, or strange, requiring interpretation, explanation, and familiarization.

Typical summer sounds include the light-hearted conversations of women working in the same or adjacent gardens. This region has a special style of calling which carries information over distances, especially up and down hills or across valleys. It is most often used to carry information from the house to the fields and back. This form of calling can convey basic information such as the need to send someone right away to fetch something, it can be a location check, a call to return for a meal, a question about who is watching the cow, or a request for water or food. This form of calling is best understood within families, but neighbors and other relatives may be used to a person's calling voice. Further east on the Black Sea Coast is a region where a special whistling language (called "bird speech") has been developed for similar geographical reasons.[1] Despite distortion from wind and distance, people are very accurate in their assessment of who is calling, from where, and for what reason. A woman's lament, heard from a distance, may be the first way that a family learns about a death. The lament will include familial terms ("Oh, my father," "Oh, my girl," etc.) which convey who has died. Locals recognize the specific lamenting voices of most individuals. One morning in the village of Gebeşli, I watched as Aunty Emine and Uncle Ferit listened intently to the sound of a woman's lament. They soon determined that the woman's cow had died, and, relieved that no human life had been lost, returned to the breakfast table.

Cows can be heard bellowing in the distance, and the sound of their bells is recognized by their owners. When cows are being driven out to pasture or home again, they are moving along quite quickly, and their bells jingle noticeably more than they do when the cows are grazing. Cows are also directed with switches and sometimes by the loud curses of their owners. Many people can tell who is passing their house with their cows without looking outside. This can be useful information because people on good terms must greet each other, while enemies pointedly avoid looking at or speaking with each other. People are especially attuned to the sounds of cows in distress, and can often tell where the cow is and what the matter is even when the cow belongs to someone else.

People also listen carefully to the sounds of cars and other vehicles and can tell a lot about who is on the way home, or leaving, or going to a wedding (minibuses are rented for weddings at a distance), or coming back from the market in a hired car. The day is divided by the five calls to prayer, emanat-

---

1. Bird language: John Freely (1996) cites without detail the *New York Times* as reporting that a certain village inland from Görele is named Kuşköy (Bird Village) "since the villagers are renowned for their ability to communicate across intervening valleys with their shrill "whistle talk" which is believed to be an ancient language indigenous to remote regions such as the Pontic Mountains" (113) Whether or not such a language has ever been a fully expressive language, it is certain that the people in the region of my research use special calls and sounds to convey information across distances and over valleys. When asked about a special "bird language" they believe it is possible, but only have experience with their own repetoire of calls limited to families or neighborhoods.

ing from the crackling speaker of the local mosque, recited by the *hoca*, the government employee in charge of the religious life of the village. This sound organizes the ebb and flow of daily life.

When there are no loud sounds, the breezes carry the buzzing of flies, the rustling of leaves in the wind, the distant sound of radios or televisions, the sounds of chopping wood or hammering nails, the scratching and fussing of chickens, and the occasional bark of a dog or cry of a baby. The sudden intrusion of a fighter plane's roar silences the songbirds for a moment. Then they resume, with their specific calls for different times of day. The warning note of a familiar bird makes people look up from their work to see who is passing or to chase a cat away from the chicks.

Listening to my research tape recordings and watching my videos, I am reminded of the sensory texture of life in Medreseönü. Sound is one of the many sensory factors which shapes local culture and colors the experience of living in this place. Each chapter of this book will begin with a passage descriptive of the local setting, to give a sense of the local way of life, followed by an analytical investigation of the culture, particularly as it relates to healing practices.

******

Total description *is a present and ever-withdrawing horizon; it is much more the dream of a thought than a basic conceptual structure.*

—Foucault 1994, p. 115

An Ethnography of Healing Practices

This book is an ethnography of healing practices in one specific geographic area. It focuses on culturally specific ideas of illness, health, birth, and death because these ideas form the warp and weft upon which the fabric of culture is woven. By studying traditional healing practices in dynamic interaction with clinical practices introduced in this century from the West by way of the Turkish national government, I learned about the cultural construction of beliefs about health, illness, the supernatural, the place of humans in the world, gender roles, tradition, and change. The specific focus on what Turkish village women and their counterparts in the health clinic know, and how they demonstrate and explain their knowledge to others, shows much about how women participate in the construction, maintenance, and redesigning of culture.

The objective of this research is not only to document actual practices, but also to describe the health care system in action, showing how people choose and negotiate care for themselves and family members. This approach should add to existing studies and help develop theory which will enhance cross-cultural study in general, and, more specifically, the study of the ways women determine and are determined by their own cultures.

LOCAL HISTORY

The ancient history of the Black Sea Coast is known mainly from Greek sources which follow the stories of the adventurer Jason. John Freely (1996) writes, "The first Greek mariners may have ventured into the Euxine (Black Sea) late in the Bronze Age, in the thirteenth century B.C., their exploratory voyages perpetuated in the myth of Jason and the Argonauts....When Jason set off on his expedition he built a ship called the *Argo*, which was endowed by Athena with the power of speech; and heroes from all over the Hellenic world, including Heracles and Orpheus, volunteered to fill the fifty seats of her rowing benches." (pp. 1–2) The Golden Fleece, the prize sought by Jason, was to be found in Colchis, an Eastern Black Sea region now in the nation of Georgia. Strabo, the Pontic historian (born 64 B.C, died ca. A.D. 25), describes the land of one of three tribes of women warriors called Amazons in the region between Samsun and Ordu. (p. 86) The point which extends out from the area of my research, known in antiquity as Iasonion Akrotirion, is still today called "Yason Burnu" or Jason Point after the story of the Argonauts. (p. 97) Travelers since Jason have kept mainly to the coast, noting the wild and verdant lushness of the hillsides, skirting rocky promontories by boat until the late twentieth century when tunnels were blasted through for the coast road. Recent finds in underwater archaeology, particularly off the coast of Sinop, promise to yield fascinating information about the history of settlement around the Black Sea, even suggesting a catastrophic flood which may be the basis for the Biblical story of the Flood.[2] More details on local history

---

2. The National Geographic Magazine has published several articles on the Black Sea, including "Crucible of the Gods" vol 202, no. 3 September 2002, pp. 74–101 Zwingle, Erla, Author and Olson, Randy Photographer; "Ancient Wrecks Await: Ballard Expedition 2003" May 2004 Volume: v. 205, no. 5 Pages: 112–129 Contributor(s): de Jonge, Peter Author McLain, David Photographer; "Deep Black Sea" or "Black Sea Discoveries: Startling Evidence of an Ancient Flood" May 2001 Pages: 52–69 Contributor(s): Ballard, Robert D. Author and Olson, Randy Photographer.(http://www.nationalgeographic.com/blacksea/).
The National Geographic Society has also sponsored some of the University of Penn-

and sources on the complex ethnic, religious, and linguistic mix of the Black Sea coast are given in the appendix.

LOCAL ECONOMY

The best-known feature of the Black Sea Coast is its lush greenness. Because of the micro-climate around the Black Sea, certain crops, notably tea and hazelnuts, can be grown only in this region of Turkey. The province where I conducted my research is called Ordu, and its major source of income is from hazelnuts, with other types of agriculture, animal husbandry, fishing, and forestry contributing also. Most of the villagers have plots of land reserved for hazelnuts, one or two milk cows per family, vegetable and fruit gardens providing most of their needs, and supplemental income from family men who travel for fishing and factory work to the big cities of Turkey and Europe. One local man worked for a two-year period in Saudi Arabia and returned to marry and live in the village. The local type of subsistence requires constant labor from those who tend the gardens and animals, and periods of intense labor for the men involved in fishing and migrant labor.

The stereotype known throughout Turkey about the Black Sea Coast is that the women do all the work while the men sit in coffeehouses and tell stories and gamble. The nature of the local division of labor brings this tendency about: women are responsible for daily agricultural work, which includes a lot of carrying, while men pitch in for the intense seasonal work of hazelnut gathering, planting, and cutting. Men also do almost all of the building of houses, transportation of goods to regional centers, forestry, and upkeep of fishing boats and nets. Meeker (2002) shows that Black Sea men have been involved in travel for work for centuries, and that "Women's labor in the gardens and stables was the precondition for men's participation in the horizons of elsewheres." (104) He shows that social prestige rests upon men's non-participation in agriculture, whereby a man will wear clothing such as pressed shirts and suit trousers even if he has no official job, showing that he has no need to perform agricultural tasks. In fact, this social logic requires women to perform the heavy tasks of carrying wood through the public thoroughfares, care for the domestic animals, and tend daily to the vegetable gardens and

---

sylvania Museum of Archaeology and Anthropology's "Black Sea Trade Project" which "uses new archaeological techniques and a holistic approach to explore the ancient colony of Sinop from mountaintop to ocean bottom." For more information, see: http://www.museum.upenn.edu/Sinop/SinopIntro.htm

fields of crops. Meeker rightly connects the local cultural importance of jealousy, public displays of arms, and women's training in the use of firearms with the absence of men from home for extended working migrations. (106) Beller-Hann and Hann (2001) link the tradition of women's communal agricultural working groups (*imece* or *meci*) to the fact that "women had moral as well as physical anxieties about working alone"—a situation which implies, in a patriarchal society such as the Black Sea village, the absence of male family members in the fields. (103)

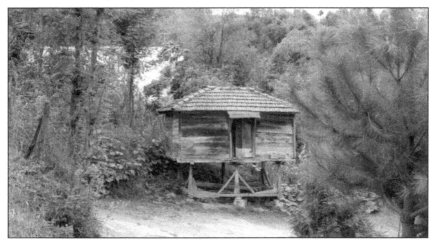

5. A Traditional Hazelnut Storage Barn

GLOBAL IMPACTS ON THE LOCAL

Although the Black Sea Coastal areas were historically well-connected through the sea trade, the Turkish coast is currently undergoing an unprecedented level of rapid globalization, being drawn into various kinds of economic relations which extend beyond the historical linkages. Owing to what is clearly a developing environmental disaster, including severe water pollution, over-fishing, and catastrophic events such as the explosion of Chernobyl (on April 26th of 1986), fishing has dropped to very low levels.[3] Many families are suffering from both the lack of fishing jobs and a world decline in hazelnut prices. Local culture has also been impacted by the influx of shuttle traders from Eastern Block countries, making temporary visits into Turkey for

---

3. From an unpublished paper by John McNeill, "Environment and Society in the Black Sea Basin: Historical and Contemporary Perspectives," presented at a Georgetown University conference on "The Black Sea in History and Politics," May 4, 2001

trade, and of those women known in Turkey as "Natashas," who became en-
tangled in the illegal prostitution which burgeoned after the opening of borders with the former Soviet Union and Eastern Europe.[4]

Labor migration to Germany, beginning in the 1970's, led to the new iden-
tity-marker *Almancı*, the term created to describe a local person who has moved
to Europe for work (the term, specifically referring to Germany, is often used
even if the person has migrated to a different European country). The Black

---

4. The term "Natasha" has been used in Turkey to refer to any unaccompanied female
traveler from the former Soviet Union or Eastern Europe. The influx of women from Communist bloc countries beginning in the late 1980's became a flood with the demise of the
Soviet Union. Although most of these women were operating small-scale businesses as
shuttle traders, bringing Soviet goods to sell in Turkey's "Russian bazaars" and taking back
suitcases full of clothing to sell at home, there were those among them who found that sex
could be traded for the capital needed to purchase such goods. Observers describe the common yet often mistaken Turkish perception that female shuttle traders from the former Soviet Union or Eastern Europe were likely to involved in the sex trade as well. This influx
produced a challenge to established norms of public behavior led to extensive discussions
of morality in the national media as well as in communities, many newspaper and television exposes, at least one film, and various protests in eastern Black Sea cities against the
traders and the prostitutes.

Hatice Deniz Yenal, in her 2000 PhD Thesis from SUNY Binghamton "Weaving a Market: The informal economy and gender in a transnational trade network between Turkey
and the former Soviet Union" makes a convincing connection between the shuttle trading
phenomenon in the post-Soviet period with the historical trade relationships in the Eastern Black Sea, which involved Genoese, Greek, Armenian, Jewish, Balkan, and Ottoman
Turkish traders in relations with Crimean, Caucasian, Persian, and later Russian markets.
(20) In her research on the 1990's, Yenal gives the example of a woman she calls Linda who
had been living for three years in the Black Sea city of Ordu when interviewed. Linda is
half Georgian, half Polish, and started bringing Soviet goods to sell in the "Russian Bazaars"
on the Black Sea Coast in 1988. After the demise of the communist system, she had to ad-
just her economic practices to buying clothing and footwear in Anatolia to sell in Georgia
and Indian clothing in Georgia for sale in Turkey. At the time of the interview she was required to return for her visa extension to Georgia once a month, but hoped to find a way
to live permanently in Ordu. (83–84). Although Yenal found that consensual sex between
tradesmen in Istanbul and shuttle trading women from the former Soviet Union was often
involved in cementing a business relationship that would last beyond a single business
trip(131), the informant, Linda, in contrast, has converted to Islam and works hard to distinguish her own story from that of women who come explicitly for the sex trade.

The subject of the sex trade, especially when it involves international travel, is notori-
ously difficult to research and document with certainty. Most observers, however, have noticed that the role of personal business initiative, which seemed to be an interesting factor
in the early activities of female shuttle traders has largely been overrun by mafia-type sex-
ring exploitation and male dominated large scale trade. While Beller-Hann and Hann

Sea coastal communities sent large numbers of men, and later whole families, as a part of this arrangement between the German and Turkish governments. The *Almancı* must then work to maintain local ties back home, using various reworked traditional strategies such as arranged marriage in order to maximize the benefits of both local land-owning and foreign income-earning.

Family loyalty, once assumed to be a natural part of selfhood often becomes strained because of the economic inequalities resulting from migrant labor and cash income. Those who work in Germany complain to each other that their families don't understand how hard and expensive it is to live in Germany, and the local family members often complain that their relatives in Germany are holding back money which they should share, or are showing off too much. Health care is an expense to which *Almancı*s are expected to contribute.[5]

While many people from the region have migrated to large Turkish cities or to Europe, land is usually kept within the family, and many family members return to the area for the hazelnut harvest which falls in August (conveniently coinciding with the European workers' holiday period and children's school vacation). The salaried city jobs bring cash to the families of the area, which has changed daily life in a number of ways. The pattern of extended

---

(2001) see a trend toward normalized relations between locals and foreigners from Georgia and beyond, as reflected in a lessening of public discord over the issue (90), it is also possible that the sex trade remains as active, but is more organized and better hidden. Istanbul has also largely replaced the cities of the Black Sea as the main nexus for trade and perhaps also of prostitution.

Human rights agencies and researchers on human trafficking have noted, for example, that Ukrainian sex rings send women to many destinations, including Greece, Turkey, and Israel in the Eastern Mediterranean, as well as nations of Europe, the Middle East, and Asia. Donna M. Hughes (2000) writes: "In some parts of the world, such as Israel and Turkey, women from Russia and other Republics of the Soviet Union are so prevalent, that prostitutes are called "Natashas." (4) Journalist Victor Malarek takes this name for his book *The Natashas: Inside the New Global Sex Trade* (2004) about the trade in women particularly from Russia, Ukraine, and Moldova.

Another consequence of prostitution across borders is the increase in sexually-transmitted diseases. Hann and Beller-Hann (1992) were told by doctors in eastern Black Sea towns that the media alarm concerning a sharp rise in the incidence of sexually-transmitted diseases is entirely accurate. (5) When I was conducting research on health care practices, AIDS was mentioned only as an outside threat, associated with the loose morals of foreigners. In remains to be seen how attitudes may change if this and other sexually-transmitted diseases become a real health concern in the community.

5. In a separate study (1997), I have described in detail the characteristics of the term *Almancı* and I have followed links from the specific Black Sea region of my research for this work to the German city of Ludwigshafen to trace links between music and sentiment in the migrant community.

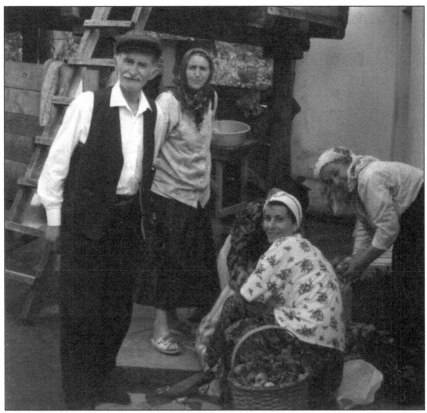

6. Everyday Work in the Village

male travel for work, however, should not be taken as a new product of "modernization" or "globalization," since it has a long local history. What is clear is that the scope and effects of twentieth-century labor migration, while building upon local traditions, have produced new social tensions along with new opportunities.

POPULATION FIGURES

The population of the province of Ordu, according to the 1985 census, was 766,348, with 268,034 living in the cities and 498,314 living in villages. The district of Perşembe is the region within Ordu which contains the villages in my study. It has 38 villages under its jurisdiction, and a 1985 population of 8,322. According to the 1993 statistics of the health clinic of Medreseönü, the town center to the villages I worked in, the population of this smaller unit is 3,832. This breaks down into the town center, six *mahalle* neighborhoods, one of which was incorporated in 1993, and one *köy* village. This study uses the English term village for all of the seven areas outside the center because they are not contiguous in the sense implied by the English word neighborhood, and each has its own mosque.

This study employs the name of the administrative center of this area, the town of Medreseönü, to refer to the local scene including the villages up the hills from it. To be specific about a particular village, the individual names will be given (fieldwork was carried out in the villages of Gebeşli, Afırlı, Çandır, and Okçulu). The town center has an elementary school, a middle school, and a new high school. It also has the seaside mosque which draws most of the men from the upland villages on Fridays for the noon prayer. Along the coastal road, interspersed with privately owned businesses, local government facilities include a wedding salon, a pharmacy, a health clinic, a post office, and a cluster of government offices.

The villages are all quite high up from the sea-level town center, so, whereas people gladly walk to town, they appreciate a ride back home up the hill, especially if they are carrying groceries. One of the recent innovations is the introduction of personal cars and minibuses to take people up and down and to weddings for a negotiable fee. This is one way for a young man to pay for his own car and to keep up with all of the area's comings and goings. Because cars and passable roads are fairly new in the area, older people do not know how to drive. Local women usually do not learn to drive, but they are tickled about the women who have learned to drive, often while living in foreign countries.

Health Facilities

As of 1990, the health facilities in the province of Ordu included the 400-bed main hospital in the city of Ordu, the 75-bed hospitals in the smaller cities of Fatsa and Ünye, and health clinics in some 62 of the region's towns. In 1980, the 200-bed Bronchial Illness Hospital of Ordu was turned over for the use of the armed forces. A new hospital is under construction. The region also has a Mother and Child Health Center, a Tuberculosis Clinic, a Syphilis Consultancy, and an Administrative Office, with two branches outside of Ordu city, for "The Fight against Malaria." I have visited both the Ordu and the Fatsa main hospitals. In Medreseönü itself, a new building is under construction to house the health clinic, which currently shares a building with the post office and the mayor's office. Money for the new building comes from a combination of government funding and charitable donations from local businessmen and locals who work in Europe. The town fire truck and ambulance were also purchased through a collection of donations from local families who work in Germany.

Local Identity on the Black Sea Coast

The phrase "local identity" suggests that location is the most important factor in identity. The phrase traditionally assumes a type of society in which people are born, live out their lives, work, and raise families all in the same location. The concept of "local identity" comes to the foreground because of contact with outsiders. This can happen when outsiders move in, or can happen when locals move out to other settings. When locals move, they may continue to identify "home" as the place they came from. In this case, they must make a conscious effort to keep the connection alive.

One generation ago on the Black Sea Coast, identity was primarily based on family, which coincided for men with the location of birth, the place where one grows up, marries, has a family, works, and is eventually buried. Women traditionally had one place where they were born and grew up and a second place where they lived with their husband and his family, had children and eventually were buried. For their whole lives, they are called *gelin* "the bride" by their contemporaries in the husband's village. These affiliations continue to be important in a person's sense of community and belonging to a place, and, although individuals may move to other places for long stretches of their lives, they often continue to identify themselves with the region and village of their birth, maintaining their connections in various ways.

Within the village context, family relation identifiers (like "my uncle's son's wife's mother") are most common in identifying people. Secondarily, place names can be used if the person is from another village or physical location of the house can be used to describe a person in the village (the one who lives over there, above the such-and-such field, next to so-and-so).

Research

Research for this ethnography of health care practices followed touristic and academic visits to Turkey dating back to 1984. In the summer of 1990, I circled the Black Sea by ship as a tourist and then went to visit the Black Sea Coast to meet the extended family of my future husband. We then had a wedding in his home town of Medreseönü the following year. The following year,

I spent a month in the villages around Medreseönü, embarking on ethnographic research involving interviews with elderly women. At this time, made welcome in the home of Aunty Emine and Uncle Ferit, I started to make video and cassette tapes about local healing practices, including traditional midwifery, bone-setting, and interviews with some staff at the Health Clinic. The summer of 1994 was spent mostly on the Black Sea Coast. Major research visits were the four months spent with my infant son, Timur (starting when he was three months old), in 1996, and the two-and-a-half months spent there in the summer of 1997. A bound copy of my dissertation was shown around the village in the summer of 1999, becoming an object of mixed pride and disappointment. The nurses in the Health Clinic were excited to see their names in the acknowledgements, quickly pointing out one misspelling and making a correction. The biggest general disappointment was the lack of photographs, but everyone who saw the book congratulated me and encouraged me to continue my work.

Family and research visits continue, as when Timur, then six years old, accompanied me to Medreseönü for the hazelnut harvest of 2002. Then, in the bitter February of 2003, I rushed back for the funeral of Aunty Emine, my generous hostess and key informant. Her heart troubles had lead to major heart surgery in Ankara in August of 2002, and it was a heart-attack that took her from us. Her funeral and the *mevlûd* ceremony held forty days later were crowded with people who remembered her caring concern, her expertise, and her helpful advice through the years. Her husband, Uncle Ferit was buried beside her in November of 2004. May God show them mercy (*Allah rahmet eylesin*).

JOINING THE COMMUNITY

In Medreseönü, my roles as a family member and as a researcher have always been mixed together. When I married a man from the region, I acquired the kinship status of *gelin*, which translates as "bride" but is a word formed from the verb "to come" (*gelmek*) because the *gelin* leaves her childhood home to live with the groom's family. It is not unusual in this region for *gelin*s to come from outside the community, but I was the first American *gelin*. Although I have been asked to find brides from my own people for the eligible bachelors of my husband's region, no further American *gelin*s have joined the community so far. Much of a new *gelin*'s time is spent with her mother-in-law, and I met various older women who would later teach me about the practice of traditional medicine during social visits with my mother-in-law. Because I was married to a man from Aunty Emine's family, and because I lived

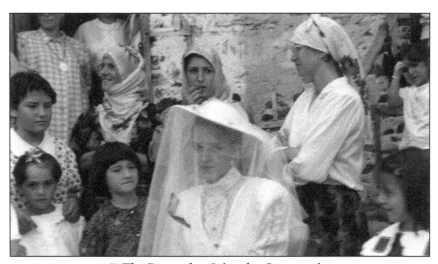

7. The Researcher Joins the Community

in her house while staying in the village, we established a relationship along the lines of mother and daughter in-law.

Personal lives and local perceptions of ethnographers always shape the research experience. The experience informing this book is thus distinct from the experience of other researchers, and can contribute to a complex understanding of Turkish culture when taken in combination with various other studies. For example, two Austrian researchers, Sabine Strasser and Ruth Kronsteiner, (1993) visited a village near Trabzon on the Black Sea Coast to study women in Turkish culture. Both were feminists who worked with Turkish women in Austria and were interested in issues of patriarchal violence and female consent. They had to make choices about how to introduce themselves in the villages where they were to stay for fieldwork. They had learned enough about Turkish culture to know that it could be problematic to be completely honest about the fact that the unmarried woman was not a virgin and that the other woman, although previously married and mother of a son, was divorced. They decided to foster the idea that the unmarried woman was a virgin and that the divorced woman was separated from her husband because of work rather than divorce. This purposeful manipulation of identity caused some awkward moments, but these researchers concluded that cultural differences make some less palatable personal facts worth concealing.

Another non-Turkish female researcher in a rural society, Carol Delaney (1991), who lived in a central Anatolian village for her fieldwork concerning gender relations and metaphors of reproduction, reports a local concern for her "wandering about too much" and for the ambiguity of her position as a woman without a male family member to be responsible for her movements (173) (for more on her treatment of the concept of patriarchal permission, see Chapter 2). Because she had been married and had a daughter, she was accorded the status of *dul kadın* (widow) and allowed to live in her own house. (166) In fact, her status as a *dul kadın*, combined with her interest in the sexual experiences of her informants, seems to have suited the needs of the women who visited her regularly. Delaney reports:

> Women spoke freely with me about sexual matters, especially at the weekly tea parties in my house, but still I found it extrememly difficult to know exactly what they meant and what kinds of activities were and are engaged in. (43)

A *dul kadın* must be particularly careful about her reputation, because a woman alone might be willing to entertain the advances of local men. Delaney solved this problem by behaving consistently and under close observation throughout her time in the village:

> On a few occasions in the beginning, men did try to visit me at night, but it was observed that I did not open my door to them. The day after one such event, everyone commented that they had seen what happened and were glad I had not let the man in. After a while people relaxed and I was allowed to have male neighbors and friends visit during the day and even occasionally at night. (183)

In contrast to these researchers, as the *gelin* of a local family, along with my own financial means and the status of a foreigner with higher education, I was assumed to be under appropriate control and was not subject to much prying into my past. Any *gelin* requires coaching in the local norms of behavior, and my conduct, while my husband was not present, was taken to be the responsibility of the members of his extended family. Any mistakes in conduct I have made thus far in the village setting seem to be written off as the errors of a well-intentioned outsider who will learn with time. With every return visit, I learn more about how the local society functions and demonstrate my commitment to the family and the area.

When going "to the field," (if a cluster of villages perched on steep hills can be called a "field") I was nervous about what my in-law's extended family would think of my research and how to explain my intentions to them. I was also unsure about how to arrange to talk with authorities at the health clinic and at the governor's office and how to collect statistics. I anticipated a big social and communication gap between the traditional experts in folk medicine and the professionals at the clinic. Because of the small size of the community, family connections smoothed over many of these problems, while traditional healers and clinical professionals were in contact with each other and even negotiated their respective roles. As a family member, my interest in health care was mostly taken as a natural part of learning the ways of my husband's community. It was important, however, to be properly introduced to the local officials, and to explain the areas of research and where results would be used. Reactions of informants to this research involved a combination of regional pride in local traditions and a slight suspicion about the intentions of outsiders. Because the Black Sea Coast is considered a "peripheral" region in the national sense of ties to the central government and benefits from government policies, locals express a frustration about being underappreciated. On the other hand, the "Fatsa Incidents" of 1979–1980[6] showed that the attentions of the central government could become repressive if local politics were seen to exceed bounds set in Ankara. Black Sea residents often convey a sense of feeling marginal in the distribution of national resources, and the people interviewed in this study, while shying away from any statements which could be interpreted as separatist or anti-nationalist, often expressed interest and pride that their customs would be featured in a book.

Ethnographic research has been an important part of the modern project of creating the nation-state of Turkey from the ruins of an empire, so no one is surprised to learn that an outsider/intellectual wants to ask questions about local traditions, whether they be a foreign anthropologist or a folklorist from a Turkish city. Traditional folklore collection has focused on men's genres of music, poetry, folk dances, agricultural practices, proverbs, stories, and songs. My interest in the women's areas of folk healing was accepted as appropriate for me, although a common misunderstanding was that I planned to practice

---

6. The reputation of Black Sea coastal peoples for boat building, sea trade, and even smuggling and piracy is a reputation which can cut both ways. In a section "The Laz" of his article about the Eastern Black Sea people, Magnarella (1998) writes "Over the centuries the Laz have utilized the fine woods of the Pontic forests to construct small boats especially suited to Black Sea travel. Their seafaring abilities helped Mustafa Kemal (the founder of modern Turkey) win Turkey's post World War I struggle for independence. Employing their small boats, the Laz smuggled large quantities of arms and munitions from Batum to Samsun, from where they were transported inland to Kemal's forces." (175) This type of activity is claimed proudly by many along the coast, rather than the few who are actual speaker of the Lazuri language, but, in the violent period of the 1970's, gun smuggling across the sea was looked upon in a different light by the central authorities. During a period of right-wing/left-wing violence, when a tailor in the city of Fatsa was elected major on a communist ticket, Ankara saw fit to send in the Third Army to crush the movement. The period is referred to in contemporary Turkey as "Fatsa Olayları," meaning "The Fatsa Events".

folk healing myself rather than just studying it. The retired village midwife, for example, examined my hands to see if they were the right type for midwifery. When I became a mother, my interest in healing practices was seen as a natural part of learning my responsibilities for the health of my family. People were generally curious about what this "American bride" was up to, patiently allowing for my slow absorption of the local dialect and customs. Those younger than me, exposed daily to standard Turkish in school and on TV, often pointed out dialectal differences or "translated" for me when their elders were speaking. As my son grew out of infancy, I was allowed to attend funerals, a ritual off limits to nursing mothers. My research was thus always shaped by my developing status in local society.

ESTABLISHING RAPPORT

Early in my research, I had anticipated difficulty in getting to know the people at the health clinic, assuming that they would be either too busy or too suspicious of my research to talk openly with me. I soon learned that the head nurse, Nurse Rahime, was the wife of the Mayor, who himself is a childhood friend of my husband. Since the wedding season was at its peak during the time I was there, and since the Mayor generally makes an appearance or even officiates at weddings, I saw Nurse Rahime in social settings which were not prearranged. She also invited me to her house, showed me pictures of her family, and was amused when I tape-recorded her mother-in-law's lullabies to a nephew. In other words, she was very friendly and open, glad that someone was interested in the health of village women—a subject about which she cared deeply. My initial nervousness about making contact with the local officials led to my inappropriate request that my husband introduce me to the Mayor himself. I had not realized that the Mayor knew me as well as he needed to because of attending our wedding two year's previously. Thus, a formal introduction between a married female (me) and the high male official would have been strained, artificial, and unnecessary. When it turned out that I could meet his wife just by walking into the health clinic, the problem was solved.

This was one instance of many in which my social and research-related expectations were challenged in the Turkish cultural setting, and my access to informants and data was guided by local norms. Over time, I was better able to follow cues about appropriate behavior and develop research methods which did not significantly disrupt the normal flow of life. The video recorder, for example, could blend in at a wedding, but caused most informants in an informal home setting to become embarrassed or to start clowning. The exception was Aunty Zeynep, the bone-setter, who demonstrated a professional manner with me at all times, jumping right into detailed descriptions of her techniques, comfortably demonstrating various procedures for the video camera using her granddaughter as a model. Aunty Emine also encouraged me to pay Aunty Zeynep for the research sessions we conducted, whereas other types of gathering information in social settings did not involve monetary transactions. For sound recordings in the context of a social visit, the start of the tape would inevitably be drowned out by the excited questions of children about the machine and its fascinating sound-activated red light.

The way that I got to know the women around in the villages, aside from seeing them at weddings, was to be taken around by Aunty Emine, who relished the chance for social visiting, in a common practice called *gelin gezdirmek* which can be translated as "taking the daughter-in-law (bride) around." This is an element in the relationship known by everyone concerned with Turkish culture to be a crucial one: that of mother and daughter-in-law. Since the traditional practice is for the new bride to go to live with her in-laws, especially until the young groom can establish his own house and security, the bride tends to spend more time with her mother-in-law than with her husband. An important social ritual after a wedding is "going to see the bride" (*gelin görmeye gitmek*) by the neighbors of the mother-in-law. In this situation, the bride's housekeeping skills, new furniture, cooking, and manners are commented upon by her new social circle. In *gelin gezdirmek*, the mother-in-law takes her bride around to see friends, family, and important neighbors such as the school teacher's wife and the *hoca*'s wife. In such circumstances, I tried to follow as best I could the rules of "good bride behavior" and was welcomed into a wide network of homes. Since showing family pictures is an important part of visiting, I could get clues about whom we were visiting and whom they were related to by looking at the pictures. Figuring out who was married to whom continues to be a problem for me, because I am used to the American-style simultaneous introduction of spouses, a technique seldom used on the Black Sea Coast. Although people would explain who was whom in crowds, the photographs were easier for me to understand. The intricacies of family relations and the gendered nature of community interactions will be dealt with in more detail below.

The Identification of Informants

The names of all informants have been changed to protect their privacy as individuals and as members of families. Translations of Turkish familial terms,

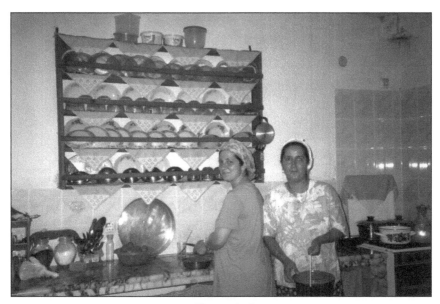

8. Village Kitchen

such as "Aunty" "Uncle" and "Granny" have been chosen to reflect local usage and generational distinctions. The Turkish term *Yenge* remains because it has no English equivalent, meaning "sister-in-law older than oneself." As the term *gelin* is used for a female in-law younger than oneself, the term *yenge* preserves both respect for elders and the cultural importance placed on the distinction between those women who marry into the family and those who are of the family. Nurcan *Yenge*, mentioned in Chapter 2, for example, is *yenge* to me because she is the wife of Uncle Ferit's brother, a member of the male line of my husband's family. We are both *gelin*s into the family, but, as she is older than me, I call her *yenge*. For these and other Turkish terms, the reader is referred to the glossary. In only one example have I tried to transcribe some of the local pronunciation, and that is in the extended interview with "Granny" at the end of Chapter 2.

RESEARCH QUESTIONS

My preliminary dissertation research in five villages on the Black Sea coast of Turkey began with the question: Is Western-style clinical medicine destroying traditional types of health care? What I found was a complex and dynamic relationship between clinical and traditional medicine, in which health care recipients negotiate with providers in choosing from a range of possible remedies to relieve their health problems. I also found that women are extremely active in this type of negotiation, as patients, as family members of patients, as clinical workers, and as traditional healers. Despite their training in clinical medicine, local doctors, nurses, and midwives are also intimately involved with traditional healing techniques and healers in a variety of ways— at times trying to stop a local practice they consider harmful while at other times trying to incorporate traditional methods and cultural attitudes which they respect and find efficacious. In this way, my initial essentializing of the clear division between a "pure" local culture and a hegemonic larger-than-local culture was, to use folklore theorist Amy Shuman's (1993) term, "dismantled." As she puts it, "What needs to be displaced is any possibility of studying 'the folk' as an unmarked, natural, authentic category....The only choice now is to study the processes of marking, claiming authenticity, and negotiating boundaries between groups or genres." (349–350)

Health and illness are personal and social issues of great importance. An illness is an incontestably real experience for a patient, one which is dealt with in culturally-specific ways. The processes of naming an illness, describing it to others, gathering advice, determining its cause, and acting to remedy it are determined by cultural norms and expectations. By studying how members of a culture deal with these issues, one can learn about the cultural ways in which an individual is incorporated into the social fabric. Arthur Kleinman (1980) provides a model of a "health care system" which is "a system of symbolic meanings anchored in particular arrangements of social institutions and patterns of interpersonal interactions." (24) When an individual is facing an illness, either as a patient, healer, or as a concerned bystander, various levels of culture always influence what is thought to be the cause, what remedies will be sought, in what order, through what institutions, with what expectations, and with what participation by others. This does not mean, however, that all members of a local culture respond in the same way to an illness. A health care system is complex and allows for many possible choices, changing explanations, new healing methods, social criticisms of individuals' choices and actions, and ways to reject failed methods. The field of medical anthropology has developed to use interdisciplinary methods to describe the many facets of a health care system. The complexity inherent in any health care system is described by folklorist and health care systems researcher Bonnie O'Connor (1995) as follows:

> Any individual can have multiple cultural memberships and influences, and any cultural group encompasses a great range of individual diversity. Cultures may be conceptualized as consisting of inter-

pretive and expressive repertoires, upon which individuals draw se-
lectively and in an infinite range of possible combinations, all of
which are subject to personal modification. Thus, while it is possible
to describe the ingredients in a cultural repertoire associated with any
given group, it is *not* possible to predict on that basis how any individual member may believe or behave." (170)

Before coining "health care system," medical anthropologist Arthur Kleinman (1975) had defined the "medical system" as that which:

> …represents a total cultural organization of medically-relevant ex-
> periences, an integrated system of social (and personal) perception,
> use, and evaluation. That is, medical systems are much more than
> particular kinds of medical facilities, practitioners, and practices.
> They are cognitive, affective, and behavioral environments in which
> illness and health care are culturally organized. Moreover, they are to
> be appreciated as such only on the local level, where they actually
> function. (596)

Kleinman has been a leader in the development of interdisciplinary theory in
medical anthropology, calling for studies which both reveal the cultural complexity of health-related ideas and behavior and demonstrate how disparate
healing practices are integrated into a coherent cultural system (1975). He has
noted a lack of attention to the individual in previous studies of health-care
decision-making, as well as an ethnocentric and Western biomedical-centrist
bias. In this study, I aim to describe an adaptive local cultural system which
has evolved to respond to human suffering. Through translated interviews, I
hope to show the riches of individual variation in one particular health care
system.

The study of health care practices in a foreign setting involves a curiosity
about other ways of thinking about the self, the body, and its place in the community and in the larger universe. Focusing on health in a new context can
make us aware of our own concepts and practices, including the ways that we
are well-served and ill-served by our own cultures' heath care systems, even
leading us into new avenues of research into health. Medical anthropology can
shed light on cultural concepts and power structures which shape the roles
available to individuals and communities. It also has a moral underpinning:
we study methods for caring in the hope that suffering can be better alleviated, in an equitable way, and that neither the symbolic power of tradition
nor the symbolic power of modern clinical medicine override the diverse physical and spiritual needs of individuals.

O'Connor (1995), in her study of "vernacular healing systems" in the United States, including the practices and health care theories of sub-groups within mainstream American culture, such as those present among southeast Asian Hmong immigrant communities and those connected with groups facing the medical challenges of HIV and AIDS, finds an interdisciplinary approach mandatory:

> It is important therefore for vernacular healing systems to be well studied, thoroughly described, and well understood in all of their aspects. This will require interdisciplinary efforts, pursued with rigor of scholarship and avoidance of polemic. Such a study must incorporate (and continue to verify) the recognition that vernacular health beliefs and practices, like conventional medical care, are systematic bodies of thought that are fundamentally rational, and which are bolstered by lengthy histories of ideas, considerable social support, and reputations for efficacy sustained by experience, observation, and evaluative processes. It must take into account patients/ own authority and agency, and be descriptive, rather than prescriptive in nature. Attention needs to be directed both to illuminating and obviating the risks some vernacular healing actions pose, and to understanding and encouraging the ways in which these systems function as significant and effective therapeutic responses. (192)

FOLKLORE

Folklorists often study verbal expressions of cultural concepts. Stories about real ailments and the attempts to remedy them are an important part of social interaction in Turkish culture. As women visit each other in the course of regular daily life, they tell stories about their own health, about the health of family members and neighbors, and even about the health of strangers whose extraordinary conditions or pitiful situations have been reported in the media. Along with these types of stories of sickness and attempts at cure, there are stories by or about healers which tell how they learned their crafts, how successful they have been with various types of ailment, and what they expect in return for a successful outcome. Doctors, nurses, bone-setters, religious healers, midwives, and those who have remedies for the evil eye can all equally become the topics of lively discussion. The traditional healers tell stories of their own interactions with clinical practitioners. Doctors and nurses in the clinics have stories about village ignorance, health concerns, and their own interactions with local culture. During the course of my research, I have collected many such stories and have examined them to see how health-care is managed and represented in the community. It is my aim to present these stories and to analyze them, in order to present a picture of the complex and constantly changing health care system of this particular cultural area.

Recent theoretical developments in the field of folklore have integrated important insights from other disciplines. My work has been interdisciplinary by necessity. The trend towards interdisciplinary theoretical work has been a boon to scholars placed in the intersections of folklore and area studies, like myself, and like those who study folklore in South East Asia. Editors Appadurai, Korom, and Mills (1991) explain:

> ... folklore has become the locus and critical nexus of important interdisciplinary debates and contests pertaining to the expressive dimension of social life ... [we are in] an era when terms such as 'genre,' 'performance,' 'tradition,' and 'text' are no longer markers of terminological common-sense but point, rather, to large areas of intense debate. The field of folklore is host to these debates and, moreover, has participated in opening them up to even larger debates in the fields of critical theory, media studies, and cultural studies. (5)

The insights of post-colonial critics and ethnographers have shown the theoretical and political consequences of doing fieldwork across national and economic borders. It has become impossible to ignore the impact of social, economic, historical, and political struggles and inequalities on the collection of cultural data. A scholar aware of her or his own implication in the messy realities of cross-cultural contact can admire the resilience of folkloric forms. Folklorist specialist on Tunisia, Sabra Webber (1991) comments that:

> Folklore, like other aesthetic forms, is rhetorical, dynamic, and adaptive. It is potentially a force for both stability and change, repression and liberation. It is a phenomenon that is manipulated by its performer and subject to negotiation by its audience within communally determined bounds. But even those bounds may be knocked askew, especially when participants have frequent and intense contact with other cultural models. Folklore enables a performer in collaboration with his or her audience to appropriate selectively ideas or practices from other groups in a manner aesthetically and practically agreeable to his or her own community. (xx)

When a folklorist tries to take the "larger-than-local" (Shuman 1993) into account, the local can seem small and threatened. In another passage, Webber finds that:

> As we try to place communities in global and historical settings, they begin to seem very much at the mercy of those larger forces—helpless and, finally, culturally nonviable. Folklore is a tool with which communities can reinforce and revitalize community identity when it seems the community should be falling apart under the onslaught of, say, western hegemony or the ups and downs of the global economy. (8)

While realizing that "folklore is a tool" for a community, we should also admit that it is a resource for Western academics, in the same way that the labor power or natural resources of poorer countries are resources for our economic machine. We may be panning for nuggets of folkloric gold, hoping to show that human creativity is inexhaustible. The paradigm of inexhaustibility has been used in a long series of exploitative ventures, such as mining and fishing, which have caused extensive damage. We cannot "extract" folklore without changing its environment. There is no such thing as "neutral observation."

At the same time, part of the drive to understand and document foreign health practices is the hope that they hold promise for human ailments across cultural boundaries. People searching for relief from illness are often quite willing to explore uncharted territories. Although certain remedies, for example, can be used for healing when learned from a distant culture, efficacy seems to be tied to the integration of patient and healer into a cultural project of healing. What Erika Brady (2001) calls the "item-centered" approach of collecting folkloric items such as specific remedies and presenting them in a list "removes the object of [folklorists'] study from the rich matrix of social context, leaving behind much of what may be relevant to an understanding of the whole picture." (9) I have described throughout various common remedies for possible comparative interest, but have focused mainly on detailing the contexts through which remedies are used in practice.

This book owes a great deal to the approach of David J. Hufford and Bonnie B. O'Connor, called "pioneers in the area of medical folklore" by Erika Brady, whose edited volume includes their joint article "Understanding Folk Medicine" in which they:

> offer a comprehensive introduction to a contemporary approach to medical folklore centered on an understanding of folk belief systems,

examining the ways in which these systems draw on bodies of knowledge and belief, support specific means of knowledge production, provide explanatory methods for causation and treatment, and supply evaluative strategies to determine efficacy. (9)

David Hufford has extensively studied folk belief systems, including medical belief systems, as well as the scholarly and medical professional debates about these systems. His work is interdisciplinary, including a familiarity with scientific and medical debates, anthropological studies from around the world, comparative religious studies, philosophy, folklore, and popular cultural debates. His theoretical contributions include the description of scholarly and medical "traditions of disbelief" (1982b), the call for the accurate and nonjudgmental collection of "core experience" (1982a)—which he also calls the "phenomenological approach" or "experiential theory," the need for scholarly reflexivity in belief studies (1995), and a recommendation of an "inclusionist approach" (1988) in the examination of belief.

This work, then, is interdisciplinary and is inspired by the efforts of scholars from a range of academic backgrounds. Rather than as a methodology or type of data, the term "folklore" has become, for me, a sign which marks a place in the web made up of shifting cultural and academic strands.

Tradition-Bearers

The fact that folklorists often collect stories from elderly informants can lead to the mistaken assumption that these types of stories will disappear with the older generation. Folklorist Patrick Mullen (1992) explores the relationship between tradition and the elderly:

Not all old people are active tradition-bearers, though; some passively carry on traditions, but the active ones value the past, maintain a connection with it, and often identify themselves as traditional performers and craftspeople. This does not mean that they live in the past; they keep traditions alive by using them as resources for coping with the present. Folklore as an academic discipline is not the study of the past but rather the study of present situations informed by the past. The people who actively bring the past and the present together in creative ways are the ones folklorists seek out in the community, and finding them is not hard because most people in the community know who they are....and they are often the oldest people in the community. This might suggest that folklore is dying out, but it is not.

Younger people are often aware of tradition but do not yet actively carry it on. (2)

In Medreseönü, young women know about remedies and practices, but the older women have more actual experience, more stories to tell, are respected for their experience (thus get an audience). They may also be in a safer position to talk about health, being more responsible for the general health of the community and less responsible for the specific health of individuals (such as babies—for whose health the young mothers are held most responsible and for whose illness they are most likely to blamed). In the next chapter, I will discuss the fact that no one wants to be blamed for a treatment that goes wrong or fails to work. The older women, with their higher social standing, are safer from blame unless their methods are thought to be dangerously backward. Many of them have reduced their performances of actual treatments because of the possibility of blame, but they freely give advice. As they grow older and amass experience, women take on a more active and vocal role in the maintenance of tradition, even as they adapt new ways to their local needs. Traditional healing practices are performed and passed on particularly by older women, although there are a few older men who are known for specific healing abilities.

The Term "Traditional"

To explain the subject of my research interests to inhabitants of the villages around Medreseönü, I used the local term "*kocakarı ilaçları*" (which means "old woman medicines"). With the health clinic staff and with city dwellers, I was more likely to use the term *geleneksel tedavileri* (meaning "traditional remedies" or "traditional medicines"), which is the scholarly term used in Turkish. When I use the term "traditional," in English, I mean to focus on the means of transmission of knowledge—in that it is passed down within a fairly bounded social group from one generation to another, from one individual to another, in a local setting, through well-established local pedagogical techniques.

I do not mean the word "traditional" to suggest a fixed or moribund set of old-fashioned ways. Rather, I mean it in the sense of "tradition" used by Handler and Linnekin (1984), as a negotiation between what people know and what they learn as circumstances change:

> We must understand tradition as a symbolic process that both presupposes past symbolisms and creatively reinterprets them. In other words, tradition is not a bounded entity made up of bounded con-

stituent parts, but a process of interpretation, attributing meaning in the present through making reference to the past. (287)

When a bone-setter gives her clients pain-killers acquired from a pharmacist, she is using a technique which has a shorter history than the technique of binding a limb with beeswax-soaked rags. The role of a healer, however, is to bring relief from suffering through a combination of medicinal and symbolic elements. By incorporating a clinical product into her healing resources, she is appropriating both the medical and symbolic power of clinical medicine. Entirely new techniques, then, can be "traditional" and time-honored procedures can easily be abandoned if their usefulness is over. Once again, from Handler and Linnekin:

> We argue that tradition is a symbolic process: that "traditional" is not an objective property of phenomena but an assigned meaning…that the relation of prior to unfolding representations can be equally well termed discontinuous as continuous. (286)

In his book on the Kung people of the Kalahari Desert, Katz (1982) clarifies his use of the term:

> The word *traditional,* used to describe the healing approach I studied in the relatively unacculturated areas of Dobe in the late 1960s, is merely a relative term, meant to distinguish the healing approach found in a primarily hunting-gathering setting from the approach of more sedentary Kung. It is hard to imagine one 'original' setting for the healing, just as it is very difficult to specify any one individual or even as the beginning of a healing dance. The context for healing among the Kung seems to have continually changed and is still changing. (254–255)

The term "traditional" should never be understood to describe a static cluster of know-how which cannot adapt to changing circumstances and which is a result of ignorance. Traditional medicine must necessarily adapt to changing circumstances because it is itself an empirical system, tested through time and changing circumstances, in which the effective elements are retained and the ineffective elements are rejected or re-configured.

The Terms "Local" and "Lived"

Aware of the potential simplification and essentialization of a culture which comes with the use of terms such as "local" or "folk," I none-the-less need a term to describe the practices and culture which occur in the region of my fieldwork. When I call a practice "local," I do not mean that it occurs nowhere else, or that it sprung up, fully-formed, in the place where it is used. I do not claim that there is no contact between the people and culture found in the area I arbitrarily marked off as "my field"—and, in fact, I try to show that a trip to Germany or to Istanbul for an operation is part of the local health care system. The people who provided me with the information I have used in this study have a sense of local identity and local culture. Neither of these concepts is fixed in stone—they can change over time, according to different situations, in response to different challenges.

Likewise, I prefer the term "lived" to describe practices situated in culture. Instead of trying to describe local culture, local belief, or local health care practices as if they existed as an ideal type, I wish to make clear that these systems are constantly in flux, being renegotiated by those who use and are used by them. I do not find the term "vernacular" (Primiano, 1995) to be preferable to "lived," for reasons delineated in Chapter 5.

The Empirical Basis of Traditional Health Care

Hufford (1995), takes pains to emphasize the empirical basis for many practices which have been labeled and denigrated as "folklore," "superstition," or "folk belief." The fact that the empirical method is the corner stone of the biomedical theory of health care does not mean that non-biomedical theories are not based on accurate and systematic observation. He writes:

> Folklife scholars have long been aware that folk traditions concerning architecture, food preparation, agricultural practice, botany, the making of textiles and pottery, and so forth, constitute impressive bodies of valid knowledge rooted in experience. (31)

As a part of the "and so forth," it makes sense to include traditional healing practices. In describing the Kung health care system, Katz (1982) shows the intelligent and adaptive uses of all available medicines:

> A practical and pragmatic people, the Kung use things that they believe work. They have been exposed to other systems of treatment, both African and Western, yet they continue to rely on their healing dance. Antibiotics may be used in conjunction with a dance, to provide extra protection or to deal with diseases particularly amenable to Western medicine, such as gonorrhea. Antibiotics are

also used sometimes in conjunction with or instead of indigenous medicinal salves. Although contact with Western medicine is still limited, the pattern of that contact is clear: the Kung integrate elements from other treatment systems into the tradition of their dance. The prevailing mode of healing remains num, though the Kung attitude remains realistic. As Gau says: "Maybe our num and European medicine are similar, because sometimes people who get European medicine die, and sometimes they live. That is the same with ours." (56)

Byron Good (1994) discusses the difficulty of studying a system which is based upon a different set of assumptions, knowledge, and belief:

> ...it is difficult to avoid a strong conviction that our own system of knowledge reflects the natural order, that it is a progressive system that has emerged through the cumulative results of experimental efforts, and that our own biological categories are natural and "descriptive" rather than essentially cultural and "classificatory." These deeply felt assumptions authorize our system of medical knowledge and, at the same time, produce profound difficulties for comparative societal analysis (3)

Within the discipline of anthropology, Good suggests that medical anthropology, in particular, confronts philosophical issues of reality and relativism because of the ways in which the truth claims of medical science (and thus of the anthropologist) are brought together with competing truth claims from other medical systems. (3) There have been anthropologists/folklorists/researchers whose personal beliefs or experiences have been at odds with mainstream explanatory models, making it easier for them to show the cultural constructedness of these models, but there remains a disciplinary reluctance to spell out such "unscientific" personal factors. What could be called the "Carlos Casteneda model" of explaining a radically different way of viewing the world from the inside, although potentially inspiring and informative, has generally been held outside the cannon of acceptable cultural descriptions.

THE TERMS "ORTHODOX/UNORTHODOX"

Much of the scholarship which has looked at differences between the biomedical theory of health care and other theories has used the pair of terms "orthodox" and "unorthodox." For example, Norman Gevitz (1988), introduced his edited volume with the following definitions:

> "Unorthodox medicine" may be defined as practices that are not accepted as correct, proper, or appropriate or are not in conformity with the beliefs and standards of the dominant group of medical practitioners in a society. Individual healers who persist in engaging in these activities in spite of the disapproval and opposition of the dominant group may be classified as "unorthodox practitioners."

And:

> ...orthodox physicians as a collectivity share certain ways of apprehending phenomena, certain ways of diagnosing problems and handling them once identified, and certain standards of conduct. They may be regarded as being part of a professional community in that they speak the same language, rely on the same general pool of knowledge, share certain beliefs, subscribe to similar values, and strive for common goals. (1)

While these terms may be useful in the study of the history of medicine in the United States, the term "orthodox medicine" does not work in the Turkish cultural setting because it conjures up historically incongruous associations with Christian religious orthodoxy.

THE TERM "CLINICAL MEDICINE"

In this study, use of the term "clinical," in distinction to "traditional," follows that of Foucault (*The Birth of the Clinic: An Archaeology of Medical Perception*, 1963/1994 English ed.), in that it describes what is practiced by institutionally-trained doctors, nurses, and midwives in the health clinic, private doctor's offices, and hospitals which serve the five villages around Medreseönü. The term encompasses the location of the healing practices (even though the clinic staff sometimes make tours of the villages to provide clinical services), the training of the staff (including the theory of a biological basis of health and illness), the costumes worn (the doctor's white coat or the nurses' uniform, as governed by national laws), and the technologies in use (pharmaceuticals, plaster casts, thermometers, stethoscopes, scales, test tubes, needles and syringes, etc). Foucault (1963/1994 ed.) analyses the emphasis of clinical medicine on the gaze of the practitioner, showing that biomedical medicine is a way of speaking and thinking, as well as a set of techniques. He states:

> The figures of pain are not conjured away by means of a body of neutralized knowledge; they have been redistributed in the space in which

bodies and eyes meet. What has changed is the silent relation of situation and attitude to what is speaking and what is spoken about. (xi)

In the history of self-described modern medicine, Foucault (1963/1994 ed.) declares a significant moment:

> At the beginning of the nineteenth century, doctors described what for centuries had remained below the threshold of the visible and the expressible, but this did not mean that, after over-indulging in speculation, they had begun to perceive once again, or that they listened to reason rather than to imagination; it meant that the relation between the visible and invisible—which is necessary to all concrete knowledge—changed its structure, revealing through gaze and language what had previously been below and beyond their domain. (xii)

When I use the term "clinical medicine," then, I mean to draw attention to the fact that it is also culturally placed within a historical, political, and economic framework. It is as constructed in discourse and practice as "traditional medicine." Biomedicine, although framed in the language of scientific neutrality and objectivity, should not be assumed to be any more or less neutral or empirically-based than any other system. As Foucault (1963/1994 ed.) shows, the strength of the clinic is a strength in discourse:

> The clinic—constantly praised for its empiricism, the modesty of its attention, and the care with which it silently lets things surface to the observing gaze without disturbing them with discourse—owes its real importance to the fact that it is a reorganization in depth, not only of medical discourse, but of the very possibility of discourse about disease. (xix)

The "Health Care System" Approach

Scholarly studies which take an anthropological or folkloristic approach to examining traditional healing practices look for the context which binds the individual practices to each other and to the culture as a whole system. Arthur Kleinman's *Patients and Healers in the Context of Culture* (1980), is a leading example of an ethnography of a "health care system" (Kleinman's term) which displays the contemporaneous, cooperative, and competing natures of the many healing practices which exist in any society. Kleinman's fieldwork examines the Taiwanese health care system, but his theoretical approach has been useful in this study of the health care system on the Black Sea Coast of Turkey. "In every culture," he says, "illness, the responses to it, individuals experiencing it and treating it, and the social institutions relating to it are all systematically interconnected."(24) Healing, as well, can be described in a broad, systemic manner. Richard Katz's study of community healing among the Kalahari Kung (1982) is another example of the health care system approach. He writes:

> I view healing as a process of transition toward meaning, balance, wholeness, and connectedness, both within individuals and between individuals and their environments. (3)

Theoretical advances in the "health belief system" approach have been made by Hufford (1983, 1988), O'Connor (1995), and Snow (1993). O'Connor (1995) summarizes this approach as follows:

> The systems approach includes healers, patients, theories of disease causation and cure, *materia medica*, and therapeutic techniques within its purview. It takes into account cultural influences, personal interpretation, intra-group variation in belief and practice, and the dynamic aspect of belief (its variability through time, across changing circumstances, and from person to person). (59)

Kleinman, with his medical background, is concerned with the perceivable outcomes of healing, which he divides thus:

> Cross-cultural studies reveal that healing refers to two related but distinguishable clinical tasks: the establishment of effective control of disordered biological and psychological processes, which I shall refer to as the "curing of disease," and the provision of personal and social meaning for the life problems created by sickness, which I shall refer to as the "healing of illness." These activities constitute the chief goal of health care systems. (82)

I am less concerned than some medical anthropologists with documenting the actual results and success rates of various techniques and remedies, so I find less need to separate the biological and social into discrete domains. In this, my approach resembles that of O'Connor (1995), who says, "I cannot speak to efficacy, except to report how users of various healing systems understand and evaluate it." (xvii)

Unlike Kleinman (p.83), I do not use the term "clinical" to refer to traditional health care practices which take place outside of the actual institution of the clinic. He makes the important observation that traditional health-care practitioners have concerns and practices which are similar to (and as important as) those of a western-style clinical practitioner. In trying to make a case for cross-cultural and ethnographic study of health care systems, Kleinman needs to sway an audience of readers (including Western medical practitioners) which has a biomedical model of health and illness. The reader of this work is presumed upon to suspend disbelief in unfamiliar practices and to weigh equally the contributions of the mostly distinct realms of traditional medicine and medicine associated with the institution of the health clinic. These realms are understood by the inhabitants of Medreseönü as distinct, as they well may be by most people, everywhere. There are points of overlap, like the bone-setter who gives out prescription pain-killers, but I want to reserve the term "clinical" for a kind of technology and explanatory model which was introduced to the area within the living memory of the older inhabitants.

LOCAL DISTINCTIONS MADE BETWEEN TRADITIONAL AND CLINICAL

The people I lived with and interviewed had a clear idea about what types of practices were officially sanctioned and in use in clinics and hospitals (*hastane, doktor işi*) and which types were "village stuff" (*köy işleri*), "old woman's medicine" (*kocakarı ilaçları*), and "herbal, local medicines" (*ottan, yandan ilaçları*). In the arenas of traditional and clinical, health care education is one of the distinguishing factors—traditional medicine is learned by people in their own local setting, from family and neighbors, usually as a part of general "know-how": learning by watching, helping to do, and doing; while clinical medicine requires a formal training in institutions away from home, involving the use of specific items of technology not in use in the traditional setting.

BELIEF, RELIGION, AND HEALTH CARE

The study of folk belief systems is essential to the study of folk medical systems. According to Kleinman (1980):

> The health care system, like other cultural systems, integrates the health-related components of society. These include patterns of belief about the causes of illness; norms governing choice and evaluation of treatment; socially-legitimated statuses, roles, power relationships, interaction settings, and institutions. (24)

Religion is an important part of the health care system of Medreseönü. In fact, all of the traditional practices could be called "Muslim healing practices" because they are performed by Muslims. Despite its secular veneer, clinical medicine is also practiced mainly by and for Muslims in Turkey.

At the local level, individuals distinguish in various ways between general wisdom handed down through generations and practices which are considered to be specifically religious. Sometimes the distinction comes from the need to be ritually clean for a procedure—such as reading a *nazar* prayer, or performing a ritual such as *mum dökmek* (described in Chapter 5). For Muslims who practice the required five daily prayers, ritual cleanliness is continuously renewed throughout the day.

Readers familiar with practices in other Islamic cultural situations will find some similarities between what they know as Muslim practice and what is described here. I have chosen not to call the healing practices in Medreseönü "Islamic" or "Muslim" because these terms are too general. While the inhabitants of the area mostly consider themselves to be Muslims, and while the textual source for Muslim belief and practice is the same, lived religion is specific to individuals and communities. There are similar problems in using the general term "Turkish" to describe health care practices in a small region on the Black Sea Coast. Chapter 5 discusses in greater depth issues concerning belief, including religious faith, perceptions of the supernatural, and ritual activity.

The Terms "Western" and "Modern"

The clinical medicine under examination in this work cannot simply be called "Western medicine" because, although originally imported from the West, it has taken root and become integrated into the local scene. It cannot rightfully be called "modern medicine" either, because that would suggest that traditional practices were somehow left in the past, over and done with, obsolete—when in fact they continue to be practiced, modified ("modernized"), and used in the present. Foucault (1963/1994 ed.) has shown that the term "clinical" itself conveys the historical, global, political significance of the world-view, discourse system, and technologies of biomedicine.

The Patient-Centered Approach

A focus on the particular moment when a patient and a health practitioner come together in the effort to solve a health problem is a convenient starting-point for studying a health care system. The risk of this narrow focus is that it privileges technologies, recipes, and specific techniques, and can get bogged down in the details of specific practices, becoming a list of items out of cultural context. Although some might like to be able to reproduce a particular practice for their own health care purposes, the interest of the readers of this book is assumed to be "academic" rather than practical. This assumption is the opposite of that of my informants—they consistently assumed that I wished to practice the techniques they were describing. While studies providing a rich description of the culture which surrounds healing practices often do not describe specific techniques in great detail, studies which stress recipes and techniques often ignore the general cultural context which makes them viable and sensible. This work aims at a balance between specific details relating to particular health concerns and a general cultural description useful in a broader context.

In contrast to an approach which only looks at the practices of specialists, be they doctors or traditional healers, a patient-centered examination of the healing practices of a particular culture reveals the world-view and priorities of non-specialists. Instead of only collecting the theoretical and abstract views of experts, who are often frustrated when the behavior of a real patient does not conform to their ideal vision, I have gathered information about how patients choose, combine, and change treatments until they are satisfied with the results. In Chapter 6, I describe the various treatments sought by a woman who could not conceive a child. This patient-centered, long-term view shows how complex an individual's use of available health care can become. If I had only interviewed the specialists who treated her, I would not have learned how she adjusted her views about traditional and clinical techniques as she progressed through a series of treatments.

The approach of this work is take specifics of healing as windows on the general local culture, taking examples from a small number of informants linked by family ties and neighborly proximity. The intent is to describe how a health care system is an integral part of a culture, and to show how an individual in a specific cultural setting seeks relief from suffering within a web of cultural meaning and possibilities.

FOCUS ON WOMEN

This book's focus on women and their roles in the heath care of their families and communities was an outgrowth of my position in the community as a *gelin* and researcher. Many examples of individual behavior are provided to counteract the possible assumption that "women" are a homogeneous group, even within local culture. For the sake of a coherent theoretical model, I do not want to disguise the fact that women have a multitude of positions and possibilities which they can negotiate and inhabit at different times in their individual lives, often in direct conflict with other women, constrained in various ways by culture in general and by particular circumstances, including economic and political factors. This attention to gender dynamics is, in part, a result of trends in scholarship in the United States, yet also a topic which often comes into sharp focus in cross-cultural encounters. My access to women's discourse was determined by my family connections to the area. My participation in the roles of *gelin*, wife, and mother, as determined by my own life history, gave me a particular place in local society. From this place, I was able to join and observe women as they interacted with the local health care system.

Anthropological Debates on Definitions of Terms "Illness" and "Disease"

Robert A. Hahn (1984), within the forum of an edited volume on South Asian Systems of Healing, extensively critiques literature on the cross-cultural study of health care systems (including Kleinman), in an attempt to reach a firm, objective, and useful definition of the terms involved for such a study. He shows the slippery nature of even careful definitions of "illness" and "disease," in which the authors' own beliefs about the reality of either are obscured in the attempt to be non-universalizing. To avoid this problem, he suggests that the common human experience of suffering be taken as a universal starting point, after which the culturally constructed natures of what he calls *Illness-ideologies* (the perspectives of the sufferers), *Disease-ideologies* (the specific perspectives of biomedical practitioners), and *Disorder-ideologies* (the varied perspectives of traditional, non-Western healers). (Hahn, 1984:15–16) This approach is useful, and similar to Hufford's "core experience" approach (1982) to study comparatively what people in various cultures report about their experiences. Hahn is still making problematic dichotomies between patient and specialist, biomedical models and "traditional, non-Western" models. Biomedical practitioners, after all, are also sufferers, a disease is a disorder in the biomedical ideal system, and the terms "traditional" and "non-Western" need to be as carefully examined as other terms in the argument. I would rather call all the perspectives *Disorder-ideologies*, which could then be subdivided into equally valid and interesting types such as individual experience-based descriptions and coping mechanisms, particular lived examples of biomedical models and procedures, and any other specific models and procedures, whether they be tied to a certain group or geographic area. In this way, the complex mix of health care strategies available to any particular inhabitant of a village on the Black Sea Coast could be shown to include elements of biomedical ideology as well as traditional ideology, all in an effort to alleviate the concrete suffering of that individual and to control its effects on the community.

The biomedical model is commonly taken for granted by researchers to the extent that it is discussed as a universal system which can be introduced, transported, taught, and used as if it remains unchanged by time, geographical distribution, and human participants. Of course there is a specific history to this universalizing discourse, which is why the biomedical ideology often gets called "Western medicine." In actual practice, however, biomedical training, technology, and the practices of specialists and patients are not as consistent and unquestioned as we, as participants in the cultural ideology of biomedicine, are conditioned to believe. There is a great deal of debate, disagreement, and change over time within any particular Western country's health care system, despite the hegemonic front presented by the community of specialists to the general public. The physical accoutrements of a clinic (white uniforms, stethoscopes, x-ray machines, etc.) may be similar across national boundaries, but the actual beliefs and practices of clinic staff may vary widely.

Good (1994) speaks of medical language as "a rich cultural language, linked to a highly specialized version of reality and system of social relations, and when employed in medical care, it joins deep moral concerns with its more obvious technical functions." He has defined illness as a "syndrome of experience," "a set of words, experiences, and feelings which typically 'run together' for members of a society." (1977:27 quoted in his 1994, p. 5)

Conclusion

In light of Shuman's recommended project (1993) for folklorists, namely to "develop and contribute to discourses on local cultures as contested categories," (362) the following chapters will describe aspects of a dynamic health care system in one interconnected group of villages on the Black Sea Coast of Turkey. Chapter 2 begins with an examination of local cultural concepts of the body itself, with the idea that it is necessary to understand how the healthy body is thought of before being able to understand ideas of illness. Some of the concepts introduced in this chapter may seem familiar and others strange, for example, the idea that filth can cause illness is fairly widespread whereas the concept of a "fallen stomach" may be new to many readers. The chapter ends with a lengthy interview with an elderly resident, who speaks about health and remedy for illness from her status as a wise woman, giving a broad range of concepts deemed important to her generation. Chapter 3 attempts to describe the traditional shape of the life of a rural Turkish woman, which included growing up in a close-knit family, leaving home at the time of marriage to live with her husband's family, and the stages of motherhood from birthing and caring for babies to passing on knowledge to the next generation of mothers. This chapter addresses the economic underpinnings of Black Sea families, the metaphors used to describe the characteristics of women and mothers, and the effects of labor migration on the traditional patterns of life. The forth chapter, "Women's Ritual and Social Lives," portrays the interactions between women and compares the importance of certain religious events in the Turkish village to similar events examined in other Muslim societies. The chapter on "Faith, Religion, and the Supernatural" looks briefly at contemporary religious discourse in Turkish society before turning to address ideas of the supernatural and the problems associated with *nazar* (usually translated as "the evil eye"). Chapter 6 is a close look at one individual traditional practitioner, a bone-setter who has lived her entire married life in this village overlooking the Black Sea. This is an example of the practical and empirical nature of a traditional specialist whose practice continues to draw patients despite a strong national media campaign against traditional "ignorance." Chapter 7 takes up one of the concerns most important to the women of Medreseönü —reproduction: including fertility, birth, and infant feeding. Chapter 8 examines the institutions of clinical medicine, from the local health clinic to the nearby hospitals, addressing their place in the range of local health care resources as well as the status and training of clinical practicioners. The final chapter looks at care for the elderly and the cultural mechanisms which come into play at the time of a death in the family. Readers may wish to refer to the glossary of Turkish terms or the appendixes on local history, population figures, and ethnic groups.

The descriptions in this work are, by necessity, simplifications of the existing range of possibilities in the health care system of Medreseönü. As O'-Connor (1995) warns:

> Any description of a belief system is to some extent a composite and an idealization...It represents only a "freeze-frame" moment in a dynamic and always-changing phenomenon...There is as much diversity within a system as there is among systems....Attempts to be too pre-

cise would distort the tremendous complexity and infinite variability of the actual picture of vernacular health belief and practice. (xxi)

This book does not, for example, trace the history of Ottoman medicine, with its roots in Classical Greek philosophy, Islamic scholarship, and interactions with a global scientific community. Tracing the origins of clinical medicine to Europe in the early 19th century is a convenient and Euro-centric simplification. At any rate, the clinic in Medreseönü is not merely an earthly manifestation of an ideal type of "clinical medicine." It is local and distinct in various ways which constantly adapt to changing circumstances. Likewise, the "traditional culture" of the region is not a pure, authentic form untouched until recently by outside forces—it also a product of change and adaptation. As with all systems, a health care system is always being re-created as it is being used. The following interviews and observations, although bound in time and place, reveal the cultural dynamism, mobility, adaptability, and perpetual creation involved in the human response to suffering.

> *Beyond estimate and analogy*
> *New poetry is uttered constantly*

—Şeyh Galib *Beauty and Love*, 881, trans. Holbrook 1994, p. 91

> *In sum, is not perpetual creation*
> *The cause of original expression?*

—Şeyh Galib *Beauty and Love*, 783, trans. Holbrook 1994, p. 91

CHAPTER 2

BODY IN BALANCE,
SELF IN SOCIETY

Lokman Hekim gelse yaramı azdırır
Yaramı sarmaya yar kendi gelsin

If the Herbalist comes, he'll staunch my wound
To wrap it, let the Beloved herself come

—Anonymous, recorded by Gündoğarken, 1999

It is mid-morning and I am tidying up after breakfast with Aunty Emine, an elderly traditional healer who has accepted me as family. I have spent the night with her, and try to help out with various chores around the house, in the manner of a *gelin*. I am on the roof, shaking the carpets over the downhill side of the house, when a woman turns up at the door with two of her grown sons. I bustle about putting the carpets back in place on the wooden living room floor and the tiled kitchen floor, while Aunty Emine has them sit down. One son leaves almost immediately. I haven't figured out why they have come at this mid-morning hour, which is not the usual time for casual visits, so I ask Aunty Emine if I should put water on for tea. She tells me to boil water and bring it to the living room. Listening in as I wait for the water, I come to understand that the woman's son has injured his wrist and his mother brought him so that Aunty Emine could look at it. When I bring a bowl of hot water, Aunty Emine pulls a new bar of soap out from the storage area under the couch and begins to massage the young man's wrist, asking where it hurts most, how he injured it, and in which direction it was pushed when it was injured. While the young man knows he hurt his wrist the previous evening, he is not sure just when and how (or is perhaps intentionally vague, as if he had been drinking or fighting when it happened). Aside from these direct questions, Aunty Emine mainly con-

43

verses with the young man's mother, who is about her age, exchanging little bits of local news. This draws attention away from the massage, and the patient begins to add bits of news to the conversation between the women. When she hits a sore spot, the patient expresses a lot of pain, but he is cheerful and joking when she moves on to another area. After the hot water and soap massage, Aunty Emine has me bring olive oil, and she continues working on the injured wrist. The patient had come in with his wrist wrapped in a cloth saturated in beeswax. She has me warm up the cloth by passing it over the gas stove burner, so that it will soften and can then be re-wrapped after the massage. She tells the woman to wrap the wrist in a white cloth, emphasizing that it should be white and clean. She says it would be best to have the wrist looked at (by implication by a doctor who would x-ray it). She found a spot where a nerve was pinched and has now softened the spot with massage. She says that there is no break, but that she can't be sure about a fracture. The patient seems more comfortable, and his mother expresses thanks as they are leaving. They did not drink tea, as it had not been a social visit. The following week, I see the young man at a distance at the local marketplace, and his wrist is no longer wrapped, suggesting that it he had recovered.

*****

On another morning, I wake up with an upset stomach. I tell Aunty Emine, who has already been up to do chores and start breakfast. She tells me that her own daughter, Şengül, visiting for a few days, had asked for a plastic bag to take with her when she went to Fatsa. "I asked her 'Why?'" she says, and laughs, "Because she might throw up!" Yesterday she had had the same problem as I have now. I gag down a spoon of ground coffee followed by salty *ayran* (yogurt with water), a remedy I had learned during another illness the previous year. This makes me throw up immediately. Aunty Emine rummages through a shelf of pills, looking for the pills she had given to her daughter yesterday. I tell her that I don't want pills because the medicine would pass to baby Timur through my milk. She says it wouldn't hurt the baby, but I still decline. Instead, I go lie down on my bed. Concerned, her husband, Uncle Ferit, comes and sits on the side of the bed, trying to diagnose my problem, saying "You didn't eat anything bad (*Yaramaz bir şey yemedin*)." He decides that I have caught a cold (*Üşütmüşsün*) I remind him that he had been scolding me the previous day for not wearing slippers. He nods, "See, you have to wear them" They ask me to come and eat breakfast. I don't, preferring to lie in bed feeling sorry for myself, my infant son beside me.

After breakfast, Şengül brings me a big cup of tea with lemon juice. I decline the offered sugar and drink the tea. A bit later, she comes in with her head covered in the style for prayer (suggesting that she had prayed over the remedy she was offering), with a small tulip-shaped tea glass filled with coffee grounds in lemon juice in one hand and a glass filled with water in the other. When I make faces and noises while drinking them, she laughs and says "*Afiyet olsun*" ("Good Appetite"). A while later, Aunty Emine comes in and sits on the bed. She checks the temperature of my forehead with her hand, and feels the pulse in my wrist. She pats my hand and asks if the remedy has made my stomach settle. She says that she had noticed yesterday that my color wasn't good. She then goes on to talk about her own health, telling me that she is not supposed to eat pickles because of her *tansiyon* (roughly equivalent to hypertension), they don't do her any good. She frets about the chores, how they make her head spin, her heart thump, and her back hurt. She is specifically complains about the hard work and lifting which are a necessary part of caring for the dairy cow. She sighs, "Well, what can I do? I have to carry on." By noon, I am fine, ready to get up, even hungry.

*****

The Body in Context

In order to begin to discuss concepts of health and illness which guide healing practices, we must examine concepts and categories that are ordinarily taken for granted. Encountering foreign ideas about the self, the body, the environment, and reasons for suffering can help up to examine our own assumptions and see them as part of our culture. This encounter can be an uncomfortable one and can lead to a rejection of the other's whole system of thought. Hearing the statement "we don't have microbes here" was one such encounter for me—anyone who intuitively "knows" that microbes are a natural part of every human environment is likely to be shocked by this seemingly irrational statement. The easy way to deal with this kind of cognitive dissonance is to reject the statement outright by questioning the rationality of the speaker or assuming that the speaker just lacks the proper education or information about "the way things really are." It is much more difficult to reserve judgment, to assume the speaker is competent and knowledgeable, and to figure out how such a statement fits into a whole realm of understanding about the self and the world. In academic and clinical realms, studies of health systems have often attempted to describe foreign concepts of health and illness in order to dismiss them or to allow biomedical health providers to circumvent them in the name of providing clinical care. This study, however, will try to describe a complete and ever-changing system of thought and action which assists individuals, families, and communities in managing health and illness. To approach this task, concepts of the body and of the physical, social, and spiritual environment must be examined.

LOCAL IDEAS ABOUT THE CAUSES OF ILLNESS

In the everyday talk about illness and its causes, people seem to attribute most problems to fluctuations in temperature. "You got cold (*üşütmüşsün*)." "You must have been sitting in a draft." "Don't walk on cold tiles without slippers, you'll get gas." (Shoes are never worn inside the house, and slippers, although always recommended, are not often worn in the summer). "Cold drinks will make your stomach sick (*miden üşür*)." "She was in the sun too long, she got sun-struck (*güneş çarptı*)." "Oh, it's too hot, my clothes are sticking and I feel like I'm suffocating (*bunalıyorum*)." "Don't sleep with your throat and upper chest (*gerdan*) exposed, you'll get a chill."

The local model of health and illness does not include a general idea of the possibility of infection by invisible biological entities. When the causes of illness are discussed, the basis of health is explained as a balance within the system of the body and soul. In part, this comes from the Greco-Islamic tradition of humors, in which importance is placed on maintaining a healthy balance between hot and cold, wet and dry.[1] As Good (1992) notes, in local

---

1. Byron Good (1994) classifies as humoral medical systems classical Greek medicine, Islamic and popular Hispanic traditions, Ayurveda, and Chinese medicine which all "conceive of the universe as made of basic opposing qualities—hot and cold, wet and dry, in the Greek system—and physiological functioning as a set of interactions among basic constituent "humors"—blood, phlegm, yellow bile, and black bile, in the Greek and Islamic case. (101) After encountering a humoral medical discourse during ethnographic research in Iran in the 1970s, Byron and Mary-Jo Good looked back to the classical Islamic medical texts in an attempt to understand the local meanings used in everyday speaking of health and illness. Byron Good writes:

"In the classical texts of Galen and Islamic theorists such as Ibn Sina (Avicenna), digestion is conceived as follows. When food is eaten, it undergoes "heating" or "cooking" first in the stomach and then in the liver, where it is transformed into the four humors. Blood is the primary product of the liver and travels from there to all organs of the body. One part of the blood travels to the heart, where it undergoes further cooking and is combined with the breath, thus being transformed into the "vital breath." This vital breath or *pneuma* travels through the arteries to each part of the body, where it interacts with the

Muslim contexts, this ancient system is variously combined with Islamic concepts about morality, ritual purity and filth, the power of the sacred word and of numbers, the presence of angels and *cin* (these supernatural beings, the "genies" of Middle Eastern tales, will be discussed in more detail in Chapter 5), and the overarching power of the Divine as the final recourse for those who suffer. The social context of the individual is also considered to be important for health, since social imbalances can bring about *nazar* (the 'evil eye' see Chapter 5). Bad behavior or ill will can strike a person down.

It seems that the traditional specialist called *hekim*, known for specific knowledge of the humoral balances, has been replaced by the clinical doctor, who is expected to have studied and mastered a complicated theoretical body of knowledge which the patient does not need to know in order to benefit. Before the introduction into the Turkish language of the word *doktor*, *hekim* was the normal term for a medical expert. Now the *lokman hekim*, who is a specialist in salutary herbs, is mostly a figure of nostalgia that comes up in song lyrics and is being resurrected in cities as herbal tonics become popular among the urban elite. In an herbal shop in Fatsa in 2004, I met a contemporary *lokman hekim*, who sells various herbs for cooking and healing remedies. He generously shared the knowledge he has gained from books and experience, sending me off with packets of herbs from local sources (dried nettles being the most prized), from the highlands (a yellow flower from the summer pastures called *yayla*, used to scent clothing in trunks and prevent moth infestation), and from inner Anatolia (red pepper and cooking spices from the Turkish South East). His customers are mostly married women responsible for feeding and caring for their families, and his manner with them was an interesting mix of Muslim propriety and light-hearted humor.

Since the 1990's, there has been an upsurge in the publication of books in modern Turkish popularizing Islamic science based on the Koran and the Hadith, including new books interpreting the rich history and wisdom of Islamic medicine. There are books available about the humoral system and herbal remedies. Arif Pamuk's *Şifalı Bitkiler Ansiklopedisi*, 1991, for example, combines explanations of the Greco-Islamic tradition through centuries of Islamic scholarship with lists of efficacious herbs in alphabetical order.

---

blood and "true assimilation" occurs nourishing the organs (Ibn Sina, Canon: 113). The liver thus produces the "dense part" of the humors, the heart the "rarefied part," and the breath produces life." (105)

For an anthropological treatment of the contemporary uses of the classical Greek and Islamic philosophy of humoral medicine in Malaysia, see the work of Carol Laderman (1983) and (1992).

While villagers may show respect for such books, particularly when things that they know already can be found in them, they rarely keep such books in their homes. This type of popular Islamic science reaches villagers through certain Islamist television shows and through formal and informal Islamic schooling, following the traditional means of oral transmission of knowledge. Young people with high-school education may own and refer to such books, and their ability to consult such sources to address a particular problem holds a higher social value than, for example, an interest in literature. Individuals are always collecting and testing information about healing practices but few claim a systematic knowledge of health and illness. As we will see in the next chapter, women gather experience in home healing practices over their lifetimes, and hold the Holy Koran as the only book needed for a healthy life.

In home remedies, found in both urban and rural settings, certain plant materials are known to be efficacious in balancing the body and managing chills and fevers. Local knowledge on the Black Sea Coast also includes information which seems to be tied to the humoral tradition, such as foods which should not be eaten in combination (fish and yogurt), should be eaten in moderation (green fruit, raw hazelnuts), or are good against imbalances of heat (blackberry and garlic, cool mud, vinegar, bitter seeds).

Aside from certain serious conditions which are known to spread through close contact (like venereal diseases, which are also associated with immorality and foreigners, see the note on "Natashas" from the previous chapter), people reject the idea that a healthy person might get sick just by being close to a sick person, especially a sick person in one's own family. Illness can perhaps come from strangers or from those with ill-will, but it cannot come from a close, caring family member. In fact, the culturally appropriate response to an illness is for family and concerned neighbors and relatives to visit the patient, sit close by, touch and massage the person, spend time in the room, and make sure the person is never alone. This contrasts strongly with the typical American cultural response of the avoidance of contact with sick people. The mainstream American fear of invisible, microbial contagion was vividly driven home to me when a visiting American friend cut his hand on a rock in the Black Sea. As every local he encountered wanted to hold and closely examine his wound, he became increasingly concerned about the cleanliness of his wound until he was almost in a panic. For the locals, an injury to a guest was a matter of great concern, requiring close attention. He was taken to the Health Clinic, where his worries about cleanliness were only compounded. As a guest, he was taken to the doctor's office before a local man who had been sitting silently in the waiting room, a pool of blood seeping from his foot which had been crushed by agricultural machinery.

Pislik: Filth

Along with temperature imbalances, "filth" (*pislik*) is also blamed for many illnesses. In this agricultural setting, excrement, both human and animal, must be dealt with by each household, independently of the types of civic facilities available in towns and cities. The Health Clinic is responsible for enforcing the sanitation rules and regulations passed down from the national and local governments. The Clinic staff may fine any household found to be fouling the creeks and rivers below their home or gardens. The disposal of filth is an issue which can cause feuds between neighbors, especially when one family lives on a slope below another. Flies, because they are attracted to filth, are considered *pis* (dirty), and illnesses can be caused when flies land on food. Parasites such as intestinal worms are a known problem, to be dealt with quickly, before their effects become serious. Local children are taught to avoid sewage outlets into the Black Sea, so that they will not swim in dirty water. Body fluids are considered *pis*, and must be cleaned with clear running water, as in the Islamically-mandated ablutions. Parents, for example, should take care to be ritually clean before holding their own infants. So while infection is not seen to be a problem within the family circle, cleanliness is an important prerequisite for family health.

Hospitals are also criticized for being *pis*, and children, considered more susceptible to filth than healthy adults, are usually allowed only short visits while adults may visit family members for extended periods. Family members bring sheets, towels, clothing, and food to patients in the hospital, in part because the hospitals lack adequate resources (for more on hospitals, see Chapter 8), but also because items from home are considered to be cleaner. The connection made between hospital care and filth is especially prevalent in poor populations who depend upon the state hospitals. The mainstream American cultural idea, in contrast, links cleanliness with hospitals—items provided by the hospital are considered sterile while those from home are considered to be potential carriers of infection.

The criticism that a person, family, or house is filthy is a very strong insult, and people often advise each other, in a friendly way, on how to best maintain cleanliness. An immoral, gossiping, or unfriendly person can also be called filthy. Illnesses, including those caused by *nazar* (the 'evil eye,'), are associated with filth. After recovery from an illness, a person should have a full body bath in order to wash away any remaining traces of it. As part of the process to remove the effects of *nazar*, the person being treated enters and exits a stable, where there is animal filth, because filth is said to draw filth to itself (*pislik pisliği çeker*). Women are held most responsible for the cleanliness of their homes, stables, and family members, and this is one of the factors which gives women greatest responsibility for the health of their families (See Chapter 3). A child's illness or delayed development can be blamed on the mother's bad hygiene or immorality.

MICROBES

Kantar sever darayı Mikrop sever yarayı
Tanır mı ondan başka Zengin sever parayı
Güve sever tahtayı İmam sever meftayı
Beşiğinden mezara Doktor sever hastayı

The scale loves the weight, the microbe loves the wound
The rich man loves nothing but money
The moth loves wood, the preacher loves the treasure
From the cradle to the grave, the doctor loves the patient

—Words by Abdullah Karaman,
Sung by Black Sea singer Davut Güloğlu, *Katula Katula*, 2003

The term *mikrop* ("microbe") has recently entered the local vocabulary, transmitted through the agencies of TV, traveling relatives, local health clinicians trained elsewhere, and through national education campaigns in schools. Aside from any scientific use of the term, it has joined the list of affectionate insults for children in everyday speech. Since the bad effects of *nazar* can result from praise and admiration, family members have extensive lists of these fond terms of insult (*çirkin* ugly, *yaramaz* good-for-nothing, *kerata* rascal, *sıska* skinny, *pis* dirty, *sümüklü* snotty, *böcek* insect, and even *sümüklü böcek* slug, and so forth). I only once heard Aunty Emine use the term *mikrop* in its scientific sense, in a case in which a child was about to suck on another child's pacifier—she warned the mother in time for her to grab the pacifier away: "Don't let her have that, it'll be microbed (*mikroplaşır*)!" In this particular case, I think the fact that the children were from different villages increased the sense of danger of contamination. People more readily accept the idea of contamination if an outsider is involved. I got a clearer picture of the place of the microbe in the local theoretical system of health and illness when, returning home from a social visit in which illness was a major topic, Aunty

Emine told me, "There *are* microbes and there *are* illnesses which can pass from one person to another, but, may God prevent it, we don't have them here." (*"Allah göstermesin, bizde yok."*)

Aunty Emine's daughter Fatma, who now lives in a central Anatolian city because of marriage, trusts her own knowledge based on the traditional model more than the *mikrop* model held by certain urban neighbors. She views them as comically meticulous and coddling. After I suggested that her child's runny nose might cause my child to become ill, she told me a story about a woman in her city who paid excessive attention to such things. The woman constantly fussed about *mikroplar* (microbes) and kept her child away from other children. The result of this concern over trifles, my informant reported with satisfaction, is that the woman's child is always sick. To further drive home the point that *mikroplar* were not involved, she explained that her daughter's nose ran only to relieve pressure in her ears (See the story of this girl's ear problems in the next chapter). In this case, my assigning of danger to *mikrop* was probably a defense against what I thought to be excessive contact between the girl and my baby, an attempt to get the mother to rein in her daughter. Her response was to tell a story ridiculing the *mikrop* model, which served to deflect my criticism and obviate any need to interfere with her daughter's behavior. Ironically, in the context of spending time with urban Turkish mothers in apartment buildings, it is I who find their attention to *mikroplar* excessive — Turkish housewives are very meticulous about hygiene and cleanliness, in general, so those who have internalized the *mikrop* model of illness seem to be constantly washing toys, bleaching clothes, wiping surfaces and children's hands, and worrying about contact with other children.

EXAMINATION OF THE BODY: DIAGNOSIS

Traditional, informal diagnosis of illness is based on patient's skin color, forehead and neck temperature, brightness or dullness of the eyes, pulse felt with the fingers on the patient's wrist, and the patient's own description of sensations. Everyone knows to look for the basic signs of illness. A specialist will diagnose with more precision, perhaps asking about specific feelings when a certain body part is pressed or massaged. An expert has more terms available to ask about sensations and more experience observing the symptoms and course of various ailments. A patient expects various technological means to be used for the purposes of diagnosis when visiting a clinic, hospital, or doctor's office — the stethoscope, the x-ray machine, the blood pressure cuff, the thermometer, and other devices associated with clinical medicine.

THE GENDERED BODY

When studying the general cultural concepts of health and illness in the village, gender came into focus as an important factor in definitions of the body. As has been the case throughout the history of American medical practice, the basic standard of humanity against which others are to be judged is the healthy, financially secure adult male. Variations away from this ideal are associated with more frequent illness. Overwork of the body, for example, can cause sweating and lead to a chill. Ageing is also seen as a process which can increase susceptibility to illness and general aches and pains. Individuals also pass through times in their lives when they are more vulnerable to illness: pregnant women, nursing mothers and babies, people who have been shocked or upset, and travelers are known to be more susceptible. Unlike men, children are not yet able to survive alone and need to learn appropriate behavior; while young men are subject to rash behavior (they are called *delikanlı*, "crazy blooded"), travel, heavy work and injury. Women past puberty have regular periods of ritual impurity due to menstruation, alternating with the potentially problematic states of pregnancy and nursing; while women past childbearing years are considered to be entering old age. The ideal male has established a family to care for him and his progeny, he has the social networks in place to procure health care if needed, he has financial stability, he is morally upstanding, and he practices the kinds of moderation in diet and behavior which maintain health. As Martin Stokes (1992) has noted "the social ideal for the male adult in Turkey is to be in a state of repose: entertainment, business, food, pleasure, and guests are all brought to him: he is never required to go and get them." (158). To translate this social ideal into health care terms, an ideal male adult should never suffer illness at all—his environment and physical maturity all contribute to balance and repose. He has established a home which provides him with all necessary care, ideally from his mother, his wife, and his children. A woman, by contrast, is considered to be "naturally" more likely to be ritually unclean than a man, in part because of her menstrual cycles, and "naturally" more susceptible to illness. The state of pregnancy, because it halts menstruation, is positively valued in terms of cleanliness, but comes with restrictions against abrupt physical movements, ritual fasting, and travel because of possible effects on the baby. A nursing mother must take precautions to avoid the ill-effects of *nazar* so that harmful influences are not passed to the baby through her milk. Gender is also a factor in a commonly noted ailment called "stomach-falling" (*mide düşüklüğü*), which can have effects ranging from a temporary discomfort to infertility (see Chapter 7 for more detail). The notion of falling can carry a moral weight (as in English a "fallen" person is morally corrupt or of low character), but it is most often used in the physical sense of something being displaced in a downward direction. Although men can suffer from and be treated for "stomach-falling," women, especially in child-bearing years, have more potential problems with various forms of abdominal falling or slipping.

While an adult male is responsible for his own ritual ablutions and behavior, a married woman is responsible for the cleanliness of her own person, of her family, and of her home. An ideal male adult avoids inappropriate contact with women by restricting his sexuality to the home, where the body can be kept clean. The ideal woman takes pride in the cleanliness of her home and family members and is careful about her physical and social interactions while outside the home. The pursuit of family health care and the responsibility for a healthy home, as we will see in the following chapter, are crucial elements of the women's domain.

Faith and Fate

Aside from the physical imbalances and filth, the local explanatory model for illness includes the overarching religious belief that everything comes from God for a reason, even if not understood by humans. The life of a human is a short span, filled with both suffering and pleasure, as decreed by God. Illness, in this broad view, is inevitable, its onset and its cure are beyond human control. Some go so far as to say that a person's entire life, including illnesses and time and cause of death are preordained, or "written on one's forehead." Others claim that God has made available in nature the remedies for all illnesses, the succor for all pain, if only humans can learn how to use them and have faith in their efficacy (see, for example, the interview with Granny later in this chapter). In the more concrete level of individual illnesses and injuries, the traditional belief often points to *nazar* as the cause of illness. (For a detailed description of the symbolic complex of meaning around *nazar* and the religious issues in local health care, see Chapter 5) Because *nazar* is mentioned in the Koran, it is a phenomenon which bridges the textually-based religious belief and the folk beliefs which are often scorned by religious scholars. When I went on a visit with Aunty Emine to see a man who had fallen off a roof and badly broken his right arm, everyone agreed that his reputation as a hardworking and capable fellow had brought the ill-effects of *nazar* upon him, causing his fall from the roof of the wonderful barn he had built himself, specifically targeting his hard-working and strong right arm.

THE INNER WOUND

Metaphors of physical and psychological suffering abound in Turkish poetry and song, in both the folk *aşık* tradition and the courtly Ottoman divan tradition. This poetic discourse continues in folk songs and in the popular music associated with the dislocations of modernity, called Arabesk (see in particular Stokes, 1992). In traditional Turkish Muslim cosmology, the individual human has been separated, even torn, from the Beloved, a layered metaphor which is typically described as referring at once to God, the human beloved, and the ruler (although I will argue that this metaphor can additionally refer to the comforts of home as personified by the mother). In this drama of existential separation, the voice of the poet longs for union, bemoans the torments of inner wounds, and begs for relief. The common metaphors of this suffering are inner bleeding (*'İçim kan ağlıyor'* 'My insides are crying blood' sings İbrahim Tatlıses), tears of blood (*'Gözlerime yaş yerine hep kanlar doldu'* 'Instead of tears blood kept filling my eyes' sings Müslüm Gürses), uncontrollable tears (*'Çaresiz ağlarım kendi halime'* 'I weep helplessly at my condition' sings Gülden Karaböcek and *'Silsem gözlerimi kurusun diye, Bahar seli gibi boşanır gelir'* 'If I wipe my eyes to dry them, they pour out like a spring flood' sings Orhan Gencebay), of a burnt heart (*'Acımadan sen benim bağrımı yaktın felek'* 'Fate, you ruthlessly burnt my breast/heart' sings Müslüm Gürses), and an inner wound not known or appreciated by others (*'Bilmezler melhemsiz yaram kanıyor'* 'They don't know that my wound bleeds without ointment' sings Orhan Gencebay, *'İçimde dinmeyen yaram kanıyor'* 'My unceasing wound bleeds inside me' sings İbrahim Tatlıses, and *'Gönül yarasından acı duyanlar'* 'Those who feel pain from a wounded heart' sings Alaadin Şensoy).

The rich poetic vocabulary about the seat of the emotions, traditionally the liver *ciğer*, but now more typically the heart or breast (*gönül, kalp, yürek, bağır, iç,* sometimes *can*) is tied to the metaphors used in discourse about health and illness through the use of phrases such as inner bleeding (*iç kanaması*), suffering pain (*acı çekmek*), ache (*sızı*), cramps (*sancı*), fever or inner burning (*ateş, iç yanması*), inner dryness (*'Kurudu gönül bahçesi'* 'the garden of the heart dried up' sings Cansever) a feeling of constriction (*'Dunya bana dar geliyor'* 'the world seems narrow to me' sings Bülent Ersoy, and *'İçim daralıyor'* 'my insides constrict' sings İbrahim Tatlıses).

In the ultimate examples of the genre, all of the metaphors combine to express an unbearable torment:

> Yüreğim yanıyor, ciğerim kanıyor
> Olmasaydı sonumuz böyle
> Göğüsüm daralıyor, yüreğim kanıyor
> Olmasaydı sonumuz böyle

> My heart burns, my liver bleeds
> If only our end had not been like this
> My chest constricts, my heart bleeds
> If only our end had not been like this

> —sung by Yavuz Bingöl,
> words by Yusuf Hayaloğlu

Other poetic terms of physical pain include various verbs expressing extreme states: *harap olmak* and *yıkılmak* to be ruined or destroyed, and *ıstırap, azap,* and *işkence çekmek* to be tortured or tormented.

The causes for this suffering can come from being ill-fated (*kara kaderli, kötü kaderli, bahtı kara*) or from suffering the blows of fate (*feleğin sillesine uğramak*) or from the ill-will of others, even of the Beloved, and include: *zehir* poison, *hıyanet* betrayal, *haksızlık* injustice, *şerifsizlik* ignobility, *acımasızlık* mercilessness, *merhametsizlik* heartlessness, *insafsızlık* cruelty or unfairness, and a host of other torments.

The only hope for cure comes from the uncaring or distant Beloved ('*Derman bana senden gelsin, Bekliyorum dertli dertli*' 'May the cure come to me from you, I am waiting in anguish' sings İbrahim Tatlıses). Words for this longed-for relief include: *teselli* consolation, *merhamet* mercy or compassion, *şifa* recovery of health, *çare* remedy or antidote, and *derman* cure. The cure is often likened to water for the thirsty, as in this seventeenth century couplet from Bâkî:

> Sehâb-ı lutfuñ âbın teşne-dillerden dirîğ itme
> Bu deştüñ bağri yanmiş lâle-i nu'mânıyuz cânâ

> We are the poppies of this wasteland,
> whose hearts are burnt black with grief
> Oh beloved, be generous as the cloud,
> don't withhold your water from the thirsty heart.

> —translated by Andrews, Black, and Kalpaklı, 1997

In the metaphorical world of poetry, then, terms of spiritual or psychic suffering and the longing for relief mirror the physical world of illness, injury,
and pain and the efforts to resolve suffering. If the ideal individual is in a situation of comfortable repose and good health, the ideal poet speaks from the
opposite state of wandering and exile (*gurbet, ayrılık*), suffering excruciating
internal and external pain, loneliness (*yalnızlık*), and unbalanced mental states
(*deli, çılgın, mecnun*), a stranger to himself and others (*garip*), separated from
the comforts of a loving home or 'nest' (*yuvasız*), and begging for relief. Just
as poetry speaks on many levels about the significance of things, daily talk
about mundane states of health also can involve multiple layers of reference
to the physical, social, and spiritual worlds.

> *'Âşık-ı dîvâneye dîvanum oldı hasb-i hâl*
> *Ehl-i derdüñ derdini eyler müdâm iş'âr şi'r*

> Poetry reveals the pained desires of the people of suffering
> For the maddened lover my book of verse
> is a declaration of bewildered love

> —from the sixteenth-century Ottoman janissary poet Yahyâ,
> translated by Andrews and Kalpaklı, 1997

BALANCE IN THE SOCIAL WEB OF SUPPORT

According to local wisdom, a sick person should not be left alone. People
should visit bed-ridden people, pat them and tuck in their bedclothes, bring
them appropriate drinks or foods, sit by them and sympathize, spend time,
talk about local events and other current health issues, give advice. Common
illnesses, however, should be treated lightly—it is considered amusing to hear
how someone was vomiting, racing to the bathroom, or tossing and turning
all night, as long as it is over. People, as they get older, are expected to recite
their various aches and pains when asked, young people should be more
stoic—after all, what do they know of suffering? After a visit to a doctor, when
asked about her health, one elderly woman practically crowed with pride: "I've
got high blood pressure, cholesterol...No diabetes, Thank God...I've got
heart problems — I've got everything!" ("*Tansiyonum var, Yağ var... Şekerim
yok, Allah'ha şükür...Kalp var—Her şeyim var!*")

In local social visiting, the first topic of conversation revolves around
health, in answer to the question "How are you?" Unlike in mainstream American culture, where this question is understood to be a formality requiring a

short, positive answer such as "Fine, and you?" this question is answered with either formulaic modesty, as in "*İdare ediyoruz.*" ("We're making do.") or "*Uğraşıyoruz.*" ("We're struggling along."), or with real information about health problems: "*Hastayım, biliyorsunuz, doktor'a gittim…*" ("I'm sick, as you know, I went to the doctor…"). Women express sympathy for each other, they solicit advice; they show off their economic means by discussing visits to expensive specialists, they discuss the illnesses of family members and acquaintances, and they compare symptoms and remedies. Of course, there are limits to the acceptable discourse about one's own health, and some women are known to talk too much about their problems.

İLGI: Caring for the Ill

One crucial concept in the local rhetoric about health care is that of *ilgi*, which can be translated as "interest" or "attention." The most commonly heard complaint about the State-run hospitals is "*ilgilenmiyorlar*" or "*ilgi göstermiyorlar*"—meaning, "they don't pay (enough) attention," or "they don't show interest." At home, a patient should be shown plenty of *ilgi*, and a family member's willingness to display *ilgi* is carefully watched by all. Daughters-in-law often have a heavy burden of health care responsibilities for their husbands' aging parents, and they can be harshly judged if they do not show enough *ilgi*. People express approval of a doctor if he shows *ilgi*, and compare doctors on this basis. People who have moved to Germany for work often compare the German system favorably in contrast with the Turkish health care system. One woman, Lale (more on her below), told me about her relatives in Germany:

Sylvia: What do they say, about the hospitals, about the doctors?
Lale: They like it a lot. They really like the doctors and nurses. The really pay attention (çok ilgi gösteriyorlar). They talk about how clean the hospitals are. I don't know… They like it a lot. They don't like Turkey.

Along with ilgi, the verb *bakmak*, which literally means "to look" but can be used in the sense of "to look after someone" is often used in conjunction with health care within the family.

TORPIL: Social Networks

Torpil comes from the French word for explosive mine or torpedo, but has come to mean "pull" or "influence" in everyday talk. To get anything done which involves an official institution and the connected bureaucracy, connections are crucial. No one in their right mind goes into an office without first having ascertained whether or not there is any existing familial bond or acquaintanceship involved or at least asking around for insider information. If a person, in casual conversation, mentions trying to get a telephone hooked up, for example, others in the room will immediately put forward people they know who know people in the telephone company, or at least who have successfully obtained telephones. A man's mandatory military service is a place where *torpil* can ease the rigors of training (if a person from the same area is found, he takes the new person's side in any jostling for power or in the inevitable fights among the soldiers). Military service is also the basis for a lifelong network of *torpil* which transcends regional affiliation—a man's military service buddies can be friends for life and their assistance can be sought when their network overlaps an issue involving their friend's needs. In daily life on the Black Sea Coast, any contact with government officials, be they police, schoolteachers, tax collectors, or doctors, *torpil* is crucial. Lack of connections means harsher penalties, longer waits, bigger fines, more homework or physical punishment in school, and worse health care.

In her book about women's labor in the informal sector of home-based piecework in Istanbul (1994), Jenny White describes this social networking as "a web of mutual support."(9)
From White:

Labor and services are not given in expectation of return, but rather in expectation of indebtedness. The labor and service which characterize a mother's relationship to her son, for example, are not only gifts of love; they also create an unrepayable debt of the son to his mother (the "milk debt"). This indebtedness is the foundation of the mother's long-term social and economic security as her son grows older and is expected to support her. While this indebtedness is consciously acknowledged and pursued, it is not perceived to be a closed transaction (i.e., a gift which must be reciprocated by a countergift), but rather a natural manifestation of the roles of mother and son. Indebtedness is the currency—the common denominator—of all these exchanges. It can be saved, stored, lose value or gain it, depending on the circumstances. I emphasize indebtedness rather than gift giving because it is precisely the practice of putting off the countergift (by which I also mean labor and other services) which joins people and groups in long-term, open-ended, elastic but durable relations... Evidence of this web of reciprocal, delayed obligations can be found in other areas of Turkish economic, social, and political life. Relations of obligation in society beyond the family are often represented metaphorically as family relations, as for example between the citizen and what the Turks call "Father State" (*Devlet Baba*). (14–15)

Social relations are thus modeled on family relations, and a Turkish person from a small community will discuss family ties when meeting a local person for the first time, usually being able to find some blood or marriage link to bind them. White describes how this strategy has been adapted for the large-scale environment produced in cities and because of increased mobility:

> When two strangers in Turkey meet, often the first thing they do is verbally sift through a list of people they might know in common. They are looking for a reciprocal link on which to base a personal relationship. Reciprocity, then, gives access to more than a particular group or grouping, but rather to a varied web of relations which are linked through reciprocal indebtedness, involving people whom the individual may not know directly. (98)

When talking about a person, the elderly women of Medreseönü always identify the person by familial relationships. Because I am accustomed to the American method of identifying people first by personal name, and because Turkish culture allows for the use of family terms for people who are not actually related, I often felt confused about whom we were discussing. In a village, everyone can call everyone else by a term which indicates a family relationship—young people call older ones "Big Sister," "Big Brother," "Aunty," "Uncle," or "Granny," and "Grandpa," according to relative age. A woman who has married into the village more often called *yenge* or *gelin* than by her personal name. When in a new situation, such as coming to a big city to look for work, villagers often try to make meaningful contact with strangers by using familial terms. A person might call an unfamiliar minibus driver *Şöför Ağabey* (meaning "Big Brother Driver"), address an older woman in the street as *Teyze* ("Aunty"), or enter a grocery story and greet an older shopkeeper as *Amca* ("Uncle"). This usage with strangers is frowned upon by upper-class city dwellers, although they use the terms within their extended family or in particular relationships which last over time.

As an example of the active use of family and social networks, I offer an account of Nurcan Yenge's visit to an eye doctor in Fatsa, the closest town to Medreseönü. She went to spend the night at a friend's house in Fatsa so that she could visit the eye doctor recommended by that friend the next day. Her eyes had been bothering her and she wondered if her headaches were related to eye strain. She got a ride with her neighbor's grandson, who was visiting from Germany and has a car. When she went the next morning, she learned that the doctor doesn't come in to his office until four o'clock in the afternoon. She had to return to the village without seeing him because she had to look after the cow. In order to return to Fatsa a few days later, she walked down to the coastal road and examined each passing minibus to find one driven by a local. Not only can a local be swayed to charge a lower fare, but he may feel obliged to help an elderly woman from his own village (also quite likely a relative) to find her destination, agree to pick her up for the return trip, and read any signs that she cannot. During her visit to the doctor, Nurcan Yenge learned that she needs glasses. Her son later stopped off in Fatsa on his way to a construction site in his municipal dump truck, in order to pick up the glasses, which he then took home to his mother that evening.

In another example, during a visit to a bank in Fatsa, the banker who is a *tanıdık* (acquaintance), asks Aunty Emine how she is. She tells him about her diagnosis of *tansiyon* (high blood pressure) and *yağ* (high cholesterol). The banker pulls some garlic pills out of his desk drawer to show her. He says they are good for *tansiyon*, don't make your breath smell, and aren't too expensive. Aunty Emine's grandson who is visiting from Germany writes down the name of the pills, for his own information. When we get back to the village, we ask around, and everyone agrees that garlic is good for *tansiyon* and *kalp* (heart). This kind of informal advice occurs often, even in a public, non-medical setting such as a bank, as long as there is some kind of network relationship involved.

People use personal references to get the best treatment they can from health care providers, whether traditional or clinical. They will say, for example, "I am the such-and-such relative of the patient so-and-so, from such-and-such village, that you treated for so-and-so ailment."

İzin: Patriarchal Permission

Carol Delaney (1993) noticed, in a Turkish village in Anatolia, the use of the concept of *izin* "permission" which implies "authorization to do something specific." (143) In family situations, the patriarch of the family is considered to be the source of *izin*. Elder women have rights of granting *izin* to younger women and children in the family, under the general rubric of patriarchal approval. This permission does not need to actually be granted for each individual case, but acting in a manner which would be considered "*izinsiz*" or "without permission," can cause familial and social repercussions. In health care decisions, *izin* may not be required, for example, for a mother-in-law to take her daughter-in-law and grandchild on a local visit to a traditional healer.

In cases where transportation is needed, however, or a visit to a state institution such as the local clinic is involved, a family consultation is ideally required, and every effort is made to locate the patriarch of the family to make the final decision. In emergencies, if the male head of the family is not available, others may step in to encourage the available family to go ahead and seek health assistance. The general talk about the incident afterwards may well contain mention of the appropriateness of the actions taken, and people present at the time of the crisis may advocate for the correctness of the decision they promoted on the spot. In the age of international labor migration, something like *izin* can be solicited by long-distance telephone, especially if an expensive health procedure may require money to be sent from abroad. In this case, the male considered most important in the decision making may the one with the best financial backing, rather than the eldest. Often, in such cases, efforts are made to get spoken permission from the eldest male as a matter of form and to avoid insult to personal honor.

Liability and Blame in the Social Network

Aunty Emine is now reluctant to get involved in serious problems or with childbirth, because she has learned that people will blame the practitioner more than fate if something goes wrong. If a person is accused of giving bad treatments, it can cause a major rent in social relations. It is much safer to give some advice and send a person off to the clinic or hospital. Even if the person doesn't actually go to the clinic, they can't later say that it wasn't suggested. Because relationships between villagers are often life-long, and because feuds are common and serious (see Chapter 5 for more on this subject), women like Aunty Emine try to avoid situations which might be used as ammunition in village strife. Some illnesses can be caused, intentionally or not, by the jealousy of other people or supernatural beings which manifests itself in *nazar*, which thus denotes an imbalance in social networks. Remedies for the effects of *nazar* may make explicit reference to social troubles or they may studiously avoid overt reference to such problems in order that they not be exacerbated.

Medical professionals in cities who serve the health needs of villagers are fairly immune to accusations of mistreatment from their patients. They have the powerful backing of state institutions. They may lose positive referrals if patients are dissatisfied, but this is unlikely to severely affect their practice. Health Clinic doctors are more vulnerable to local opinions because their practice depends more on building trust in the local community. However, if they lose their reputation for efficacy in one setting, they can transfer to another posting.

GENDERED RHETORIC:
WOMEN AND MEN TALK ABOUT ILLNESS

When women in Medreseönü talk about health care issues, they always use concrete examples taken from their own personal experience. Even when asked a general question like, "What should a person with a sore throat do?" women will give advice using personal pronouns: "You heat *taflan* leaves and press them on your throat," or "You should get him/her to drink hot water with honey and lemon juice." They often continue with examples taken from their own sphere of knowledge, "I gave so-and-so from up the hill some *taflan* leaves from our tree because her kid was sick, but she didn't use them right away and they turned brown—then they're no good." Or, "So-and-so from over in Afırlı makes a really good *pekmez* (a concentrated mulberry syrup). You can put that in hot water and give it to your baby. Before you go back we'll ask her for a bottle. Last year she didn't give me any, but she'll give you some." It is very difficult to solicit general opinions about doctors or various healing practices—every question is answered with personal examples: "I don't know much about doctors, but my mother-in-law went to one in Ordu for her diabetes. He gave her medicine. She used it all and now she needs more. My husband is supposed to bring some when he comes back from Istanbul." or "Dr. Gündüz (the local clinic doctor) is nice. He is not from here (*buralı değil*), but he likes it here. Maybe he'll get married and stay." Or "She (a local woman) gives shots to anyone who needs one. She is good at it. It doesn't hurt when she does it—she's got good hands. My husband had to get shots, so he went to her. When he's down by the shore road, he'll get one of the nurses to give him the injection, but he usually gets her to do it up here."

Women tell about problems with health in a framework of relationships. When they give an example, they never just say a person's name (in fact, it is often hard to learn someone's name without directly asking), rather they say how the person fits into the web of relationships which connect the person to the speaker: "So-and-so's girl, you know, who married our uncle's son." Without specific stories of the treatment of a family member or neighbor, women are unwilling to make a judgment about a particular remedy. I had been told about a spring where people used to go to get water for various ailments. When I asked about it, women had heard of it, but since they

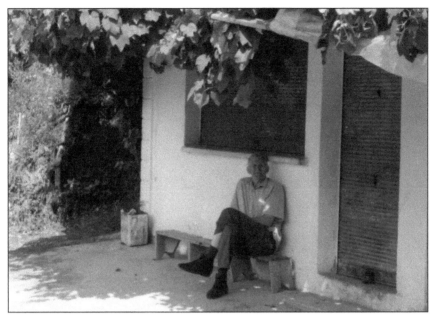

9. Ready to Tell a Story

didn't know anyone who had gone recently, they wouldn't say what they thought about its efficacy. Women also tend to use family members and neighbors as examples rather than themselves, unless they are the only relevant case of a particular ailment. Women talk about health in a conversational way, adding information to that of others, contributing supporting or detracting examples, and easily shifting away from health to other topics.

For women, the topic of illness and injury is an everyday one. Women share information about themselves and others, making casual recommendations or conjecturing about why a remedy didn't work or why a person got sick. Although they pay close attention to the morality and behavior of others, they do not often claim that an immoral person deserved to become ill—illness is usually thought of as an unfortunate state that everyone, saint or sinner, must experience at some time. One exception to this general view is the case of a local woman with a severely handicapped son. If pressed to explain this boy's state, most women blame the father, who is a known theif, as the reason for this misfortune. For the most part, illness is seen as the will of God, a trial to be endured, which will pass only when God wills, although God has made available every kind of comfort for those who know how to find and use the bounties of creation and their God-given intelligence. Women can pass along specific detailed remedies or describe exact procedures, but they assume these are being learned in order to help specific people with specific problems. They see no point in general theorizing about the serious and everyday issues of health and illness, especially when there is always so much work to be done.

Men, on the other hand, are much more likely to make general pronouncements about efficacy, often supporting their claims with ideas heard from others, from TV, or from newspapers. They create a stage for themselves, filling the available space with their tales. They tell stories about health problems and resolutions, which are rhetorically formed in chronological order, with beginnings, plots, character descriptions, building up of narrative tension, and a resolution, perhaps with a moral. Men give detailed information about means of transportation, the exact costs of things (including a figuring of old amounts to current value based on inflation), place names, and numbers. Men are often the main protagonist of their own stories.

When I was tape recording in a group which included men, a man would often start a story, recognized as such by everyone in the room, and would tell the entire story with few interruptions from others, until the end was reached and a point had been made. During such story-telling, women would shoot glances at each other and at me to provide silent commentary on the story and to check if I was actually interested.

The husband of Aunty Zeynep, the *kırıkçıkıkçı* (the bone-setter discussed in detail in Chapter 6), told a long, complex story about his own long-term illness, although everyone knew I had come to interview his wife. His story can be summarized as follows:

> When he was about 30 years old, he decided to go down from Çandır to the Sahil mosque in Medreseönü. When he got in there, in the middle of the prayer, a green light surrounded him—he doesn't know how he got out of the mosque and how he got his shoes, but he fainted outside. Some people picked him up and took him down to the sea, where they dunked him in the water. He revived and they took him to a restaurant to eat some yogurt. Then he went to the doctor, who laughed and said "Didn't I warn you?" and gave him a shot in the arm and in the leg. But he didn't get better, so he was told to go to Istanbul. He had to take a *paytun* (horse carriage) to Samsun and then a train to Haydarpaşa. He was looking out of the window on the train when a bearded guy, a *hoca* (religious teacher), asked him if he was sick (*hasta*). He said no, the *hoca* asked twice more, and twice more he denied being sick. The *hoca* insisted that he was sick. The *hoca* was from an important mosque in Istanbul and offered to

heal him for a certain price, an offer he declined. In Istanbul, he went to a hospital. He had a hard time finding the hospital because he didn't know anyone in Istanbul. A young man reading a newspaper at the hospital had him wait with him and then got him in to the doctor before the other patients. He had five treatments and stayed in the hospital a long time. He was even visited by a professor from a medical school. He began to believe the *hoca* he had met on the train after having a dream in which two men and a woman were swinging him in a blanket like a baby. He wanted to leave the hospital, but they didn't want him to leave. They had his clothes and he didn't have any money. Anyway he got some clothes and got away from the hospital and went home. At home, he tried to find a *hoca*. He finally found one who told him that he had come very late, but wrote him a *muska* (amulet with a written prayer). After seven years of emptiness (*Yedi sene boştum*), he was finally cured, thanks to the *muska*. He ends the story with a comment on how the times and morals have changed for the worse.

His story builds upon various traditional storytelling devices, including a problem which motivates a journey, a green light (a common device in Muslim stories of spiritual pleasure or affliction), a mysterious bearded *hoca* who asks a question thrice and is thrice given a negative answer (incorrectly), a meaningful dream, a futile, expensive, and confining procedure leading to an escape, and a supernatural cure. This was clearly a story, and was listened to by the audience until the end. During his telling, the only contribution made by Aunty Zeynep was a sigh and the phrase "I suffered a lot (*Çok çektim*)." Aunty Emine once interjected "I was the same," as if to tie the story into relationship with her own experience. Later Aunty Emine explains to me that his illness had been a *ruh hastalığı*, or "soul (spiritual) illness," the everyday term for mental illness.

In Chapter 6, we will hear a story from Uncle Ferit, husband of Aunty Emine, about a *kırıkçıkıkçı* (bone-setter) who stole patients from the doctor and walked out on his own heart operation. The storyteller makes no special claims to actually know the people involved. The point of the story seems to be to show that a traditional healer was superior to the doctor, and the story itself has typical story elements like surprise, plot-driven tension, and its relief.

The fact that it is mainly men who tell this kind of story does not mean that women never tell complete stories which involve health and illness. As an example, we will hear a story from Granny in Chapter 5, which resembles Aunty Zeynep's husband's story in that it is about a supernatural affliction which happened to her in her own youth. I have also been told that women tell more stories in the winter, when they have more time. It can be said, then, that the issue of health and illness is generally an everyday topic among women, who are most concerned about people they actually know and how suffering can be alleviated. When they are asked specific questions by a female researcher (and one who is integrated into the community through family ties as I was), they continue with this general conversational tone, giving examples mostly from their own families. According to several Turkish men I asked, men do not talk about health as much among themselves as women do (as women are held more responsible for managing health care within their families). When a female researcher asks a man about health and illness, the situation is more particularly framed as distinct from everyday talk (being an unusual one), and the man is likely to come up with a fully formed story, perhaps one which concerns an extraordinary event in the teller's life, or one which illustrates a moral point or a value judgment about health care options.

In local women's discourse, men are assumed to be outsiders to women's conversation. The appropriate family relationships must be foregrounded in order to include men in a mixed discussion. When I am visiting a house and baby Timur wants to nurse, the women tell me I can go ahead because "No one is at home." ("*Evde kimse yok.*")—meaning no men are home. In terms of privacy for women, men are the marked category.

Interview with Granny

For the purposes of this study, I'll call this woman "Granny" from the Turkish *Nine* (Nee-neh), which is a diminutive word for a grandmother. The mother of Aunty Emine's neighbor Nurcan Yenge, Granny was 87 years old at the time of the interview. She comes from a Black Sea village above Fatsa, but visits her daughter and grandchildren in Medreseönü regularly. Aunty Emine's daughter Fatma, whose three-year-old daughter was very interested in the tape recorder, was also listening to Granny while going about her own business, and asked an occasional question. Granny's daughter, Nurcan, also interjects when her chores brought her within earshot. In my transcription of Granny's Turkish, I have tried to indicate some local pronunciation, such as the pronunciation of the letter "k" as "g" and the shortening of verb endings. During the interview, I held my 17-month-old son Timur in my lap. Because he was slightly feverish and somewhat fussy, Granny addressed his particular health needs in the course of her general comments on health care.

In her speech, I observed an underlying theory of health and illness which involves a contrast between good and bad air and which seems to base decisions about appropriate foods and healing substances on their heating or cooling properties. Granny is fully aware that the health care practices of her youth are quite different from the health care methods of today, and that many younger people reject various older ways. She is amused by the dependence that the younger generation has for the clinical institutions and specialists, considering the new methods often to be a waste of money.

In Granny's discourse, the basic discomforts of the body seem to involve excess heat and sick blood, which can be relieved by cooling air and mud or plant remedies, or an incision and a poultice to allow a "sweet air" to bring relief to a painful head. She realizes that her old ways involving naked mud baths might seem scandalous to the youth of today, and her talk of that method is punctuated by giggles. I have placed the word "relief" after the translation of the word *hava*, because, although *hava* literally means "air," Granny uses it in the sense of something that brings relief, like fresh air, a sigh, or the relief of pressure built up. In other situations, *hava* carries a negative connotation, such as when it strikes a person like a draft that brings on a cold.

I have taken out only the sections in which Granny talks about childbirth and the "fallen stomach," because I will cite them in the Chapter 7.

*****

Granny on the Old Ways

Granny: They used to make a pill from the plant tops, we'd swallow it. On the road, in the fields, there is a flower that grows, in the grazing pastures…

Fatma: What for? For what illness? What was it for?

G: It stopped malarial fever (*ısıtma/sıtma*), for catching a draft (*hava çalması*), They would let in the air. When a child like this (indicates 17-month-old baby Timur) got a fever, so…

Sylvia: What did they use for a fever?

G: For fever, they'd put the yellow flowers' water out in the clear/cold night air (*ayaz*). When that flower's water was boiling…

S: Is it Chamomile?

G: No, like red-ish, they smell sweet, those flowers. We would boil them with water. We'd leave them out in the clear night air, on top of the house. Then later, we drank it, so, we did it that way.

S: Doesn't anyone do it, now?

G: Now noooo one does it, oh! They go straight to the doctor! Someone's got a headache—(goes right to) the doctor. Now, no. I'm surprised at this, so...Then there weren't so many illnesses. Those things (like the flower water) went in the place of medicine, they were effective, it was good. Well, they would get together to work in the fields (*imece yapardu*), of course, in the villages. Someone has a headache, right? Right away they would shave a tiny place right in the middle of the head, right at the base of the hair, with a strop razor. Now they have *jilet* (safety razor). Just like this, they would shave a little place. You know how there's a blackberry, that you'd eat when it's black, they would crush it with garlic, we'd crush it with garlic. In the little shaved place on your head, they would make a little scratch, so it would sting a little, in order to give a little air to the inside, give a little sweetness (or relief). They would cover it with that (the blackberry and garlic paste), and that *mübarrek* (the blessed soul/brain, created by God), would get air (relief).

S: Right on the top of the head? In the middle?

Granny: Yeah, here, right here, (she indicates on Timur's head) Just a little in the middle.

S: Right where a child has a soft spot?

G: Yeah, right in this soft place. Before, that's how people passed the time. When you were sick, that was the doctor, see? For us...

S: Is it good for anything else, other than headache?

G: That wasn't for headache! It was for a fire, a fever, a flame. They did it for feeling hot. For a headache...This is old-time business (*bu eski işler işte*), so, now they'd take a headscarf or a handkerchief the right size for the throat, it could be a man, it could be a woman, they'd squeeze it like this. From there (indicates forehead), a blood (vessel) would come up, and if it was cut, the pain would go. In the old days it was like that, *gülüm* (she is calling me her "rose"). Now I am bewildered, neither suffering ends, nor illness lessens. God forgive me! (*Şimdi şaşırıyom, ne dert tükeni ne hastalık eksiliyor. Tövbe estağfurullah!*) And they say old-time people...(*eski toprak insanlar*: literally "old earth/soil people"). With the food (*gıda*—nourishment), people passed the time, with the old ways (*eski işlerde*). What do I know...Illness was like that.

Granny's Mud Remedy

G.: Now a big illness happens, I can't get up, right? They would say, she got a draft, a situation would arise in a person. (*hava çalıyor derler bi haller olurdu.*). You'd go to the outlet of a pool, a little pond (at the base of a spring), they'd dig there, like this, you'd dig...And they'd lay you down there (she giggles), in the water, in the mud, completely naked, and you'd feel pleasure, like going in the sea. So, we'd lie down in the clay, in the mud. That's how you'd feel contentment. You'd lie there until you got cold, just like that remedy where you go in the sea and stay until you are done. But that clay, that mud is cold of course. And you are burning, "I'm sick!" I lay myself down in the mud. I lay down, just like this in the mud and buried myself like that. That's how I got contentment. Indeed, I lay there until I got cold and started to shiver. Now, if you say, "I'm cold, get me out," I'd get up from there, I get up from the mud, and I'd go to the mouth of the clear spring, of the pool, and there I'd rinse the mud off really nicely and wash off like this. Then put on clean clothes. Really clean. It is said, now...I don't know how it's done nowadays, (but) from that (procedure) a person wouldn't have even a bit of illness remaining (*Hastalığı mastalığı kalmi*). You would rise up like a saint (Pir gibi gabarırsın). Like you were never sick, never had an ache. Oh Majestic Lord of the World! Still I sometimes long for it. If something like this happens to me, I'm in flames, I go right away and lie down there. Now I have a fever, I'm burning this much, "Ah!" I say, I'm looking for a breeze over there, Now what am I going to do with a breeze? I'd better go to a hidden place and lie down right in the mud! I'd feel content like that. It would get rid of my draft. Actually, it's a habit, this. I long for those things.

S: Don't you do it now?

G: I don't, there's no one who does: "Oh my gosh — Don't go in! You'll catch cold! Merciful God, You'll get sick!" Now, give it up. I don't know, my rose (*gülüm*)...What do I know. Actually, you should do what people are used to in order to get their air (relief)...What do I know. Now they don't let you do anything. "Oh gosh! You'll catch cold! You'll get sick! You'll get worse!" Well, Thanks to God, a Thousand Thanks to God, Oh Prophet of God!...Now I miss that air (relief), I miss those states. Now, what do I know...You've seen those wild plants? Some of those bitter plants' tops, the flowers, the seeds—If I swallowed some of them, I wonder if it wouldn't be good, I say, for example. No way now! "You'll be poisoned, you'll die!" they say—what if...Then a person can't do anything, can't be comfortable. Thank God, a thousand thanks for these our days! That's how I'd get my air (relief)...What do I know. Now it's like this. Be it a baby or kid, be it yourself, say you've got a cold, you're burning. Then you take vinegar, you dip a rag in vinegar and you put it around on yourself like this (indicates rubbing it on her forehead, under armpits, across her chest), you lie down—all over yourself. That, blessed thing, will take away your fever. That's how I get air (relief), nourishment. I'll spread it on me, when it is evening, when I'm going to bed—on wherever hurts. That's just what I do, I get comfort, it gives me air (relief).

S: Where do you spread it?

G: Just where it hurts.

S: What do you spread? Vinegar?

G: Yeah, vinegar, what do I know, whatever works, I'll spread it a little with a rag. What do I know, when it burns, I'm feverish, I'll sit down and spread it this way and that. If I get cold, I wrap myself. The flame inside, I don't know… that's how we are, dear (*yavrum*, lit.: "My cub"), May God do what's good.

S: There is everything in nature, but we don't know.

G: Yeah! There is everything. Actually you should be your own doctor, after a certain point.

(Here, her daughter interjects that she had heard about women who collected three kinds of nettle and an herb and made a tea which was healthy, we all agree that nettles are good, especially for cancer. I remind them that the previous year I had taken a whole bag of nettle tops for my mother, which seemed to help.)

S: I heard that in Erzurum they roll babies in the snow, so that they get resistant to cold, they don't get sick after that.

G: They wrap (swaddle) the baby in snow, that's what they do, so the baby gets resistant. We say "He'll catch cold!" But it's good for the kid, that is actually good…I don't know.

S: Do you ever go to a doctor?

G: I go, I don't have much to go to a doctor for, maybe once in a year.

S: What did you go for?

Nurcan: Do you do any of those village cures?

Granny: Oh, you mean village medicines, no, I don't do anything like that. No, Thank God, wherever I hurt, like I said before, I rub myself (with vinegar). If the fire gets worse, I'll take myself to a warm water (spring) and go in. I help myself out as much as I can stand, that's just how I do it.

S: In the old times, was there someone who made those medicines?

G: Well, just like I told you before, from the fields, from here, from there…

S: Everyone did it?

G: That was the medicine. Just that. That's what people would do. That's what everyone did. The old folks, the older ones.

S: Because a bone-setter was a particular person.

G: That's a particular thing, of course, a strong person.

S: But everyone made medicine from plants…

G: They didn't do that (bone-setting). For a pain like that here or there, aches and pains, they would boil nettles and kill it. They would put some in water and wrap it loosely around (the ache)—you know how it stings? So that it wouldn't sting you, they would kill it (by boiling). They would hope for a remedy. Thank God, they would make it pass. I don't know. Thank God, a thousand thanks!

Granny Visits the Doctor

When asked about her recent visits to a clinical doctor, Granny shows frustration that the doctor does not share her concern for the "flame inside" her. He uses various diagnostic techniques and prescribes medication, as expected, but does not manage to explain the source of the flame. She does not follow the doctor's orders in terms of medicines, but decides she might be better off with the herbal remedy.

S: Why did you go to the doctor?

G: Me? Inside me, there was a flame...What do I know? I was uncomfortable right here (indicates chest). I was ill. In my stomach, like this. To find out "What's inside? Look—Am I alright?" I did that last year at hazelnut time, you know. I was ill. The guy said, there is nothing like that inside, he said. So he put this thing like a machine, you know like this (imitates a stethoscope), he goes around like this, and he hears inside with it, he says. He said "I see a swelled liver." What else did he say to me..."You have a weak heart." he said. Then saying "Take this, take that," he gave me medicine. I went again and he said it was a little bit erased. Now...I said "There's a flame inside me, I'm burning. What is this fire?" If you ask me, they couldn't understand it. That fire is still here just the same, this flame stays the same. I took the medicine he gave me. I took some, I didn't take others. Nothing. Now, I say to myself, if I just boiled those old herbs, I say to myself, if I just put their water in the clear night air, *anam* ("oh mother!"), and drank it, I say inside myself. If these flowers of mine would just open, if they had already been open, I would have tried it. I'm going to drink those flowers, God willing. If I see them, I'll do it. You put them where no one will disturb them, in the clear night air. Let them sit. I'll bring you some, God willing. It's a summer flower, I haven't seen it. It used to grow in pastures. It smells sweet. That flower isn't around.

Granny on Plant Remedies

G.: "Medicine from plants, from whatever's around." (*Ottan yandan ilaç*) They'd say "Medicine from plants, from whatever's around." From plant leaves...

S: Do you know cherry laurel (*taflan*)?

G: Wouldn't I know that? Cherry laurel...

S: What's it good for?

G: Your throat gets sore, it swells. In that case we'd wrap it. That day, you were there, you saw the cherry laurel. Thank God, Thanks a lot!

S: Does that cherry laurel fruit have any value? Against illness?

G: Cherry laurel fruit is very good. You should eat it. It is very healthy. Some get fussy, they say, it makes our mouths black (the fruit stains the teeth and tongue). Actually, you shouldn't do anything...

(Then another woman interjects from another room that she saw a program on TV about how cherry laurel is good against cancer.)

G: From the water (of the plant), the laurel plant (*defne*) water, cherry laurel plant water, everything is medicine. What do you think the doctors make medicine from anyway, dear, they make it from plants, from whatever's around! Now, they say (complain) that everything is bitter. For example, laurel leaves are bitter, cherry laurel leaves are bitter, too. Everything comes from them, Thank God! Wherever there is nourishment, of course, there is medicine. Thanks to the Lord. Everything is medicine. Whatever comes to us gives us relief. I especially love lying in that mud! Whatever draft I had, that would take care of it. (She gives a prayer of thanks and recites the articles of faith) They'd call it "the reason" Whatever we heard, we'd do. Thanks to God. Now what I have, most likely, is a shortness of breath, when you feel faint, I've got something like that. Thanks be to God, it's not a strong pain here or there. Just my back hurts, of course, lasting from the old days when I carried this and that, right? It's old age, what can you do? An eighty-seven-year-old person!

S: *Maşallah.* ("What wonders God has willed"—said when something is remarkably good)

G: Thank God for this my day. Eighty-seven is no joke! God forgive me!

S: Eighty-seven!

G: I am eighty-seven. Thank God I can walk this much. May God never prevent me from praying five times a day. May God give you a thousand strengths, dear. What's one to do? I'm depending on God. Be grateful (she prays).

Talk Turns to the Fussy Baby

G.: Now, this baby... (indicates baby Timur) This vinegar is really good. I'd take this baby (and treat him with it), and he'd be fine, don't worry at all. Do it when he's about to go to sleep at night, nice and light, like this. He'll be like a saint (*Pir gibi*). Don't get him cold, don't sleep up (on the roof), don't give the baby a cold.

S: Wouldn't the air be good for him?

G: Air is good, supposedly, he may get a cold. He's a baby, right? Not like us. Not like you. He's a baby, little. My God, may God do the best. May his fever pass. Don't worry. Fever makes a person uncomfortable.

S: He whines a lot.

G: I can't wear anything (when I have a fever). I have so many various things, so many clothes, but I can't wear them, they stick to my back. What can I do, dear. (She prays).

Granny Calls Aunty Emine to Confirm the Old Headache Remedy

G.: Still, the old ways were good. Thanks to God. If your head hurt a little bit, they'd squeeze your throat until a vein popped up on your forehead. They'd cut it with a razor. What can I do? May God give your sweet mother the best of health, may he pardon her. My God, don't make such suffering, don't make people suffer it My Lord, (she prays).

S: Now, a vein pops up, and then...

G: Yes, you just make a little cut and blood shoots out of that vein—whoosh!

S: Does it really come out or is it a feeling?

G: It comes out! Blood comes out. Now Emine (Aunty Emine, who has come into the room) knows about this stuff.

Aunty Emine: What stuff?

Granny: You know, how in the old days, when our heads would ache, we'd cut it with a razor, like this...

Aunty Emine: It burns...

G: It would come out, it would squirt out like this. You get relief. The sick blood comes out. (She thanks someone for bringing her tea)

Granny Speaks of the Changing Times

When speaking of the changing times, Granny focuses on new types of suffering where modernist youth and clinical practitioners would focus on improved diagnosis and treatment. For her, time has brought about new sicknesses, an increased need for money, and a new fussiness in the younger generation. All of which, however, are somehow to be understood as God's will.

G.: What can I do? We got along that way. Now, with the slightest little thing, they run right to the doctor (*Yallah doktor'a!*) I call it "Ask and give money." (She recites the articles of faith) That's what I say. Look at my old days, I say... "Ask and give money." Now if you say, "Let's do this..." "Oy! That won't do!" they say, "Are you trying to kill my kid? Are you trying to kill yourself?" A whole lot of fussing (*bir sürü tantana*). When in fact, it was good. Now can you be trusted? They have ninety types of suffering—some have cancer, some have tuberculosis, a lot of things to worry people...What do I know? (She prays).

(a person calls her from another room, and she gets up) I'm coming! Granny is greatly admired by all in the village, not only because she is sweet-natured and modest (an attribute which is conveyed in her frequent use of the phrase "What do I know?"), but also because she has the Koran memorized and is known to read the *nazar* prayer and other prayers with great efficacy, both for people and animals. She never used written amulets (*muska*) herself, and tells me that she cannot effectively read the *nazar* prayer over herself. When the call to prayer is heard, five times throughout the day, she removes an antique silver pocket watch and checks the time. She almost never misses a prayer, and peppers her speech with pious phrases and whole prayers.

In the flow of her recorded interview, Granny shows the typically female style of speaking about health and illness, in which personal ailments are listed and specific remedies are offered for ailments at hand. Instead of the more typically male discourse involving specific dramatic tales of illness, Granny gives general information and couches it in religious expression of faith and modesty. Her talk about the "old ways" is a part of her normal conversation with other women. As the visiting elderly mother of a *gelin*, she realizes that her knowledge may be valued or dismissed by the audience and calls in Aunty Emine, a *gelin* of long-standing local reputation for health care knowledge, to confirm her report of the old technique of incision for sick blood. Granny knows about my own mother's suffering from cancer, and brings her into the discussion.

THE DYNAMIC INTERACTION
BETWEEN TRADITIONAL AND
CLINICAL HEALING PRACTICES

The interview with Granny, an elderly village woman, about traditional healing practices shows not only the way in which traditional knowledge is transmitted to and challenged by the younger generation, but also that Granny's experiences involve both traditional and clinical health care practices in a negotiated, contested, and adaptive way. Granny has traditional remedies at her disposal, but she also seeks clinical help. She picks and chooses from among available resources and values treatments which bring relief. When she gives advice to a young mother, she is helping build a repertoire of health care practices which a woman needs to properly care for her family. She proposes practical remedies, warns that a baby is not the same as an adult, and prays for the baby's health. She only speaks to the particular discomfort of the moment (the fever and whining), assuming that other situations will be dealt with in a similar conversational way as they come up.

I would like to give one more situational example of the interactions between traditional and clinical medicine to close this chapter. When a woman came to the bone-setter in the Turkish village where I was conducting research, she set in motion a chain of responses which exemplifies some of the complexities of the local health care system. The woman had fallen and hurt her ankle, then had waited a week to see if it would get better. When she came to the bone-setter, she was hoping that she would not have to go to the doctor because of the expense and inconvenience involved. The bone-setter diagnosed a broken ankle and reprimanded the woman for not having come right away for treatment. The ankle was tremendously swollen and discolored, and the woman could no longer carry on with her daily work. The bone-setter agreed to attempt treatment, but guessed that the woman might have to go to the doctor for a more complicated operation because of elapsed time, in which, in her terms, "the flesh boils in the bone." The bone-setter, through the use of hot beeswax compresses and manipulation of the ankle, got the swelling down and the bone in place. (For a more detailed description, see Chapter 6) The bone-setter, a woman from the same village familiar with the rigorous requirements of daily agricultural life, worried that the woman would not rest properly and would re-injure her ankle. She agreed to give the patient pain-killers, which the local pharmacist regularly supplied to this traditional healer, only if the patient would promise to stay in bed for a prescribed period. The threat of having to be transported to the doctor for what would perhaps become a costly operation was used to gain compliance. When the woman left, the bone-setter grumbled with authority (much in the manner of clinical practitioners) about patients who do not immediately seek appropriate treatment and do not comply with "doctor's orders."

From this example, we can see that the patient had a range of options: to do nothing until the problem became unbearable, to seek traditional help from an expert in the same village, and to go to the doctor in town. O'Connor (1995) prefers the term "order of resort," to the older term "heirarchies of resort" (Romanucci-Ross 1969) to describe "the sequential patterns of selection and use of health care resources." (26) She finds that:

> This usage [of "order of resort"] denotes a simple chronology in the selection of therapeutic modalities, and removes the implications both of serial replacements and of "upward mobility" through the therapeutic ranks. (27)

Among the villagers I questioned, expense and convenience were strongly determining factors for ordering health care choices. People tended to try the lo-

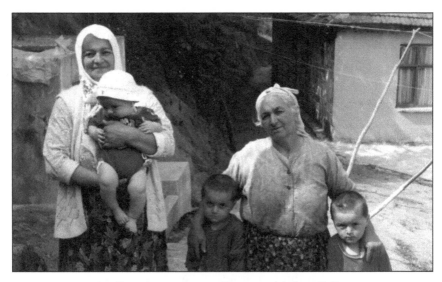

10. Bone-setter Aunty Zeynep with her Gelin,
Timur, and Twin Grandchildren

cally available and non-cash treatments first, going farther afield and tapping more deeply into their financial and social resources if dissatisfied with the initial treatments. In local terms, an "emergency" meant that a car was needed to transport the afflicted person, with very little time to discuss options or to minimize expenses.

The bone-setter in the above case also had the choice to refuse or attempt treatment, and she felt comfortable using the pharmacist and the town doctor as back-up resources. The bone-setter has both traditional techniques and clinical medication at her disposal. She had a certain kind of authority over the patient because of the severity of the problem, yet she also had sympathy for the financial worries of the patient and understood the patient's need to balance the requirements of farming with the requirements of healing. If the outcome is a success, then the healer's reputation will be enhanced. If the outcome is a failure, then the healer has made it clear that the patient waited inappropriately before seeking treatment and perhaps did not comply with the rest requirements imposed by the healer. The story of the interaction between this patient and healer is then told around the area in many versions, to prove different points, and influences future health-care decisions in the community. In the next chapter, we will take a more general look at the lives and expectations of the women in this village.

CHAPTER 3

WOMEN AND SEPARATION: LEAVING THE NEST, BUILDING THE NEST

Yüksek yüksek tepelere ev kurmasınlar
Aşrı aşrı memlekete kız vermesinler
Annesinin bir tanesi hor görmesinler
Uçan da kuşlara malum olsun
Ben annemi özledim
Hem annemi hem babamı
Ben köyümü özledim

They should not build homes on high hills
They should not give daughters to faraway lands
They should not despise a mother's favorite
Tell it to the flying birds
I miss my mother
Both my mother and my father
I miss my village

—Anonymous, as sung by Candan Erçetin, 2002

Aunty Emine's daughter, Fatma, has married a Kurdish man from a central Anatolian city and comes back to visit her parents almost every summer, usually around the time of the hazelnut harvest when extra hands are most needed. Her husband has become quite wealthy, so they drive to the village in a private car and spend plenty of money on the woman's family while they are visiting. For example, going to a restaurant is a big luxury (and a waste of money, according to the older women—not to mention possibly unhealthy because the kitchen would not be as clean as a home kitchen), so the son-in-law tries to take his in-laws to a restaurant at least once during his visit. If he cannot convince them to eat out, he'll buy groceries, including staples to last for months, and meat to be prepared during his visit. The couple also buys things to fix up the parents' house and to pay off any accumulated debts. Aside from this type of spending, they also bring gifts of new store-bought clothes and sweets. In the past, both Aunty Emine and Uncle Ferit have gone to their daughter Fatma's house to be treated by medical specialists at the expense of the son-in-law. This situation is considered to be the sign of an especially dutiful daughter and an exceptionally generous son-in-law. Under typical conditions, such spending is expected from sons, and the daughters' husbands are not obligated to spend money on their parents-in-law.

The visit at hazelnut time is special because it is the time when the largest number of people is back in the home village from elsewhere, typically from jobs in Turkish cities or in Germany. The weather is usually dry and warm, although cool at night. Most village weddings take place in the weeks leading up to the harvest, and people joke that families are gathering new brides for the labor-intensive work of hazelnut picking. For those who live in cities or in other countries, the summer visit to the village is a refreshing change and a chance to catch up with the village news while reaffirming local bonds.

Married women who return from their husband's home to their parents' village for the hazelnut harvest come to help their family but also to see childhood friends. In the reunion of old friends, there are plenty of opportunities to demonstrate how well one has done after leaving the village. Every possible indicator of wealth is examined by those in the villages, starting with the means of transportation used by those returning: Is it an inter-city bus? Which bus company? Is it a private car? What brand? Is it Turkish or foreign? Will they give us a ride up the hill or have they gotten too proud? What are they carrying—lots of bundles and gift-wrapped packages? Did they bring a TV? How are they dressed—are their children dressed modestly or have they been spoiled by city life? Will they come visit us or have they forgotten their old friends? Will they bring us anything? Will they come to our daughter's wedding? Will they give gold jewelry gifts? Will she have her hair done at the hairdresser's for the wedding? Will she wear a city headscarf with her fancy clothes or go bare-headed like we all used to do? Will she work in the hazelnut groves like before, or has she become soft and proud?

Although there is much interest in visible signs of wealth, outright prying and unambiguous boasting are socially unacceptable. When Fatma visits her home village, her old friends can see that she has done very well for herself. To find out details of her life, however, they listen for clues in the stories Fatma tells during social visits. One of the most important signs of a woman's maturity and economic stability is her ability to care for the health and well-being

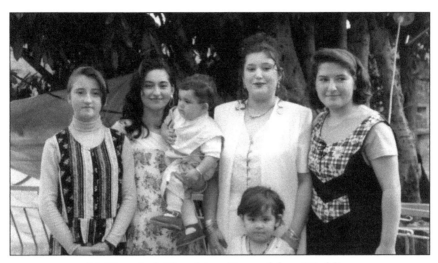

11. Nazmiye's Daughters Dressed for a Wedding

of her family. When Fatma tells stories about her father-in-law's many trips to specialists for his health problems after an accident, she is not directly boasting, although the implications of family wealth are clear. It is normal to speak about the health of family members, and Fatma's Kurdish father-in-law's story is particularly interesting because he has been to Mecca (and is thus a *hacı*), is over eighty years old, and survived being run over by a tractor while he was doing work that even young men would find difficult. When the doctors in the Anatolian town of his birth could not sufficiently remedy the complications stemming from the accident, his sons flew him by private plane to Ankara to be seen by the nation's top specialists. The care and expense lavished on this revered father demonstrates the fealty and success of his five sons, and, by extension, the sons' wives. Listeners in Fatma's home village do not personally know this man, but they have heard about him over the years. While the ostensible point of the story is to express concern over the old man's health and to share a story about family health and loyalty, the underlying appeal of the story is in its detailing of fantastic expenditure. As is common in stories told in the village, actual monetary figures are given for various procedures or related expenses. Because of the high rate of inflation, each figure is often translated into the current lira amount so that its impact is not lost on the listeners.

At another time, we were at work in the kitchen when a woman stopped by to ask for a recommendation for a woman with bronchitis. Aunty Emine and Fatma were both present and agreed that the best remedy is mint tea with one slice of apple in it. Red currant tea was also mentioned, but it is a store-bought remedy in this area rather than a home remedy. As the woman thanked them and left, Fatma began to tell about her toddler daughter's diagnosis of bronchitis and her initial motherly attempts to remedy it. As the girl's pain resisted the basic home remedies, Fatma began to take her to doctors. Each doctor diagnosed the girl's illness as bronchitis. At one point, the girl was kept in a breathing tent in the hospital for three days. When this still did not solve the problem, Fatma took the girl to the doctor at the Medical School (*Tıp Fakültesi*), who is of higher status that the doctors she had previously seen. When that doctor also diagnosed bronchitis, Fatma protested, "Excuse me, Mr. Doctor (*Doktor Bey*), but this girl's *ears* are hurting!" The doctor checked her ears and had to admit that Fatma was right. The story ends with Fatma's chuckle, "I am my own doctor—all the women come to ask me about their illnesses."

From this account, we can see a mixture of pride in being able to afford the finest specialists and pride in self-reliance. The father-in-law was publicly cared for by the males of his family, who took him to male specialists. His health and daily comfort were the private concern and topic of conversation of his wife and daughters-in-law. Fatma told his story as an example of how her husband's family could afford to care for their esteemed elderly father. When it came to the story of her own daughter, however, Fatma was the most active character. Even in a fairly gender-segregated town in Anatolia, she was able to take her daughter to a series of male specialists. She was able to provide the support which is required for a family member to stay for three days in a hospital, which, in most Turkish hospitals, entails bringing food, bedding, and clothes from home. As the final triumphal note, she was able to prove her own private knowledge and training through experience to be superior to even the expert in the Medical School. Although the ear infection was successfully treated with antibiotics procured with that doctor's prescription, it is Fatma's correct diagnosis which is foregrounded in her story as the deciding factor in her daughter's return to health.

✳✳✳✳✳

Women's Labor in the Turkish Family

The patriarchal nature of the Turkish family has been widely noted (see Abadan-Unat 1982, Beller-Hann and Hann, 2001, Tapper and Tapper, 1987, White, 1994, and the articles collected by Kağıtçıbaşı, 1982, Rasuly-Paleczek, 1996, Stirling, 1993, and Tekeli, 1995). Patriarchal family structures of various types have been observed in most societies of the world, and are well-documented in the circum-Mediterranean and in the wider Muslim world. Within Turkish rural society, varieties of family practice are commented upon in terms of strictness and loyalty. From the Black Sea perspective, Fatma's husband's family is considered to be typically Kurdish in terms of overly strict control of women. The fealty of the husband and his brothers to their father, however, is praised as the reason for the family's financial success.

What I find interesting, given a patriarchal structure which extends from the macro level of nation-state and international finance to the intimate relationships between individuals, is the close observation of actual behavior, which can reveal a wide range of female participation, negotiation, and adaptation within the limits of patriarchy. One of the ways women participate and shape their own lives is through their unpaid labor within the family. To the casual Western observer of Turkish urban life, the Turkish family structure may seem to resemble the "nuclear family" in the West, with husband, wife, and children living without other relatives in the same household (usually an apartment). Although this "modern" model is becoming the standard living arrangement, even in many rural areas, the traditional family living arrangement is larger: one household will support a mother and father, their unmarried daughters and young sons, and at least one of their married sons with his wife and children. Even if a young couple lives in their own apartment or home, the pull of the traditional family structure remains strong—for example, family members may visit for long periods, and a son will expect his wife to help his mother if help is needed. The *gelin*, or daughter-in-law, is still judged for her respect and attentiveness to the needs of her mother and father-in-law. Jenny B. White (1994) provides insightful descriptions of Turkish family structure. Because of her interest in economic relations, she is able to portray family relations as a web of mutual indebtedness. She describes the general cultural basis for the relationship between a mother and a son (which she calls the "milk debt", as seen in the previous chapter):

> ... the close relation in Turkey between mother and son, for example, is based on a mother's labor and moral contribution to her son's welfare and on the son's inability to repay his debt to her. The son attempts to repay his debt, but as he is not able to do so, the debt he carries is converted to homage, respect, loyalty, and so on, the intangibles which make up the symbolic capital on which a mother bases her future well-being and which give her considerable power and authority over her son. (100)

In fact, it should not be surprising that the most symbolically charged female role in a patriarchal society is the role of mother. The mother and son rela-

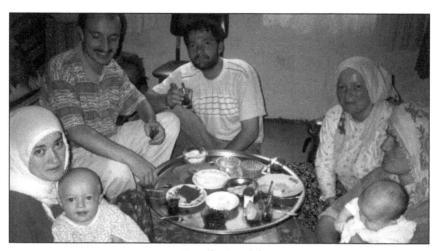

12. Family Breakfast

tionship determines the relationship between a mother-in-law and a daughter-in-law:

> The gelin ... gives a great deal of time, labor, service, and often material benefit to her mother-in-law. Nevertheless, this does not give the gelin power over the mother-in-law; quite the contrary. On the one hand, the gelin is in an inferior position to the mother-in-law in terms of social hierarchy. A gift of labor from an inferior to a superior would not incur debt but rather would be an expression of a patronage relationship. On the other hand, ... the gelin must be seen as embedded within a set of interrelated relationships rather than as an individual in a hierarchy. Her relationship with her mother-in-law can only be understood within the context of her husband's relationship with his mother. The gelin is part of a triadic relationship including her husband and his mother, and her labor and services are an expression of the son's debt to his mother. (100–101)

Although married daughters are mainly responsible for their husband's parents and the welfare of their own children, they can still feel drawn to help their own parents, especially in a time of illness. Whereas many parents-in-law complain if their *gelin* spends too much time with her own family to the detriment of her husband's, serious illness is usually considered to be a valid reason for a woman to go to her parents' home to help them. White looks at these relationships in the context of economic labor-sharing, but her insights are equally valid in the case of the non-paid labor associated with family health care arrangements:

> A mother has a moral and emotional claim to her married daughter's labor, especially if she has no grown sons, but this claim may not be accepted or acknowledged by the daughter's husband and his mother.... [Their] bond of affection and caring leads to the expectation of assistance from daughter and a sense of obligation of daughters to their mothers. (49)

It can be said, then, that the position of an individual woman in a family is determined by cultural as well as individual factors. Women's labor is particularly important in family health care, and any one woman's health-related labor can be claimed by family members in various ways. Again from White:

> [Previous examples] illustrate the contradictions that emerge from the redistribution of a woman's labor at marriage and the strategies families use to retain a woman's proximity and access to her labor. The inherent conflict between her mother's moral claim and her mother-in-law's customary claim to her labor is negotiated by adjustments and strategies of time and space. These strategies also reflect the relative advantages of class, wealth, status, and strength of the families involved. (48)

In a woman's life, then, there are several phases. First there is the period of care and training in her parents' home; followed by separation from that home at the time of marriage and a transfer to her husband's home. Traditional Turkish wedding rituals include a special "henna night" (*kına gecesi*) held by the female relatives and friends of the bride. Although the night can include happy visiting, dancing, and joking advice, the dramatic pinnacle of the evening is when the bride, dressed in her wedding finery, is surrounded by her closest female relatives and friends who sing poignant songs of separation. The bride and her well-wishers are expected to be moved to tears, and particularly sad songs are brought out until this result is achieved. During this ritual, henna is applied to the bride's hands to produce a red stain, associated with good fortune and fertility, which will last for a week or so into her new life. The bride's hands are then bound with clean cloths to keep the henna from staining her clothes through the night as the stain takes effect. This binding renders the bride helpless to care for herself, giving her relatives one last chance to care for her before she leaves for good.

As the excitement of the wedding and the henna wear off, the bride must begin to make a place for herself in her new family. The early period of marriage can be fraught with tension, as the young woman herself is no longer cared for by her own family and must take on responsibilities for work and caring in her husband's home. In this, the new bride is both a potential resource and a potential rival for her mother-in-law. In women's discussions of life and its challenges, the relationship between mother and daughter-in-law is a common topic. If a husband is harsh or difficult, it may be at the insistence or with the support of his own mother. A woman's best resource in the early stage of marriage is her natal family: father and brothers if direct confrontation is required, mother and sisters if social pressure and conversation during social visiting is sufficient. For this reason, brides who are taken by marriage far from their natal homes are pitied.

The expectations surrounding marriage and family relations play a role in negotiations for marriage partners. A wealthy and socially powerful family tries to arrange marriages for daughters which keep them within the sphere of family influence. A poor and socially down-trodden family may have to send daughters far away to difficult situations over which they will have little control. Young women contemplating marriage often compare the benefits of marrying an eldest son, and only son, or a youngest son in terms of how much they would be likely to remain under the control of the mother-in-law. An eldest son may have best access to the family resources, but his wife may be the one most tied to the service of her in-laws. An only son's wife will always be beholden to her in-laws, as there will be no new *gelin*s to take over these responsibilities as time passes. A youngest son may live apart from his parents, or he may be the only one left to care for the parents if his brothers have set up homes elsewhere, in which case his wife will have the most responsibility for caring for his ageing parents.

The second phase of a woman's life, then is the protracted period in which she slowly gathers strength in her new home, gaining the respect of her new family, bearing children of her own, successfully managing a home, entering the social network of her new setting, and showing her expertise in the care of her family. Even in the increasingly typical nuclear family, a woman is judged for her respect and concern for her husband's parents and extended family, as well as for her husband and children. With the increase in education for women at all levels of society, a new *gelin* may use knowledge acquired in school and in the broader world outside the home in the power dynamics between herself and her mother-in-law.

While the importance of male children in a patriarchal society has been broadly observed in terms of the continuation of the male line, Jenny White (1994), because of her attention to the inner workings and economic dynamics of the family, has been able to explain the importance of male children for

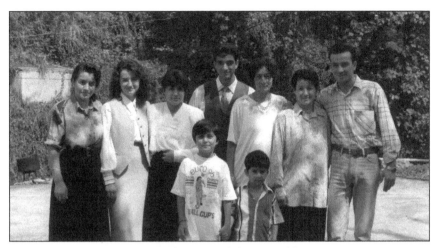

13. Family Dressed for a Wedding

the women of a family. The birth of a boy is cause for celebration for his father's family, but the relationship built up over years between a son and his
mother is crucial to her security later in life. To progress down the path of life
from daughter to *gelin* to mother-in-law, a woman needs a son. While the relationship between a mother and her daughter is often warm and enduring,
the expectation of marriage and the certainty of separation lead to the traditional saying "a daughter is a guest in your home". A woman who has only
daughters is consoled by others with the suggestion that she will acquire
*damat*s (sons-in-law), who will care for her. Obviously, this model leaves no
room for women who never marry or never bear children.

     In general, then, women in traditional Turkish marriage patterns leave one
nest, where they had been surrounded by the care of mother and sisters, and
take up residence in the nest of another woman, the mother-in-law. The relationship between mother and daughter-in-law is the family relationship most
often remarked upon as difficult in popular discussions of family. As a woman
matures, learns how to care for her own children and eventually takes on the
care of her ageing parents-in-law, her position gains centrality and prestige.
Part of a woman's integration into the new social situation is her education in
"the way we do things," for which her mother-in-law has the most important
role. She, too, is expected to bring techniques and recipes from her own home
which can entertain or be adopted by the women around her. As a woman
gains power and makes her husband's nest her own, she can increasingly negotiate for the privilege of visiting her natal family and of having her own relatives visit her. In cases of marital strife, a newly married woman can be very

much alone, especially if her family lives far away. This painful state of separation is poignantly expressed in Candan Ercetin's version of the folk song quoted at the head of this chapter.

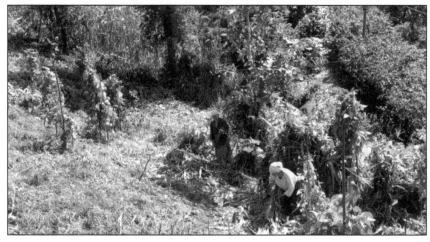

14. Women at Work

WOMEN'S AGRICULTURAL WORK

In a Black Sea village in Turkey, women's cooperative labor arrangements are an important part of daily life. The most common photograph taken of Black Sea women is of several women returning from the fields with enormous baskets strapped to their backs. The baskets are usually filled to far higher than the women's heads with firewood, leaves and grass, or agricultural produce such as corn, tea, or hazelnuts. They may be accompanied by one or two family cows, which have been grazing while the women work. Women are seen on the roads in small groups because they travel together for security and fun, but also because they often work together. The tradition of cooperative agricultural work is called *imece*. Although men can initiate or participate in *imece* arrangements, their projects are more likely to involve construction rather than agriculture. Women are the main participants in communal efforts to harvest a particular crop at the appropriate time. In central Anatolia, the harvest of large fields of a single crop (like wheat, for example) can require the participation of all members of the community. In contrast, except for the harvesting of hazelnuts, in which everyone takes part, the varied staple crops of corn, beans, and vegetables are generally harvested by women. Bellér-Hann and Hann (2001) discuss the value of *meci* (the Eastern Black Sea form of the word *imece*) as shared labor and a way for women to avoid the dangers, whether physical, supernatural, or moral, of working outside alone. (103–104) Women, particularly sisters or sisters-in-law, also work together to gather firewood, cut and carry fodder for animals, and carry manure to spread at the bases of hazelnut trees. If a visitor arrives to find that work is in progress, such as tearing the husks off of hazelnut clusters or separating the nut meat from the shell, she can choose to participate or not, as long as she wishes those busy with the task ease in their work (*"Kolay gelsin."* "May it go easily.").

WOMEN AND MONEY

The women who live in the villages I studied do not participate in the regular rotating savings and credit associations of the type observed in many places in Turkey.[1] Many women develop relationships with particular merchants in the open market or in grocery stores so that they can get credit in lean times. Cash assistance between neighbors is rare, but every family would contribute to a family known to be suffering from poverty. Milk products in excess of a family's needs must be shared (they spoil with time), and women distribute them carefully to foster good social relations. If a poor family is not present at a feast, excess food may be sent in baskets to their home after the guests leave.

The gifting of gold bracelets and coins is still an important part of wedding ritual, and the gold given to the bride is her own to use as she sees fit. Contemporary engagement celebrations and weddings on the Black Sea Coast, either in a village setting or in the coastal wedding salon, typically include a lengthy presentation of money and gold to the couple. For this, a male who is not the father of either bride or groom acts as a master of ceremonies, taking a microphone and calling people up to the front of the gathering where the new couple stands. Cash is pinned to the lapel of the groom and to a red ribbon draped over the bride's shoulders (the older tradition of pinning directly onto the dress can be dangerous for the fabric of the modern satin wedding gown). Gold bracelets, necklaces and sometimes wristwatches are fastened on to the wrists and necks of the couple. Although the value of cash gifts is traditionally announced by the master of ceremonies into the microphone, there has been

---

1. For studies on women's rotating credit associations in Turkey, see Bellér-Hann and Hann (2001), 100–102 and Tapper (1983), as well as Khatib-Chalidi (1995) on Turkish customs of women's coffee days in Northern Cyprus. The urban *kabul günü* is described by White (2002) p. 94, and the credit exchanges called *altın günü*, are detailed in White (1994) pp. 9–10.

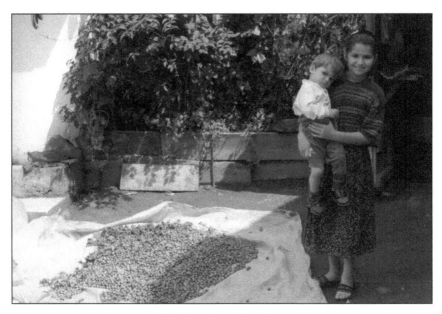

15. Hazelnuts Drying

a slight modification recently to allow the presentation of envelopes containing unknown values, which are collected in a fabric sack held by a family member. People explain that this allows individuals to give according to their budgets, rather than being publicly shamed for giving too little or seeming boastful by presenting a large gift. One of the tasks of the master of ceremonies is to foster a friendly sense of competition between the two families joined by the marriage and among those attending, encouraging gifts which will set the young couple up in life. In a village wedding, almost every household presents something to the new couple, and the generosity or stinginess of guests and family members is the source of talk in the weeks and years to come.

Since hazelnuts are a cash crop, and some hazelnut gardens may be given to daughters, the cash from those gardens is also theoretically under her control. Families traditionally provided all of the labor needed to pick their own groves of hazelnuts. Increasingly, family cash is sent from those working elsewhere to pay for seasonal workers. If the workers do all of the picking, they may be hired with a supervisor and expected to provide their own food. In the case of most families in the region where this research was conducted, the family works alongside the hired hands. In this case, they are fed by the family, housed for the nights in season, and are likely to be locals rather than workers from Anatolia. In Aunty Emine and Uncle Ferit's home, two local men, an uncle and nephew, were hired to help the family with the hazelnut harvest. They slept in a cabin-like room on the roof of the house, with sheets and bedding provided by the family. They ate the same food as the family, but often on their own portable table at a slight remove from the family (in our case on the open roof). As unrelated men, they were kept at a distance, where they smoked and talked with the men of the family. But as workers and guests, their comfort and sustenance was of great concern to the women of the family. Workers from Anatolia, often referred to as Kurds or gypsies (although this may not reflect their actual ethnic identities), are only hired by owners of large groves. They tend to travel in groups and be hired in groups under the direct supervision of their own manager. They are kept away from the family life of the locals, and viewed as potential trouble-makers.

MILK AS A RESOURCE

Milk from the family cow is completely the work of the female head of the household. She decides where the cow should graze (although it is often children or even the husband that must take the cow to graze), and is responsible for milking it and caring for its health. Beller-Hann and Hann (2001) find a similar situation further east on the Black Sea Coast: "Milking is normally considered a woman's job, for which even unmarried girls are not considered to be qualified, although they may have to deputize for their mother on occasion." (118) Milk, yogurt, and cheese from the family cow are resources a woman uses to cement social relations, exchange for other goods, and feed

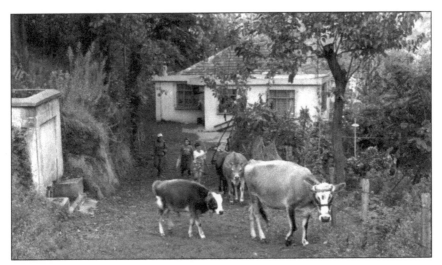

16. Walking the Family Cows

her own family. The fact that *nazar* can harm lactation in both humans and animals makes it a problem which directly concerns women and their dependents. The importance of milk from the family cow to the very survival of the family is well described by David L. Ransel (2000) in the case of rural Russian and Tatar cultures. Ransel's detailed ethnographic account is based on interviews with three generations of women about changing health care practices and it examines factors linked to infant mortality and survival. He provides an illustrative story told by a seventy-three year old Russian woman about the criticism she suffered from a doctor in the nearest city when she refused to stay at the hospital with her ailing youngest son because her cow was about to calve. To the doctor's question, "What's more important to you, your son or a cow?" she replied, "The cow is a second mother to me; she feeds everyone." She continued, "After all, how was I going to manage without the cow? What was I going to feed the children with?" (186) This woman's dilemma and the doctor's lack of sympathy for the realities of village life could have been taken from stories told on the Turkish Black Sea coast. There are many points of comparison between Black Sea village culture on the southern coast that could be made with the cultures of these northern neighbors, but only a few of them are to be addressed in the following pages.

THE FAMILY AS PRIMARY CARE UNIT

Carol Delaney (in Stirling, 1993) notes the importance of the Turkish village in the national system of caring for citizens:

> Women are also the ones who primarily care for the sick and ederly; in a very important sense the village is the nation's welfare agency. Relatives from city and town come to the village when they run out of money or work, or when they are sick. Children of villagers living in the city were sent back to the village for the summer. Widows were taken care of and not always by relatives. (p. 151)

The ties between city dwellers and the village are ties of family. In the Turkish Black Sea village, and arguably in a much larger cultural context, the family is the primary care unit for a patient. Kleinman (1980) asks readers to consider the family a "health management group" and to pay attention to a patient's interactions with this little-studied "practitioner." In comparing the type of care provided by a family group, he identifies several characteristics: small group dynamics, continuous relationships over a long period of time, informality of etiquette, and a different kind of ambivalence in attitude than patients feel when dealing with ritual or clinical practitioners. (306–307) In examining the Taiwanese health care system, Kleinman observed the importance of the relations between a patient's family and the medical practitioner, and asks us to consider it as a "distinctive therapeutic transaction" in its own right. He finds:

> The family commonly interacts with other practitioners, and in many cases *family-practitioner interactions* are as important as an occasionally more important than patient-practitioner interactions.... The *family* is regarded as *most responsible* for the patient's care, but individual autonomy of family members in health decisions varies with their age and status in the family and with the family's degree of modernity. Responsibility for the entire course of sickness and care is a major factor distinguishing family-patient transactions from other health care relationships, most of which are fragmentary and oriented to a single aspect of care. (309) (emphasis in the original)

This observation fits well with the primacy of family care in the villages studied here, with the exception that the family generally holds a stronger position than the patient in making decisions. O'Connor (1995) notices a similar communal decision-making process in the Hmong culture, which has come into conflict with biomedical concepts of "patient consent" in the immigrant community of Philadelphia:

> For the Hmong, as for most southeast Asian peoples, it is not the individual but the *family* that is the locus of identity, action, care, and decision making (Tung n.d.). The self is collectively developed and conceived, within the structure and mutual obligations of multigenerational family relations and clan affiliation. In traditional Hmong terms, there is no equivalent to the willful, self-interested, and individuated self that is so deeply ingrained and idealized in contemporary American culture. (85) (emphasis in the original)

A family is not considered to be properly fulfilling its duties if a patient is turned over to a practitioner, a clinic, or a hospital. The patient not to be left alone in these settings—the family must show its *ilgi* by having at least one family member accompany the patient as much as possible. With a traditional healer, this is usually not an issue, and the practitioner may even request the help of family members on the spot or for follow-up care. The only exception comes with gendered talk on topics such as reproductive health, in which case only family members of the same gender as the patient and practitioner may be present in the therapeutic interaction. In clinical settings, patients are examined with at least one family member present (there are compelling moral reasons for monitoring the interactions between a male doctor and a female patient, for example), and the staff at hospitals often try to control and limit the family presence to certain hours and to one or two close relatives at a time. It is common for a family member to sleep in the same room and even the same bed as a patient in a hospital, for the purpose of caring for the patient's needs for food and help to get to the toilet. A hospital is not considered to be a safe enough environment in which to leave a family member, especially one who is sick and less able than usual to function alone. In short, rather than a model of family care in which a patient is first cared for by the family in the home and then *leaves* the family to go to health care practitioners, the village patient is accompanied and supported by the family at every step. The family unit is not just primary in the sense of being the initial resource used in a time of illness, but holds the main responsibility for an individual's health throughout a single illness and over the course of a lifetime.

An individual with a problem will first tell her family about it, and if it continues, the family will discuss options as a group and participate in getting the patient to the appropriate health care provider. As an example of this family group discussion of health problems, I offer the following account. As we were sitting drinking tea one afternoon, visiting the mother-in-law of Aunty Emine's daughter, a woman came to the door with a problem she wanted advice about. She was a daughter-in-law of our hostess, and her daughter, nine years old, had a high fever and a scratchy throat. The woman explained that her child had fallen ill after eating ice cream, which had caused her throat and stomach to catch a chill. The first suggestion from the group of women was aspirin. The woman didn't have any herself, and no one volunteered to get some from their own homes. Then, someone suggested a bath in cold water to bring down the fever. Another woman protested that this would only make things worse, and that the only good way to bring down a fever is to press vinegar-saturated cloths under the child's arms and on her chest. One woman tentatively suggested a trip to the doctor (which would have entailed calling for a car, taking the sick child down the dirt road to the clinic, and waiting for the doctor), but another woman squelched that idea immediately, "Don't take her — What use would it be?" ("*Götürme, ne gereği var?*") The child's health is a concern for all of the women in the family, as well as for the visiting women. Everyone gives advice, but a child's fever is considered a fairly common, short-term illness, which does not require emergency measures such as calling for a car or even breaking up a tea-party to get aspirin.

In Turkish culture in general, women are held mainly responsible for the health of their families. Women are meant to monitor the health of family members, especially the very young and the very old. Health is a major topic

of women's daily conversation, and unsolicited advice is extremely common—
"That boy is sick, you'd better wrap him up better and give him some mint
tea." "Don't sit by the open window, you'll catch cold." "Isn't she too skinny?
You should give her a glass of milk every day." If there is illness in the family,
blame can easily attach to the mother or wife of the patient—"Did you see
how she lets her kid run around without slippers?" "He probably ate something bad (presumably ill-chosen, ill-cooked, or left out to spoil by his wife)."
"She's always visiting and chatting, she doesn't keep her house clean, her kids
are always sick." This possibility of blame ensures that health is a common
topic of conversation and that women take care to show their ability in managing illnesses as well as in preventing them. When illnesses occur, factors such
as the weather or *nazar* can be brought up as probable causes to deflect potential blame away from the woman considered responsible for the family's
health. Men in the family seem to offer advice or tell related stories about
health if they happen to hear a complaint or a question about treatment, but
they only become actively involved in the treatment of a complaint if they are
known for particular expertise (such as prayer reading and blowing) or if
transportation is needed (such as a car to ride to the hospital). Women decide
among themselves what should be done in a particular case, while men are
most often passive recipients of their mother's or wife's ministrations or mostly
silent facilitators in the transportation of a patient to a specialist.

Women are also the active tradition-bearers for health care. Although men
may have wide-ranging knowledge of traditional remedies, it is the women
who are asked for help from suffering. They keep their own knowledge alive
through everyday use and discussions with others. They regularly collect and
use herbs and plant material. They give advice freely to family and friends on
all health-related topics. They also initiate procedures in which a male expert
is required. For example, women initiate the request for a baby's father or
grandfather to perform the ritual of tying the baby's legs together with a red
cord and then cutting the cord, which is to make the baby walk quickly and
well. A man must do the tying, cutting, and throwing the cut pieces of string
to three places (a running stream, a busy crossroads, and the mosque yard on
Friday—all places of much motion—if the Friday mosque yard is considered
the same as a busy crossroads, then one piece can be buried at the foot of a
tree, in which case the wind in the tree is the agent of movement), but the
grandmother of the infant decides when it is time to perform the procedure
and the mother holds the baby during the procedure, carrying the baby three
times around the yard of the house.

A challenge to the women's roles in carrying on and carrying out traditional
healing practices has come from the textually-based Islamic revival movement,

which will be discussed in Chapter 5. Young men and women, in the name of religious purity, criticize the practices done by pious elderly women who, in turn, consider what they do to be within the bounds of a good Muslim life. The everyday practices of illiterate Muslims, especially women, are considered by the forces of Islamic revival to represent the old and mistaken ways of ignorance. Whether traditions are attacked or valued, they are particularly associated with older women.

Young women with education and exposure to other ways have confided to me that they think little of most old-fashioned health care techniques, although they value herbal remedies and special foods from their home village. Young men seem to challenge old ways at every turn, especially when talking to outsiders. When it comes to actual times of illness, however, most trust their health to whatever their mothers or other female relatives deem fit for them.

MOTHERS AND METAPHORS

Çiçek gibi tazecik
Fresh as a flower

Kıymetli bi tanecik
A precious little one

Ana sütü gibi tertemiz
Pure as mother's milk

—words by Nazan Öncel, sung by Tarkan, Dudu, 2003

Milk

Carol Delaney notices the metaphors of the "seed" (the active male role in procreation) and the "soil" (the passive female nurturing role) of a traditional Anatolian village and convincingly shows the ways that these metaphors support and reinforce patriarchy. The metaphor of "milk" as a mother's nurturing power can be seen as one which promotes the position of women (as long as they have children) without disturbing the patriarchal structure. Ethnographers who have focused on infant feeding in diverse cultures have often noted the symbolic power of mother's milk and concern about threats to its supply. D.B. McGilvray (1982), for example, finds in Sri Lanka a parallelism between the attribution of semen (both male and female forms are considered necessary for conception) as a transformation of blood and the attribution of breast milk as a transformation of blood. After weaning, a mother is encouraged to feed her child with her own hands, so that a "maternal" substance, along with maternal affection, can be transferred to child. (p.61–62)

In a study of kinship in Islamic law, in particular as followed in Shi'ite Iranian practice, Jane Khatib-Chalidi (1992) explores the category of "milk kinship," in which a woman suckles a child that she did not bear. The relationship which results restricts the woman's family and the infant's family to certain behaviors appropriate to blood kinship, with the major exception that they do not have inheritance claims upon each other. In practice, it was difficult to find an appropriate milk mother for an infant because families did not want to unduly restrict the field of possible spouses for their children in the future, and because the qualities of the milk mother were thought to pass on to the child. Khatib-Chalidi cites a manual by Ayatollah Khomeini on the subject: "She should be intelligent, of good moral character and attractive. A stupid woman or one who is not a Twelve Imami Muslim should be avoided; also one who is ugly, bad tempered or illegitimate." (117) Thus a woman who might make a good milk mother might also make a good mother-in-law. In the Black Sea village where I conducted research, milk kinship was recognized, but considered an old-fashioned practice that might not actually be taken so seriously as to prevent a marriage. Now that artificial foods are available and commonly used to substitute for mother's milk, the possibility of an infant being given to a woman other than the mother in order to survive has gone and the practice of using milk kinship to cement family relations seems to have vanished.

Mother as Bearer of Burdens

The most common image of the Black Sea woman in the Turkish national media is that of a woman with a basket strapped to her back, piled much higher than her head with sticks or fodder. Because of the typical division of labor discussed in the first chapter, women are much more likely than men to be found carrying such loads. In addition, the most common way to carry a baby to and from the fields is to wrap him in a blanket and strap him to the back of his mother or an adolescent girl using the same woven straps that would tie on a basket. The burden of the daily agricultural work (gathering food or fodder), the care of the home (collecting firewood), and of childcare (carrying babies) are all thus female burdens. Bellér-Hann and Hann (2001) find the metaphor of the basket to be a particularly salient referent for the female on the Black Sea Coast. (113) They found local sayings that affirmed the patriarchal structures such as "A woman is a basket. You empty it and then fill

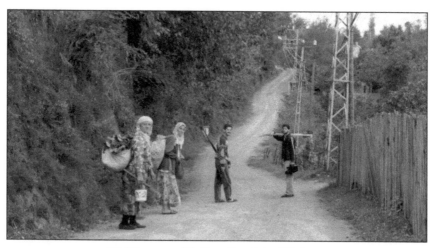

17. Women with Bundles, Men Without

it again." as well as sayings comparing a woman to an agricultural field such as examined by Delaney (1991). Although men may be seen carrying baskets at particular times such as the hazelnut harvest, and although they are often to be seen affectionately holding babies and speaking with children as they sit, they are not expected to be "bearers" in the symbolically female sense. So feminized is the Black Sea basket that Bellér-Hann and Hann can claim with justification that the local sense of manhood is based on a refusal to carry them.

While the basket metaphor refers to female labor, the image of a woman with a basket on her back can read both negatively (the Black Sea woman is oppressed and treated like a pack animal—the slant used in the national media) or positively (the Black Sea woman is free to move about without male accompaniment and contributes in important ways to the economy of her household—the slant most used by Black Sea women themselves as they contrast their freedom to that of Anatolian women). A discussion of metaphors in the context of reproduction follows in Chapter 7.

Mother as Beloved

The Turkish poetic tradition has a complex history involving heroic epics, folk and minstrel forms, and the elaborate courtly divan poetry. It could be said that poetry has always been the most highly esteemed art form of the Turks, and that skill with the spoken or sung word is still the most widely admired type of artistry. The Ottoman poetic tradition has been denigrated in modern times for reasons spelled out by Holbrook (1994) and Andrews (1997). However, any treatment of contemporary Turkish metaphors would

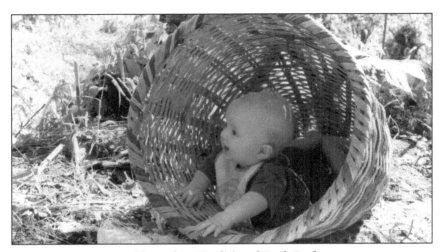

18. Timur in a Traditional Back Basket

be lacking without at least a brief examination of the important poetic traditions of the previous centuries. In an attempt to link contemporary metaphors
with Ottoman *divan* poetry, I will claim that the poet, speaking as the "Lover"
and addressing the "Beloved," may at times be demanding the attentions of a
mother as provider of care and object of desire along with the commonly recognized multi-layered referents of the Divine, the human beloved, and the political or spiritual leader. Andrews (1997) leaves room for such an interpretation when he claims that Ottoman poetry was "capable of fashioning the most
intricate metaphors, the most perplexing ambiguities, and the most mind-
boggling hyperboles." With these codes employed in such a highly developed
poetic craft, "poetry becomes a vital synthesis of the emotional content of relations to the ultimate temporal, spiritual, and personal foci of desire."(7)

The recent work by Andrews and Kalpaklı, *The Age of Beloveds: Love and
the Beloved in Early-Modern Ottoman and European Culture and Society* (2005)
examines the Ottoman poetic cosmology of desire and paints a detailed portrait of the gendered realms of this courtly tradition. There are particular cultural and historical reasons for a lack of specific reference to women in most
divan poetry (including a respect for the privacy of the female realm of family and a poetic tradition of extolling homoeroticism), and so it is difficult to
find direct references to mothers in Ottoman poetry. When asked about the
possibility of a metaphorical linking of mother to the Beloved, Andrews directed me to a story, reported by Aşık Çelebi, about a young man who was
devastated when his widowed mother announced that she would re-marry.
This young man left his family's home and walked to Istanbul, where he de-

veloped a poetic career under the name of Āhī. His mother's name was
Meleke, meaning angel, and so the following poem seems to put the poet's
mother in the place of the traditional Beloved:

> *Truly, in this world, fairy-faced angels are many, and yet,*
> *When you are gone my eye perceives no angel, no fairy.*

—Āhī, Translation by Andrews (2001) p. 88

Andrews provided several examples of poems in which a young son is the
Beloved for his mother, including one by a female Ottoman poet, Mihrī
Hatun, on the occasion of an illness threatening the life of a young prince.
Since the typical Beloved is a comely young man, the prince and his attributes
are suitable topics for such poetry.

> *May pain be distant from that graceful body*
> *It is fitting that his enemies suffer in the house of grief*
> *Why does fever grip you? Let it seize the heathen rival.*

> *Health is fitting for you, and for your enemy pain and humiliation*
> *For your mother['s sake], to whom you are unique and precious,*
> *May God grant you your due, greatness is fitting for you*

—excerpted from gazel #23, translated by Mashtakova (1967)

A woman from the royal harem, Nisā'ī, wrote an elegy after the murder of
prince Mustafa, son of Süleyman the Magnificent, in which she blames the
Sultan's Russian wife Roxelana or Hurrem for plotting the death of a rival to
her own son Selim. In this poem, Nisā'ī imagines the grief of Mustafa's mother
Gülbahar:

> *His throne and lineage were destroyed by suspicion and surmise*
> *What did that pearl-drop do, oppressed and innocent as he was*
> *His mother burns like Jacob [with grief] at separation [from him]*
> *What has the compassionless Monarch of the World*
> *done to Sultan Mustafa?*

—from Mehmed Çavuşoğlu,
16. Yüzyılda Yaşamış bir Kadın Şair Nisāyī.
Tarih Enstitüsü Dergisi IX

(1978): 405–416, translation by Walter Andrews (2005) p. 248–249

Although we have only a few examples of divan poetry which refer to mothers, the metaphorical longing for the care of a mother is much more common in contemporary folk music and *Arabesk* music lyrics, which share a fund of metaphorical riches with the *divan* tradition. In these songs, explicit reference can be made to the mother of the singer/poet/self. In fact, the traditional refrain of *"aman"* "mercy" can even be replaced by *"annem"* or *"anam"* "my mother" so that the singer is heard to be asking his own mother for the kinds of attention and help that the traditional poet seems to be asking from the Beloved. Perhaps the poetry of the wandering *aşıks* (usually called bards or minstrels in English) is more likely to contain the metaphors of loving mother and snug home. These metaphors have taken on a whole new symbolic life in the poetics of a rapidly modernizing society characterized by changing family dynamics and internal and external migration. Songs of exile and loneliness can evoke the lost ideal comfort and belonging by referring to the far-away home, comparing it to a nest for a weary bird or a port for a storm-tossed boat. These songs express the longing for compassion and care which is missing when the person is away from home:

> *Bu nasıl zalim yaraymış aman annem*
> *Beni senden ayırdılar aman annem*
> *Beni yardan ayırdılar ben öleyim*

> What a cruel wound this is, Mercy Mother
> They tore me away from you, Mercy Mother
> They tore me away from my sweetheart, it's best if I die

> Anonymous song from Harput
> —Erkan Oğur, İsmail Demircioğlu

The cry of a suffering individual for mother can be likened to the cry for the Beloved, in all of its possible manifestations (the earthly beauty, the all-powerful patron/ruler, the Divine). In fact, song refrains often directly address some aspect of this source of cruelty or mercy: Ya Rabbim, Aman Allahım, Ya Mevlam, Aman Tanrım, Ey yarim, Aman canım, Ey paşam, and Annem (Oh Lord, Mercy Allah, Oh Master, Mercy God, Oh sweetheart, Mercy my soul, Ah my lord, and Mother). In fact, the mother figure may stand for the most certain source of compassion in a cruel world, appealed to in situations of exile (*gurbet*) or imprisonment, when fate deals a cruel blow, when a folk hero is wounded in battle, when a lover is separated from his or her beloved.

MIGRATION AND EXILE: GENDERED *GURBET*

İçimde bir sızı var
Göğüsümde büyür anne
Koskoca bir şehirde
Yalnızım yine anne

There is an ache inside me
It is growing in my chest
In a huge city
I am alone again, mother

—words by Şinasi Kula as sung by Yavuz Bingöl, 2002

Köyüm cennet ne işum var burada
Ah nasil pişmanım kalmişim darda
Hiç gözüm yok ne şöhrette ne şanda
Naçar kaldım bir acayip diyarda
Bedenum gurbette ruhum sılada
Köyüm cennet ne işum var burada
Yere batsun gurbet el da para da
Of Allahım of kalmişum arada

My village is Paradise, what am I doing here?
Oh how I regret being stuck here in hardship
I have no desire for fame or glory
I'm left helpless in a strange land
My body is in gurbet, my soul is visiting home
My village is Paradise, what am I doing here?
May the land of exile and its money sink into the ground
Oh dear God I am stuck in between

—words and vocals by Hülya Polat, 2002

Men in the traditional life pattern were expected to have periods of wandering away from the nest of their father and mother, for work, study, or spiritual questing. The period of wandering or working far from home is popularly referred to by the poetically rich term *gurbet*, which contains a sense of loneliness, exile, separation, and separation from loved ones. After a period of *gurbet*, men were expected to return and take up the patriarchal center of the nest. As we have learned from Meeker (2002), men from the Black Sea coast

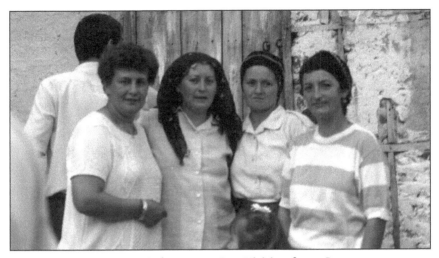

19. Four Married Women, One Visiting from Germany

have a history of travel for work which goes back centuries into the shrouds of time. Magnarella (1998) also expounds on the travels of Black Sea men:

> Historically the rugged topography had limited agriculture, and alternative land-based industries have been virtually absent. Hence many Black Sea men have had to search abroad for work. Owing to their legendary reputations for seaworthiness and bravery, they were eagerly recruited into the Roman, Byzantine, and Ottoman armies and navies. They are still actively sought out by the Turkish navy and merchant marine. Black Sea men have also emigrated to major cities in the Ottoman Empire, Persia, Russia and Poland to work as cooks, bakers, restaurateurs, and pastry chefs.... Today every Turkish city and many European ones have at least one bakery, pastry shop or restaurant run by Black Sea men from Turkey. (178)

When migrating for work in large cities in Turkey or abroad, men faced a challenge when the time of separation extended far longer than comfortable for them or for their families in the village. Some men set up nests in exile, often with foreign women. Many married in the village and left their wives and children with their parents. Some men, it is widely reported, did both. Over the long term, however, the ideal nest which would see to the needs of the male head of the household and his children was not well served by either of these methods. In the past thirty years, as the time in *gurbet* exile lengthened and family expectations changed, more men brought their wives, children, and parents to the new location.

Women, in the traditional model, rather than wandering, were expected to transfer from one nest to another, through marriage. The traditional wedding ceremony includes the poignant ritual of separation from the natal home and womenfolk (the *kına gecesi* with its sad songs and ritual marks of blood-red henna), a procession from the bride's natal home to the groom's home (often dramatized as a capture by the groom's family, which on the Black Sea requires the firing of weapons into the air), the transfer of dowry goods such as towels and bed sheets to the new home, and a series of visits paid to the new bride in her mother-in-law's house. Wandering freely may be a metaphor of girlhood in the safe environs of home, but it not a part of adult women's traditional activities. For example, Hülya Polat, in her song about *gurbet*, reminisces about the paradise of her childhood village: *Doğan güneş tepelere vurunca, Köyümde yürürdüm dere boyunca* (When the rising sun hit the hills, I would walk along the the length of the river in my village). She characterizes *gurbet* as *dar*, a word meaning narrow, which can refer to economic poverty, restricted movement, ill-health, and a feeling of oppression.

As we have seen, in the agricultural life on the Black Sea Coast, women often form groups to go out to work in fields and gather firewood (see Beller-Hann and Hann (2001) pp.102–105), which is in part a way to protect them from what could befall them if alone. From the vantage of *gurbet*, however, the traditional *imece* of laughter and mutual assistance can create nostalgia for the friends, hills, fresh air, and freedom of village life. (Of course, outside of poetic metaphor, many women and men in *gurbet* explicitly extol city life despite its difficulties and are not nostalgic in the least for agricultural work.) In the poetry of exile and longing, the kinds of movement brought about by internal and external migration are shown as challenges to gender roles and family relations, and as threats to everyone's peace of mind.

In the metaphors of separation from the home, a man in *gurbet* is in a position more drastically removed from the traditional life story in which, even if he traveled for work as a young man, he would expect to live out his life in his homeland, surrounded by the care of his mother, wife, and children. A woman in *gurbet* is like a traditional bride married far from home. Although she is expected to feel sad at being separated from her family, she is also meant to find fulfillment in her new family, raising her children in her husband's family nest.

The next chapter returns to the village setting to describe the forms of religious rituals and social relations which shape and give meaning to women's lives, including the very popular recital of an Ottoman poem celebrating the birth of the Prophet Mohammed, the rituals of daily prayer, and various forms of everyday sociability.

CHAPTER 4

WOMEN'S RITUAL
AND SOCIAL LIVES

Here Amine made ending, for the hour
In which should come the best of men had sounded.

"I thirst," she cried, "I thirst, I burn with fever!"
A brimming glass to her at once was proffered.

White was that glass, than snow more white, and colder;
No sweetmeat ever made held half such sweetness.

"I drank it, and my being filled with glory,
Nor could I longer self from light distinguish.

On pinions bright a bird of white came floating,
And stroked my back, so strongly yet how kindly;

The Sultan of the Faith that hour was given,
And drowned in glory lay both earth and heaven."

Now pray to him, make peace and full submission,
That paradise be yours for your contrition.

—The Birth of the Prophet Muhammed,
described by his mother Amine, in the *Mevlidi Şerif*
by Süleyman Çelebi, (early 15th century)
translated by F. L. MacCallum, 1943

A bright summer's day dawns early. Aunty Emine has already been down
into the gardens for the fresh cucumbers and peppers which are now frying
on the stove outside the front door. I'm too late to put the tea on to boil, but
I can get the dishes and glasses ready on the *sini* tray for our small number.
While baby Timur lies on a cloth wedged between floor cushions, on the side
away from the stove of the table set outside the doorway, Aunty Emine, Uncle
Ferit, and I sip our tea with the fried vegetables, olives, helva, and fresh bak-

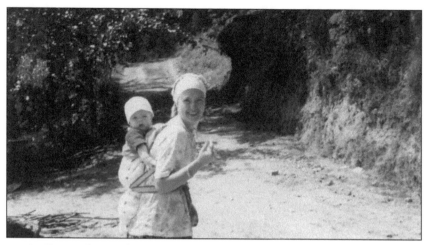

20. Researcher and Son—Dressed for Work Rather than for *mevlûd.*

ery bread delivered by truck to the dirt road intersection closest to the house. Although there is plenty of work to be done before noon, today has a special feel. In the afternoon, we will go up the hill to the next village, closer to Aunty Emine's natal village, to a *mevlûd* hosted every year by a pious family in honor of their deceased family members. Uncle Ferit has already put on his best white shirt. He'll spend the morning in the coffeehouse further up the hill and then come down to meet us at the *mevlûd.*

My morning chores include washing the breakfast dishes, removing and shaking the couch cushions and carpets, sweeping the rooms of the house with a straw broom in the direction of the central hall, and then sweeping the gathered dust out the front door and down into the rubbish pile below the house. After the carpets are back in place, the furniture is repositioned around the main living room, the shelves and television are dusted, and all windows are opened so that fresh air flows through the house. Aunty Emine has some business in the vegetable garden below the house which she tends carefully and with bountiful results. Knowing I am alone, the *gelin* from next door pops her head in for a quick chat between her own similar chores. Her husband is at work and cannot attend the *mevlûd* this afternoon. She'll go with her mother-in-law, leaving her son with a neighbor, as he is too active to sit quietly through the whole event. We'll see each other there, but probably at a distance, since her mother-in-law and Aunty Emine are out of sorts with each other, preferring to avoid each other in public. The social strains of village life lead to rifts, feuds, and reconciliation over time. As *gelins*, we must loyally observe the example of our elders, but we can reach out to each other in the few moments when we are left to our own devices. Good deeds and shared resources between families often reduce the sting of a social rift, allowing women to discretely remain friends even if their husbands are at odds, or children to visit each other even if mothers are not on speaking terms. As soon as they enter the village of their husbands, *gelins* must find allies, friends, and confidants without violating whatever social divisions are current. Over a lifetime, a woman works hard to maintain her social network so that she has friends to call on in hard times, supporters in a feud or dispute, and a wide range of people who think well of her. Women whose husbands are badly behaved or dissolute have an extra burden when forging a social network, and are generally pitied by other women.

Aunty Emine returns from the garden, we have a quick snack before we dress to go out. Because the *mevlûd* is a religious event, Aunty Emine makes sure I am appropriately dressed. I wear a long skirt that is wide enough to sit comfortably on the ground, a long-sleeved shirt, and a brightly colored flowered cotton head-scarf draped so that it covers my hair and neck. Aunty Emine wears a store-bought set of matching skirt and long-sleeved shirt, with dark knee-high hose and covered-toe shoes. Over her cotton headscarf, she ties a store-bought polyester headscarf, a gift from one of her daughters. With a handbag and sun parasol to complete the outfit, Aunty Emine looks more like a city dweller, while I look more like a villager, especially when I tie Timur to my back for the walk up the hill. Timur's outfit is a new American set, with a white sailor's hat to shield him from the sun. Aunty Emine has me pin an evil eye bead onto his clothes behind his shoulder because there will be many people looking at him this afternoon.

We set off up the hill, at a leisurely pace so we do not overheat and spoil our clothes. When we reach the first crest, we can see that there is a haze over the Black Sea, a sign of continuing hot weather which may bring the hazelnut harvesting time faster. Aunty Emine tells me a bit about the families in the houses we pass, usually in terms of their kinship with people I have met. Timur, who fussed a bit when I tied him onto my back, has fallen fast asleep. Aunty Emine checks that his skin is not exposed to the sun. Before long, we are approaching the house hosting the *mevlûd*. A dirt road leads down to the level area in front of the house. Many people have already arrived, and we are greeted and taken into a back bedroom, which seems to me to be full. Women shift to make room, and I peel my sweaty son off of my back so that I can sit with him in my lap. Without much talking, the women seated on the floor of the room greet Aunty Emine and cast appraising looks at me. I feel quite wedged in, between the shoulder of a large woman in a typical woolen vest and a pile of bedding covered in an embroidered cloth. Timur sleeps on.

The microphone is switched on, adjusted, and then, with appropriate prayers to start, the *mevlûd* recital commences. The man who is reciting the poem about the birth of Prophet Mohammed is out of our eyesight, sitting with other men in the place of honor in the main room. The poem is in Ottoman Turkish, scattered with pious Arabic phrases, and the older women in the room seem to be following along, speaking blessings aloud as various names are mentioned, including the Prophet and his mother, Amine. At certain times during the recital, everyone stands to face Mecca for a prayer. At the climax of the recital, with the section which is translated above, the women turn and stroke each other down the back, in symbolic unity with the white bird that brought relief to Amine in her birth pains. At the end, greetings are exchanged between each person in the room. The poem ends, and the reciter calls for blessings from everyone gathered for a list of individuals, from the Prophet and his family to the political leaders and soldiers of the nation, to the deceased members of the host family. The microphone is switched off, and the gathered women exchange short greetings as they shift to make room for the meal which follows the recital. The meal will be served to four groups at once in our room, with preference given to elderly women and esteemed guests. The tray table tops are brought in already set with utensils and food in common bowls, and placed on folding legs so that the women seated on the floor can comfortably eat from them. The trays are removed and brought back for the next groups of women in the room. The menu includes the wheat pudding called *keşkek*, a specialty served at all occasions which require the feeding of large groups of guests, as well as rice-stuffed collard leaves, meat stew, and plum *komposto* with a beautiful pink color and whole fruits floating in it. The *komposto*, eaten with a spoon from a bowl, is the main liquid refreshment, although water in glasses is provided on request.

After the meal, the women sit back and begin to converse in earnest. Health concerns are a major topic, as in all gatherings of women. Women have come from villages all around, and have much catching up to do. Weddings, deaths, the movements of family members, and new family members are discussed. Everyone wants to learn more about Aunty Emine's guests—does the foreign *gelin* speak Turkish? Is she a Muslim? What is the baby's name? These questions are mainly answered by Aunty Emine, although a few older women put questions directly to me to see if I can understand them. Then the topic shifts to more complicated local matters, and I nurse Timur under a blanket, careful to keep the process out of sight.

On the way out of the house, Aunty Emine thanks the host family and asks that their pious deeds be rewarded by God. Uncle Ferit joins us at the road, and we walk back down the stony road in the twilight, chatting about various

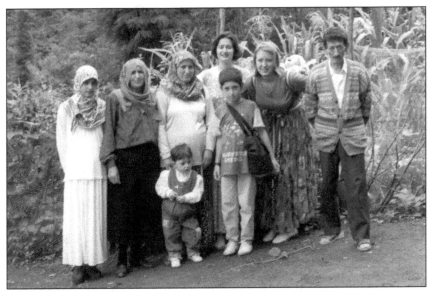

21. Aunty Emine and Family Dressed for Social Visiting

bits of news learned during our visit. Not wanting to let go of the sociability of the afternoon, we stop by to drink tea with a neighbor on the way back. She had been unable to go to the *mevlûd* so Aunty Emine summarizes the event, praising the family for their piety and willingness to hold a yearly *mevlûd*. She approvingly reports on the voice and phrasing of the reciter, the taste and quantity of the food served, and the care with which the female members of the family served their guests. The moon is rising as we get back home, a warm wind blowing across our faces.

✶✶✶✶✶

RITUALS CELEBRATING THE BIRTH OF THE PROPHET: CROSS-CULTURAL COMPARISONS

An examination of recent literature on Muslim women's spiritual and ritual practices, from Malaysia to Yemen and from Sudan to Bosnia, suggests that there may be some points of similarity worth exploring. In particular, celebratory poetry on the birth of the Prophet Muhammed, including the Ottoman Turkish poem from the early fifteenth century called the *Mevlidi Şerif,* seems to have been incorporated into ritual practice in Ottoman lands and beyond. The pre-Ottoman Arabic poetry on this topic, as well as pre-Islamic traditions celebrating the nativity of Jesus, contributed to a rich poetic vocabulary and an array of ritual behavior, some of which continues to be important today. The popularity of *mevlûd* (also: *mawlid/mevlit/mevlût/mevlut*) has brought down the wrath of extreme purists, who find the *mevlûd* to be impious because is it not supported by Koranic reference. As we shall see, despite its appeal to women, or specifically because of it, the *mevlûd* has been the target of Islamic reformers, such as the Wahabbis in Saudi Arabia.

Anthropologist Tone Bringa (1995) describes the Bosnian rituals of *tevhid* and *mevlud*, comparing and contrasting them to the Turkish rituals described by the Tappers (1987). Her description of the women's *tevhid*, given in a home for the benefit of the souls of family members of that household, resembles to a remarkable degree the *mevlûds* I attended in Black Sea village homes. The photographs provided by Bringa, could have been taken in Medreseönü, so similar are the styles of headscarf, sitting on the carpet in close proximity, and the hand gestures in prayer. (p. 190–191) The only striking difference is that I did not see the use of extremely long wooden prayer beads, although prayer beads of regular length were shared around the room, and long wooden prayer beads are available and may be used in a similar way in other parts of Turkey. Likewise, Bringa's photograph of women seated on a hillside outside a tomb is also evocative of women's gatherings on the Black Sea Coast. Although tomb visiting is not a part of local custom in the area I studied, the women who sit outside during a *mevlûd* given at a home sit in groupings and wear clothing very similar to the Bosnian women studied by Bringa.

Bringa describes the two types of religious gatherings in the Bosnian countryside:

> …the tevhid is the most frequently held ritual in the region and, of all religious activities, the one in which a woman most often engages. Indeed, the tevhid is the most frequent legitimate occasion for women (or wives) to socialize outside the immediate neighborhood and the village. However, it also means socializing exclusively with and primarily as Muslim women.[1] the tevhid in Bosnia thus has a

---

1. Although the Black Sea coast of Turkey used to be home for a mix of religious communities, in which attending or hosting a *mevlûd* recital may have played a role in the demonstration of a Muslim identity and a way to build a specifically Muslim sense of belonging, that function does not seem to be important currently. The presence of a non-Muslim, as in the case of anthropologist Delaney (1991) at a *mevlûd* in Central Anatolia,

similar position to the mevlud in the Turkish town studied by the Tappers (1987), with the significant difference that in Turkey the mevlud associated with death are mainly by and for men. (Bringa, p. 194)

It seems that Bringa is misconstruing the Tappers' division of types of *mevlûd* and male and female participants, although there is some ambiguity in the Tapper (1987) article about whether men or women hold *mevlûd* ceremonies more frequently in conjunction with a death. When speaking of men's *mevlûds*, they report:

First, the greatest number of men's services are directly associated with death. In the evening after a funeral, a mevlud will be performed in the home of the deceased.... On the anniversary of the death of a senior man, a mevlud may be held in a mosque, in which case an invitation is extended to all men via the local newspapers.... Secondly, the joyful life-cycle ceremonies of circumcision and marriage may be begun with a mevlud performed by men.... Thirdly, mevluds are performed on the occasion of the five Kandils, the major Islamic festivals recognised in most parts of Turkey, when mevluds are also broadcast nationally on television; locally the services are sponsored by the town religious establishment and are held in the main mosque in association with evening prayers. (77)

As for women's *mevlûds*, the Tappers claim:

Mevluds for women almost always occur in the context of death— immediately after a funeral, and then on any or all of the following occasions: the 7th, the 40th, the 52nd days after death, and annually on the anniversary. They are held in private houses where invited congregations may vary from a dozen women to a hundred or more, averaging around fifty. (77)

In short, it seems that *mevlûds* are most commonly held in connection with a death, with men's *mevlûds* held either in homes or in a mosque, and women's *mevlûds* held only in homes. On the Black Sea coast, the *mevlûds* held in commemoration of a death are generally held in the home of the deceased, and include both men and women, kept to separate rooms, while *mevlûds* performed in mosques are mainly for men (although women may lis-

---

is likely to draw comment and frame the event specifically within the boundaries of Islamic practice. She was allowed to participate only after performing the ritual ablutions (*aptes*).

ten from the balcony or from behind screens at the sides or back of the mosque). Likewise, as in the case of the tevhid in Bosnia, the *mevlûds* held in homes in the Black Sea villages are major social events in women's lives, bring together important strands of family, community, piety, and the hope for personal and communal salvation.

According to the Tappers (1987), the most elaborate type of *mevlûd* recital attended by women in the Central Anatolia town of Eğirdir is a type which I have not come across in the Black Sea villages of my research focus—the *mevlûd* following the women's Friday morning prayer meetings (they use the term *tasbih namaz*). Various elements of the *mevlûd* recital they describe are very similar to the *mevlûds* held in homes to commemorate a deceased family member. In the section quoted above of the *mevlûd* of Süleyman Çelebi where the prophet's mother Amine (Turkish form: Emine) describes the birth, the Tappers describe a communal performance:

> As the time of birth approaches, Emine cries out with thirst and is offered sweet ice-cold water which fills her with light and joy; at recitals commemorating a very recent death, tall glasses of sugar water or very sweet lemonade (*cennet şerrbeti*, lit. heavenly cordial) are then given to the congregation (though on other occasions, for both men and women, packages of sweets may be distributed, "for respect" (*hürmet*), in their place. Then, at the moment of birth, when the white bird comes and strokes Emine's back, all the women stand facing Mecca, while the cantor sprinkles rosewater over them. The women then imitate both Emine and the white bird: they are in any case covered with waist-length diaphanous white prayer scarves and they now move through the room stroking each other on the back. When the flurry of movement and contact is over, women return to their places and the cantor recites the standing prayer...For women, the birth section of the mevlud may be one of several highpoints. (80)

In a more recent chapter on religion in provincial Turkey, the Tappers (1991) provide the following analysis of the importance of *mevlûd* in building social identity:

> *Mevlûd* rituals provide a good example of a compartmentalized religious activity that none the less allows for complex, varied statements about social identity. The *mevlûd* poem is a narrative account of the birth and life of the Prophet, and *mevlûd* recitals are arguably the most prominent religious services held in Turkey today. When they are performed in private homes as part of marriage and circumcision cere-

monies, they have a confirmatory character and are particularly associated with men, as are those recitals sponsored on Islamic festivals by
the local religious establishment and performed in local mosques to
coincide with a nationally broadcast *mevlûd* on Turkish television.
Most *mevlûd* recitals, however, are part of funeral and mourning rituals, and have a piacular character.[2] Women are particularly associated
with these mourning *mevlûds*, but this very fact emphasizes the com-
partmentalization of religion in town life. Men tend to adopt the 'official' line in which the *mevlûd* poem and the associated hymns are said
to be 'beautiful but unimportant' because they are not in the Koran.
Indeed, for most men the only value of the *mevlûds* lies in the extent
to which they serve as occasions for Koranic readings. Women insist
that their services, and the rituals and hymn-singing associated with
them, demonstrate that they are more caring and consciously religious
than men. But the women's piety, and even the threat it may pose to
state secularism, are dismissed by the men as spurious, and the traditional stereotypes of women's social and religious inferiority are confirmed. (64)

This analysis is able to show the complexity and variety of identity claims, both
between national and local forms of loyalty and in terms of gender distinctions.

WOMEN'S CARING ROLES EXTENDED
INTO THE AFTERWORLD

The social duties involved in attending a mevlûd after a death can be seen
as extensions of the social duties a woman must fulfill in everyday life. When
she joins a *mevlûd*, a woman is careful to greet everyone appropriately, even
perhaps to peacefully acknowledge those with who she may be involved in a
family feud. In the *mevlûd* itself, she prays for the soul of the deceased and
for all of the deceased in general. Prayers are solicited for the Prophet and
his family, for the saints, for the nation and its leaders, for the soldiers in
military service, for those present and those related to the gathered participants. In the informal conversation after a *mevlûd*, women ask each other
for news, sympathize for losses, ask advice for illnesses, plan visits, discuss
weddings, and generally see to social bonding and the maintenance of com-

---

2. The distinction between "confirmatory" and "piacular" is from E. E. Evans-Prichard.
Neur Religion, Oxford: Oxford U. Press, 1956, p. 198ff.

munal ties. In village society, praying for the dead is an extension into the afterworld of the everyday tasks of women, and can be seen as a part of female caring. Women's roles in caring for the elderly and for the deceased are addressed in detail in Chapter 9, but here it should be noted that participation in a *mevlûd* bridges this world and the next in terms of care for family and community. In everyday life, a person gains the approval of her neighbors by sharing food with those who are hungry, helping lighten other's burdens, brokering peace between enemies, and doing good deeds. Likewise, a person attending a *mevlûd* is said to be gaining approval in heaven, both for herself and for her family members, living and dead. As Bringa describes in the Bosnian case:

> For the woman [attending a tevhid] herself the most important aspect of the tevhid is fulfilling her responsibility to care for the spiritual well-being of deceased persons with whom her household had close social relations, whether they were relatives, neighbors, or friends....there are several dimensions to a tevhid as practiced and understood by women in the village. First, praising the oneness of God and expressing one's membership of a Muslim moral community. Second, the remembrance and honoring of dead relatives and neighbors. And third, the earning of *sevap* on behalf of the dead whereby one assists the deceased in the other world, and increases not only one's own chances of well-being in the afterlife but also those of the other members of one's household. (194)

Just as a woman must care for the needs of her family and neighbors in this world, she must care for the spiritual needs of family and neighbors who have passed on to the next. With the appropriate behavior, a woman can see to the physical and spiritual health of her entire family. While the benefits of attending a *mevlûd* are certain, hosting a *mevlûd* is a central event of a woman's religious life. The spiritual health of the deceased becomes the responsibility of the hosting household, in which the heaviest burden of the preparations and smooth progress of the ritual falls upon the women of the household.

In the region of the Black Sea Cast of Turkey that I studied, the *mevlûds* held at home, whether to commemorate a deceased family member or given in fulfillment of a promise because a large wish was granted (son returned from war, a home built, an illness overcome), involve equal numbers of men and women. A male *mevlûd* reciter is most common, and women and men sit in separate rooms of the house, with men in the main visiting rooms and women in the kitchen and bedrooms. In a large *mevlûd*, the house may be filled to capacity, so guests sit outside in the courtyard or on the roof of the house on cushions provided or cloths they have brought themselves. The amplified microphone carries the reciter's voice to all.

If food is to be provided as a part of the ceremony, the women of the household are responsible for gathering enough cutlery, bowls, and *sini* (portable metal tray table tops with folding legs which reach the proper height for eating while seated on the floor) in advance to provide for all the guests. The sharing of a communal bowl of several types of food by unrelated women around a single *sini* is part of the religiously valued communalism of the *mevlûd*. Younger men and women, primarily of the host family, make sure the guests are served in order of social rank. The young men serve and clear the men's tables, while the young women serve and clear the women's tables and wash the dishes. Often the washed dishes are needed again for another round of serving guests. The proper guest etiquette is to eat quickly without being greedy or jostling the others at the small tables. A polite diner takes small quantities from her own side of the communal bowl and leaves choice bits for elderly guests. Not much conversation occurs at the tables, except for general compliments on the food and the event, but the women who have eaten move to the edges of the room and begin social talk in earnest.

In *mevlûds* held forty days after the death of a woman, visiting women may occupy the central rooms of the house, sharing the main guest room with the male reciter and male relatives of the deceased. Visiting men in this case keep to the courtyard and roof. I have only attended a *mevlûd* for a woman, in which women filled the house, and a general *mevlûd* given annually for all deceased members of a particular family, in which the main rooms were occupied by men and the other rooms by women. I would guess that a forty-day *mevlûd* for a man might have more men in the main room, perhaps with some older female relatives, if they were not participating in the preparation of the food and drink to be offered. In general, I would generalize from what I have seen that if male visitors are to be seated in the main room, then female visitors will be seated in women-only rooms in the rest of the house. In the outdoor, overflow areas, men and women separate into clearly defined groups.

In the Central Anatolian village studied by Carol Delaney, the *mevlûd* performed forty days after a death, and somtimes on some anniversaries of a death, was held in the village mosque, with men listening from the main level and women in the balcony. She reports: "This was the only other occasion, besides evenings during Ramazan, that women were allowed in the mosque; and perhaps partly on this account women were quite enthusiastic about mevluds." Delaney's experience leads her to discredit the Tappers' (1987) idea that this ritual represents an exaltation of birth and motherhood. Since normal births are not commemorated, the *mevlûd* as practiced in this place seems to her to be commemorating a "second birth" through death as well as the particular individual birth of a prophet. It seems to me, based on my own field experience, that women may indeed find the story of a marvelous birth resonant with their own experiences as mothers, especially as this poem is usually the only piece of religious literature in circulation which uses the Turkish language rather than Arabic. It may be that the story of the Prophet's birth fits within a patriachal cultural framework validating male over female, but it is also a story in which the mother of the Prophet, Amine, describes her own experience of birth. It may be that the quite powerful and independent female cantors observed by the Tappers in the town of Eğirdir are able to foster an interpretation of the *mevlûd* recitation which promotes a Amine/Emine as a positive female spiritual role model. They write "In their services, which almost always occur in the context of death, women create and confirm the promise of individual salvation which is offered to all Muslims. The women's mevluds do this by exalting childbirth and using an ideal of motherhood to establish an intimate link between the mevlud participants and the Prophet Mohammad." (84) They also point out that men criticize women's *mevlûd* as overly emotional and excessively melancholy. (81)

In Eleanor Abdella Doumato's recent study *Getting God's Ear: Women, Islam, and Healing in Saudi Arabia and the Gulf* (2000), the gendered nature of communal prayer in the mosque is contrasted to prayer at home and rituals outside the mosque:

> In spite of their exclusion form the experience of mosque culture—indeed, perhaps because of it—women have engaged in rituals of spirituality and community outside the mosque. In Bahrain and Kuwait, in Basra and Musqat, and in towns of the Hejaz as well, women have come together to celebrate the Prophet's birthday, saint's days and feast days, to make votive offerings in exchange for favors from God or the saints, and to mourn, not only the deaths of martyred saints but those of their own loved ones. Given women's separation from the mosque, these rituals may have been the most significant experiences of religious ritual for women, and given the limitations imposed by modesty and separation values, these outside-the-mosque rituals may also have represented the primary venue for women to experience community outside the family. (p. 111)

Doumato's comparison of Saudi women's ritual practices in Saudi Arabia and in the Gulf States shows that the specifically Saudi Wahhabi proclivity for restricting ritual practice outside the mosque has served to de-legitimize and reduce women's religious activities. She places these religious restrictions in a general context of increased state control and technologies of modernization such as educational programs and media campaigns. In contrast to the Gulf societies in which *mevlûd* rituals continue, Wahhabi restrictions have eliminated this practice in Saudi Arabia, with subsequent effects on women's religious activities. Doumato finds:

> The loss of ritual activity is a loss of women's space, space outside one's home, in the homes of others, in cemeteries, in public meeting halls, and at shrines... In Najd, the narrowing of women's ritual space could only have narrowed their experience of community and their sense of legitimate social space as well. (215)

Although there have been state-led and other top-down reforms of Islamic practice in Turkey, and although women's shrine visits have been the focus of negative attention by students of the *Imam-Hatip* schools (see Chapter 5), practices such as the *mevlûd* which are done in the home have not been attacked in the Wahabbi manner. The religious lives of the rural women on the Black Sea coast would be severely curtailed, and their social networks threatened, if such an attack were to occur. Turkish society has tended to view these rituals as harmless displays of women's piety, perhaps criticizing the events for encouraging "typical female vices" such as gossip or emotional outbursts. Like rituals specifically linked to women everywhere (the American middle-class women's book club or versions of the Tupperware party may be compared to *mevlûd* in this context), male ridicule and denigration are more likely than outright condemnation of the practices.

DAILY PRAYER:
STEPPING OUTSIDE THE SOCIAL

Ethnographic observers of Muslim women's lives, who may have easy access to the large social events such as *mevlûd* and who often list daily prayer as a normal part of Muslim life, have begun to describe daily prayer in richer detail. Doumato (2000) in a section called "Outside the Mosque: Ritually Imperfect Prayer" describes the important distinction made in most Muslim societies between an ideal of communal male prayer and the duty of private prayer:

> Whether in the nineteenth or twentieth century, in Bedouin or town communities, in Wahhabi regions or not and whether performed inside a mosque or inside a home, prayer performed correctly and in unison with others is prayer that is most highly valued by the com-

munity as a whole. Women replicate the actions of men but in ways that are ritually imperfect: women's prayer at home is performed either alone, in the company of children, or with whomever is present, such as visiting friends or family, and even when in the company of others women have tended not to pray in unison. Women offer prayers irregularly, being exempt from prayer when menstruating and after giving birth, and are less likely to use correct formulas because they are less educated than men and pray without the benefit of an imam to guide them. Prayer at home is not an experience of the mighty and the low, rich and poor, standing shoulder to shoulder as an emblem of mankind's equality before God, as the prayer books say. It is not an occasion to meet and socialize with others whom one wouldn't otherwise meet, nor is prayer at home an occasion to connect with the political life of the larger community. (p. 110)

Performance of *namaz*, the Muslim prayer performed five times daily, is not considered a social occasion, whether for women at home or in a back room of a house while visiting, or for men at home or in a mosque except on Fridays at noon or on holidays. Rather, it is meant to be a peaceful time of contemplation outside of daily life. As Delaney puts it:

> *Namaz* is also likened to a stream of pure water into which the believer plunges and cleanses himself, and the preformance of it five times a day is felt to guarantee admission to Paradise. During this brief time no one may interrupt the person praying, for that would cause a change in focus from the spiritual world to the earthly one and thus profane and invalidate the *namaz*. Even small children learn to keep their peace. Although this is one of the few times women are left alone and can withdraw into themselves, it is not a time to devote to their own thoughts but a time for those thoughts to be directed to God. (292)

At home, family members may pray more-or-less at the same time, but they do not pray in unison. They may pray in any room not needed for the normal flow of activity. Several family members may pray in one room or more, with the only stipulation that women should not take up a position for prayer which is in front of men. Youngsters unsure of the proper ritual may pray next to an elder, following his or her movements, but actual instruction in proper prayer is given in classes at the village mosque. Young children of either sex may attend pray in a mosque with their father or other male relatives, in which case they are expected to remain quiet and perhaps to follow the movements of prayer. Girls who are learning to pray also learn the proper way to cover their heads in the appropriate fashion for prayer, even if they are not cover-ing their heads in daily life.

If a pious person is visiting another household, he or she may ask for a prayer carpet or ask to be shown a quiet room for prayer. Good hospitality re-quires the provision of running water for ablutions, a clean towel, guest slip-pers or sandals if the running water is outside, a clean prayer carpet, and a peaceful room. True piety is assocated with modesty, so people should not make a big fuss about the fact that are about to pray or have just prayed. Like-wise, while people should take care not to speak to a person praying or dis-tract them from prayer, the person praying can be seen to be violating the spirit of prayer by becoming annoyed or speaking to anyone. As White (2002) describes: "If other women were present in the house, as they often were, they might join [the hostess], or take turns.... If they needed to retrieve something from the room, the other women, hushed, tiptoed respectfully around the kneeling figures." (88) The social behavior surrounding prayer time at mosques on Fridays for men, on religious holidays for men and women, and after the recitation of a *mevlûd* is an exceptional rather than normative conjunction of prayer and sociability.

Women's Daily Social Interactions in the Village

Along with ritual and religious behavior, village women are involved in many levels of social behavior, ranging from the least formal types of interaction such as flopping down on the couch with a few family members to watch the latest Brazilian soap opera—without even changing out of work clothes—to the highly formalized evening tea visits in which all members of a family, spruced up and on best behavior, visit another home, perhaps even with the intention of sealing an engagement of two young people. In between fall the less formal women-only afternoon teas, busy market day intractions, visits to new brides or new babies, calls upon the sick or elderly, trips to clinic or hospital, and visits to distant relatives or friends, even including trips outside the country. White (2002) describes in an urban setting the tradition, common on the Black Sea coast, of visiting a bride-to-be in order to view her trousseau. (p. 92) Communal social events include circumcisions, engagements, weddings, funerals, *mevlûds*, agri-cultural or construction labor groups (*imece*), and national or religious holidays.

In contrast to Turkish women in towns and cities, Black Sea women of the villages I observed do not have regularized ways of borrowing or lending cash. While credit can be obtained when needed, and while maintaining good re-

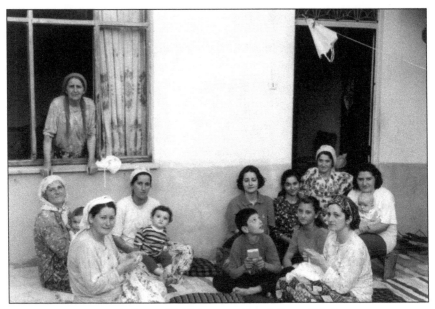

22. Informal Visiting as a Break from Work

lations with neighbors is a good strategy for preparing for the possibility of bad days, finacial security seems depend more on agricultural goods than on cash. A woman's reputation for helpfulness can rest on sharing food, milk, and advice alone, whereas a man's reputation may have more to do with the cash he can provide a friend in need. The major public display of cash gifts is the wedding, in which gold or paper money, either openly or concealed in envelopes, is presented to the newlyweds.

The social occasion which is most similar across city-town-village divides is the women's tea, in which a groups of women, usually with their children and female relatives, visit a hostess in her home for an extended social visit. This requires the preparation of tea and of something to eat along with it, store-bought buiscits being the very least trouble and a grand selection of home-cooked savories and desserts being the pinnacle of female hospitality. Along with talk about daily matters, health issues are often discussed, with lively debates about various methods being a good part of the fun. Younger women tend to be more reserved, often engaged in handicrafts such as embroidery for their trousseau or in replenishing the tea and passing around the sugar. Women with special topics to discuss in a more private fashion can remove themselves to the kitchen with the pretext of helping out. I have noticed that the television is almost always on for evening, mixed-sex tea visits but more often turned off during women's afternoon teas. The exception to this is when the time of the tea coincides with a very popular soap opera, in which case, it becomes a topic of conversation and lively banter. A large tea gathering will be prepared for in advance and the telphone or child messengers will be used to invite other households. A tea visit may occur spontaneously, however, in much the manner described by Delaney (1991):

> When a guest drops in for more than a brief chat, the hostess must drop what she is doing in order to make the guest welcome. Tea must be made, food brought, the fire stoked, and beds provided if necessary. Sometimes visits have been previously arranged, but more often they are unannounced....Americans are used to making plans and schedules, to being notified of visits, and to making and keeping appointments. In Turkey, by contrast, an unannounced visit is not thought of as an intrusion, but is an expected and desired part of domestic activity. One's own plans are dispensable, and those of others take precedence; particularly is this true for women....Yet this hospitality is not as altruistic as it may sound, for having guests and being known as a hospitible person or household is also self-serving. A visit sheds honor on the host and raises his status in the eyes of other villagers. (194–195)

In the Black Sea village, afternoon teas are mainly women's gatherings. At a similar lull in the chores of the day, men are most likely to be drinking tea in a coffeehouse. If a male member of the household is at home when female guests are arriving, he is likely to exit immediately, perhaps asking for a glass of tea through the kitchen window to drink outside, perhaps heading off to a more suitable male environment such as the coffeehouse or mosque.

Carla Makhlouf (1979), in her study of North Yemen, describes a social event called the *tafrita* which seems to share some characteristics with the rural version of tea visiting in Turkey:

> The social conditions of *tafrita* are such that they seem to stress nearness and community rather than discordance. Since it is common for over fifty women to be sitting on the floor in a room of three by six metres, perspiring and smoking together, one obvious result is that status differences will appear to be less relevant....What this crowdedness emphasises is, if not the equality, at least the sense of community of the participants. (26–27)

As she describes it, the *tafrita* is a common all-female afternoon event (there are special *tafritas* given for births or marriages) which includes removing the

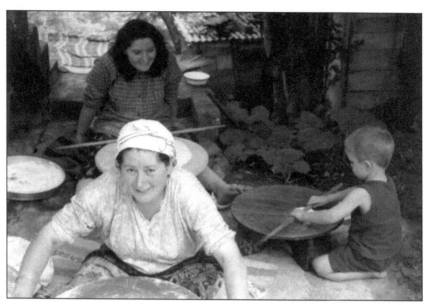

23. Nazmiye & Helpers Rolling out Dough

outer garments at the door, chewing qat, smoking from a waterpipe, drinking tea and eating snacks, music and dancing by some of the women. Men are absolutely excluded (except for some singers or comedians). It is considered a pleasant time, following the chores of the morning the family noontime meal, and constrained by afternoon and evening prayer times. Men are usually having a social time of music and qat chewing among male friends at the same time in a different location.

CHANGING SOCIAL BEHAVIOR

After being separated from her natal home, a newly married woman must carefully establish visiting patterns, based initially on the social network of her mother-in-law. In the village, the morning of an average day may allow for movement along the roads, on the way to fields, to gather firewood, or to graze the cow. *Gelins* who are neighbors or who pass on the roads may have a chance to arrange for social visiting when work is done. The telephone is increasingly a part of these arrangements, in that women may call before visiting to see if the time is convenient. A Turkish woman, who was born in the village but has moved to one of the nearby towns due to marriage, also must establish her own networks, typically starting with the women of the households in her apartment building. At various times during the year, she will visit her home village or the village of her husband, taking her children to visit their grandparents. During these visits, her mother or mother-in-law will arrange for visits so that the bonds between the city dweller and her village relatives and friends can be maintained. Makhlouf (1979) notes the changing attitude about the formal social visiting of *tafrita* as young women come to find it boring. In the Turkish case, younger village women are not in charge of the "guest list" for a tea visit, and not expected to express strong opinions in these gatherings—so are likely to remain quiet and may find the main discussions boring (although there are many cases in which younger women listen intently to topics under general discussion, saving up information for later use). In the urban environment, younger women have more say about whom to visit and what topics to discuss, tending to gather in groups more tightly organized around a certain age-group. In the context of a rapid modernizing Yemen, Makhlouf found that:

> Those among my informants who were employed outside the home all said that they rarely went to *tafrita* and only on very special occasions so as not to hurt people's feelings. Schoolgirls too try to avoid formal visits; they prefer to be among themselves rather than to go to *tafrita* where older women are present....For modernising women, *tafrita* is no longer experienced as the most enjoyable and exciting part of the day; it has become a social duty that cannot be completely avoided, a concession made to friends and relatives—and tradition. (p. 75)

It may be that the changing social landscape has altered the traditional shape of the *tafrita*, allowing women to gather in groups reflecting more exclusively their own generational concerns. In Turkey, the traditional avenues of sociability may have altered, but women still find it important to maintain ties with the people from their families' places of origin and to establish new networks of friends and allies. For example, market day down by the shore road, which used to be a high-point of a village woman's social calendar, is no longer so crucial either in terms of buying provisions or of meeting friends and learning news from more distant villages. When they go by car or minibus to a local town center, however, women often go to a familiar or recommended store-owner, following traditional patterns of social networking. White (2002) finds new forms of social interactions in an Istanbul neighborhood—political party work, piece work in the global clothing trade, and classes in a woman's center—but the importance of the bonds formed with other women remains. And even in the most modern of social gatherings, even if the options and vocabulary are new, health care remains a topic of importance to women.

The next chapter looks at the ways that faith and the discourses of religiosity shape villagers' world views. The specific concept of *nazar* (the "evil eye") will be used as an example of how supernatural influences impact health concerns.

CHAPTER 5

FAITH, RELIGION, AND THE SUPERNATURAL

They pounded and mixed the pain
of the universe and called it "love"

—Fakhruddin 'Iraqi in Chittick and Wilson 1982, p. 39

The night is lit by a full summer moon, so we can easily make our way up the dirt road without flashlights. Aunty Emine, Timur, my five-month-old son, and I are going to visit close neighbors who are also related in that the hostess is the sister-in-law of Aunty Emine's daughter Nazmiye. The road is steep, so we arrive laughing and panting, looking forward to a night of relaxation after a normal hard day's work in the gardens. Aunty Emine has changed her blouse and headscarf for visiting, and I have my baby wrapped up and tied with a home-woven strap to my back, where he struggles and pounds my shoulders with his fists. "He'll get used to it," Aunty Emine tells me, "Soon he'll be going to sleep while you walk." Indeed, most of the village babies happily travel to the fields this way, unless there is someone at home to watch them. The young mothers often have a heavy workload and need to have their hands free and their babies secure as they do house chores and fieldwork.

I have put on a cotton headscarf with embroidery edging, a gift from a sister-in-law. I long ago gave up trying to coax my hair into its usual style in the house's one tiny mirror, and felt I might look tidier with a headscarf that shows off my earrings. Before I lived in the village, I had thought the Islamic head covering for women was intended to conceal the beauty of the wearer by covering her hair. To my surprise, whenever I put on a headscarf, women told me how well it suited me and showed my face. With no makeup and no hair over the forehead or cheeks, facial features are shown for what they are. Local wisdom has it that a person's moral character can be seen from the face, and a good person's forehead is open (açık, meaning both uncovered and clear) and shines with spiritual light. A headscarf, then, is not just an indicator of religious piety, but also a beautifying accessory and a convenience.

The village style of wearing a headscarf is very different from the newly popular urban "Islamist" style, which involves a large (and usually expensive) polyester or silk scarf that completely covers the hair, neck, and shoulders, and is fastened with a straight pin under the chin. These scarves do not have added embroidery edging, which is what makes the village scarves a personalized sign of the wearer's taste, skill in handicrafts, and even mood. The urban scarf can show a wearer's taste and economic status, and women have developed a wide range of ways to show individuality through color choices, draping styles, and even fashionable pin-heads. Urban women who wear this type of headscarf often have the traditional cotton one on underneath to secure the slippery fabric and to keep on when they take off their large scarf upon entering indoor women's space.

We are greeted at the door by the whole family, in this case, the wife, husband, two children, and the wife's mother who is visiting. We are led into the living room, which is brightly lit and filled with the sound from an impressively large TV set. Television is a constant presence in village houses in the evening, and this home has the advantage of a hilltop location and a large antenna which brings in more of the new channels. Until the 1980's, Turkey had one, then two, and at last three state-controlled TV stations. Since the privatization of the mid-80's, an explosion of stations has led to the availability of foreign programs, religious shows, pornographic films, and sports events, including NBA basketball. Now every village home has a TV and everyone is saving up for a better antenna.

When we have settled down onto couches arranged along the walls facing the TV, our hostess asks us each how we are. In this ritualized exchange, the appropriate response is self-depreciating, using phrases which can be translated as "Well, scraping by," or "We're making do." In village visits, everyone participates in one inclusive conversation around the room. If there are any private discussions to be had, women can follow the hostess to the kitchen or men can go outside together. Timur is let loose to crawl on the floor and quickly becomes a topic of conversation. The hostess asks Aunty Emine how he is doing, and she relates that he is not eating well, has been fussy, and does not sleep for very long. As an American mother, I want to protest that he is doing just fine, but as a Turkish *gelin*, I know not to say anything. I have been previously warned not to tell anyone that I am nursing my baby, or to let anyone see leaking milk, for fear of *nazar* (the "evil eye"). Old women sometimes lovingly call a baby "ugly" so as not to attract *nazar* upon a beautiful baby. In this neighborly visit, saying how well a baby is doing could be dangerous, attracting the jealousy of others and tempting *nazar*. Babies who have been thriving have been known to suddenly take a turn for the worse and become very ill—symptoms pointing to *nazar*. In the general flow of conversation, someone suggests that the *"nazar* prayer" be read over the baby as a precautionary measure. For this, I hold the baby in my lap and the old woman who is the mother of the hostess sits beside us. With the TV blasting, the gossip and joking continuing full swing, this woman murmurs under her breath and occasionally blows on the baby. As she is doing this, she often yawns, a sign that *nazar* is present in the baby and is being treated by the prayer. The verb to describe the recital of the prayer means, "to read" although people recite it from memory and are often illiterate. When I ask about the prayer, which comes from the Koran, the hostess recommends that I not have it read over the baby too frequently because he might get used to it and then suffer in America where only a few people would be able to perform the prayer. She has relatives in Germany, and knows that they don't want their babies to become dependent on the *nazar* treatment when they are in the village.

*****

FAITH

I have structured this chapter around "faith," a simple term which tries to cover complex subjects such as religion, ideas about the supernatural, and theories of a person's place in the universe. These subjects are at once the most crucial to understand when studying a culture and the most difficult to describe accurately. Putting "belief" or "faith" in its own chapter is a choice molded by a disciplinary history which follows the rationalization of discourse in western thought. Good (1994) traces the history of this trend in anthropology to differentiate knowledge (what we know to be true) from belief (what the people we study mistakenly believe to be true). He convincingly shows that the scientific discourse of biomedicine has such cultural authority for anthropologists that it can be used as the picture of reality against which other cultures' ideas about reality can be tested and found incorrect. (refer to Chapter 1 "Belief, Religion, and Health Care")

In an important sense, belief is a part of all healing practices and *all* health care systems are based on faith. All are based on theories of how suffering is caused and how it can best be alleviated, theories derived from and shaping observations, taught in various ways, and shared in varying degrees throughout societies. The adherence to a microbiological theory of health and illness is as much a belief as adherence to a religious doctrine. For some, the idea that illness is caused by invisible germs which are indiscriminate in their attacks may seem completely irrational and not borne out by the observation and experience of both laypersons and trusted experts.

The separation of religion from other forms of discourse and daily practices is also problematic, revealing a split which resembles the knowledge/faith split. For people with a religiously anchored world-view, the microbiological model may be fully compatible with their faith—it is quite common for the existence of microbes and the availability of the means to cure damage wrought by them to be an integrated part of an overarching faith in a Supreme Being. The use of a conventionally secular service such as clinical medicine does not prove that a patient has a secular world-view. To repeat Snow's succinct summary (1998): "for many people *all healing* is faith healing."

In this chapter, then, I will briefly review some of the recent scholarship on belief which is significantly different from older forms of scholarship which were dismissive of the beliefs of foreign cultures or of poor or otherwise marginal groups. Then I will give a brief overview of various types of religious behavior observable in Medreseönü and suggest some of the ways that the local belief system helps to integrate both the good and the bad in human behavior into a meaningful system. Then, I will outline the types of supernatural beings and occurrences which are a part of the traditional world-view of the people I interviewed. Next, I will show that there is a general feeling that the supernatural is drawing away from regular daily life, becoming rarer, and outline the local explanations of such a reduction of supernatural influence. I will also mention the interaction between the local traditional ideas about Muslim practices and the newly strong Islamist interpretation of correct behavior. Finally, I will use the belief in *nazar,* the "evil eye," as a concrete example of how belief in the supernatural works in daily life, describing its place in Muslim belief its effects, diagnosis, treatment, prevention, and impact on social relations.[1]

Suffering is a part of life which often challenges peoples' belief systems, leading them to look for answers for life's most difficult questions. Because of human creativity and the tendency to search in ever widening circles for relief until it is found, suffering can cause people to expand or change their beliefs. Conversion to a new faith, returning to a family tradition which one had discarded, coming to believe in something one had disbelieved, reaffirming a be-

---

1. The reader is referred to Ransel (2000) for a fascinating and extensive examination of the "evil eye" in both Russian and Tatar cultures. The incredible similarities deserve careful study, which is sadly beyond the capacity of this author at this time.

lief or set of practices one had allowed to lapse, and combining elements of different cultures' beliefs to create a personally coherent belief system (as in the integration of "Eastern" and "Western" wisdom in many "New Age" beliefs), are all types of changes in peoples' belief systems that can be given impetus by a bout of personal suffering.

Timothy C. Lloyd (1995) divides the work of one folk expert into "life-cycle work, which balances supernatural knowledge with practical action, and emergency healing work, which draws more upon practical experience alone." (69) This distinction may be especially important in the transmission of knowledge, in that certain techniques can be taught even to a person who does not share a similar belief system In terms of the world-view of the practitioner; however, I would argue that the emergency work in Medreseönü is integrated into the system of supernatural knowledge just as much as life-cycle work. For the pious, religious faith is always a part of explaining and treating illness. Awareness of the supernatural can become heightened in emergency situations, and death or serious illness often cause an increase in religious activity and the use of supernatural explanatory models. Leonard Primiano (1995) suggests the term "vernacular" to describe religion in its lived form, "as human beings encounter, understand, interpret, and practice it." (44) He hopes this term will be more satisfactory for the study of human belief than the previous scholarly terms "folk," "popular," and "unofficial" which all gave the impression that there exists a pure form of religion, on a high, official plane, which is then adulterated when it is touched by ignorant believers. Because of the history of the European Christian debate over the use of Latin or the various vernaculars in church services, I find the term "vernacular" to be as tainted with bipolar implications as any of the traditional high/low, official/unofficial classic/folk, or textual/popular terms. I find "lived religion" or "belief system' or "religion in everyday life," to be adequately neutral and applicable cross-culturally.

Evelyn A. Early, in her study of women in a neighborhood of Cairo (1993), defines her approach to the study of religious practices:

> Throughout this study I refer to the Islam practiced in baladi quarters such as Bulaq Abu 'Ala as "popular Islam" in the conventional anthropological use to indicate everyday religious practice, which mixes scriptural and local traditions. It does not mean that "more formal" of "more orthodox" Islam is "unpopular." Nor should it be forgotten that many baladi Egyptians follow many devotional conventions stipulated by "orthodox Islam. (85)

Because a scholar's personal beliefs may, even unbeknownst to the scholar, affect her or his interpretations of the religious beliefs of others, the terms "folk" and "popular" have been applied to religions merely because they are different from the religion of the observer. For example, if Protestant Christianity is the mainstream religion of scholars in the United States, it is not surprising that various Catholic beliefs and practices have been studied as "folk religion." Vernon Schubel (1993) has shown that both Western and Sunni Muslim scholars have treated the beliefs and practices of Shi'i Muslim believers as "folk" or "popular," even though the Shi'is base their religion on equally serious attention to the Muslim holy texts and traditions as paid by the Sunnis. According to Schubel:

> It is tempting to organize the study of Muharram rituals around the bipolar opposition of folk tradition versus classical Islam. Many "rationalist" Muslims themselves deal with the material in this way, poking fun at their coreligionists' "superstitions" while arguing for the rationality of Islamic law....To my surprise, as I asked deeper and deeper questions of the people I was writing about, I discovered that much of what I thought would be indigenous folk religion has its root in the classical tradition. (160)

and:

> The study of Islam needs to take the context of Islamic practice seriously, because Islam is both a transcendent reality and an articulated series of responses to it. (162)

The dynamic and interpretive nature of a belief system is described by Primiano (1995):

> The process of religious belief refers to the complex linkage of acquisition and formation of beliefs which is always accomplished by the conscious and unconscious negotiations of and between believers. This process acknowledges the presence of bidirectional influences of environments on individuals and of individuals on environments in the process of believing. Within the human context, manifold factors influence the individual believer, such as physical and psychological predispositions, the natural environment, family, community affiliations, education and literacy, communication media, as well as political and economic conditions. (44)

Primiano's concept of "the continuity of creative self-understanding, self-interpretation, and negotiation by the believing individual" resembles Schubel's claim that:

Like all religious people [the Shi'i Muslim] are engaged in a complex balancing act by which they exist in a multiplicity of roles simultaneously, all the while striving to remain true to what they see as essential to their religion. As they do this they are in effect continuously creating a new tradition. (162)

Schubel's approach to studying a set of Shi'i religious practices in Pakistan resembles that of Bowen (1993), Hufford (1992a), Primiano (1995), and Snow (1993), in that he tries to work from a position of respect for the knowledge and practices of actual believers as they negotiate their lives based on their faith.

MUSLIMS AND ISLAMISTS

Since the late 1980's, a revivalist type of Islamic interpretation has had a strong impact on Turkish politics and society, after decades of Kemalist secularism. It is promoted by Islamic pedagogues, who use a network of İmam-Hatip religious schools to propagate their brand of strict adherence to the rationality of Islamic law and the absolute letter of the holy texts. Although this type of revivalism has occurred with regularity throughout Islamic history, the "Islamist" style of political engagement is thoroughly modern in its uses of media and rationalist ideology. I call this group "Islamists" because of their conscious self-identification with an international Islamic front, which has political and economic as well as religious concerns. This term is in contrast to "Muslim," (although one can certainly be both Muslim and "Islamist") which connotes a self-identification as a believer in the Koran and prophecy of Mohammed, with whatever daily rituals and beliefs an individual associates with that identification.

Bowen, in *Muslims Through Discourse* (1993), delineates a split in the Indonesian Muslim community between "modernists" and "traditionalists." (see especially pp. 21–25) The modernist approach to Islam emphasizes the "self-sufficiency of scripture and the moral responsibility of the individual" while the traditionalist approach values the history of religious interpretation of scripture and doubts the ability of each individual to correctly interpret scripture without referring to traditional scholarship. (22–24) This split becomes most interesting for our purposes is in regard to healing practices. Traditionalists tolerate much more variety in ritual and in the daily practices of Muslims, as long as their intent (*niyet*) is pure. Modernists, on the other hand, suspect many daily practices to be mistaken or even sinful and encourage religious education to correct them. As Bowen puts it, "Traditionalists' idea that scripture offers alternatives is in direct contrast to modernists' conviction that scripture offers only one correct set of ritual forms." (24) Bowen gives an example of an elderly healer who has become "puzzled and a bit worried. Once sure and proud of his vast command of spells (one for nearly every purpose), he had recently begun to doubt whether such spells were a proper part of a good Muslim's life." (76) Because of increasing international travel and communication, Muslims from all countries have been able to meet, study scripture together, and compare regional customs. This has led to an increasing standardization of Islamic pedagogy and a perception held by young, active, internationally-connected Muslims that the local traditional knowledge and practices of their elders are, at best, old-fashioned and peculiar, or, at worst, fundamentally wrong and inherently sinful. Elders are no longer considered to be righteous storehouses of religious knowledge. In fact, because their traditional knowledge is, for the most part, founded on oral tradition, they are often likely to be silenced in an argument over religious detail when an educated young person refers in a convincing way to the texts and written interpretations of Islam, or to opinions in the international community of Islamic scholars.

Building upon her long-term relationships with informants in Ümraniye, Istanbul, White (2002) shows in great detail the diversity of lifestyles chosen by residents of *gecekondu* or *varoş* neighborhoods of Istanbul, areas which have lent political support to parties associated with Islamic trends. Moving past the assumptions made by many political commentators of simple black-and-white divisions such as Kemalist/Islamist, rural/urban, or modern/traditional, White shows that individuals, families, and communities steer their own paths through these overarching metaphors of state and society, combining opposites, blending elements, and strategically availing themselves of a wide range of options, which can expand or shrink with economic fluctuations and change due to external factors such as regime change or internal ones such as individual life cycles.

In a family she has known for over ten years, White observed that two of three daughters chose,

> what Deniz Kandiyoti has called the patriarchal bargain (1988, 275): submissiveness and propriety, symbolized by veiling, in exchange for protection and support (*himaye*). Their change from modest peasant dress to *tesettür* at marriage displayed their virtuous character and respect for religion. It also indicated their new status as married women, the economic solvency of their husbands, and their hus-

band's regard for them, since *tesettür* coats and scarves are more expensive than other types of clothing they would ordinarily wear. [She then compares wearing the *tesettür* as a symbol of wealth to the older custom of wearing gold bracelets from the wedding] (p. 66)

This is a similar development to that observed by Early (1993) in urban Egypt, which she described under a section heading "The Islamic Revival: A New Personal Piety:"

> By 1980 the religious conservatism was more apparent than it had been in the mid-1970s. One marker was dress. I saw a few women at the extreme end of the dress spectrum with floor-length capelike coasts, their gloved hands sometimes appearing through slits in the side. Head coverings left only their eyes uncovered. When I left Egypt in 1977, even the first stage of Islamic dress, a head scarf and long sleeves, appeared mostly among afrangi Egyptians, but by 1980 it had emerged in the baladi quarters as well. In Bulaq, baladi women still shed their religious dress at the door, just as their mothers and sisters had shed the traditional melaya liff. In contrast, middle-class women tended to wear religious garb at any time outside their bedroom, in case an unrelated male came to visit. Baladi women treat all males in their building as "kin-like," and as they shed their meelaya liffs to wear house dresses without embarrassment, so they shed heir head scarf and long sleeves. (120)

At times, popular practices are challenged or forbidden by religious authorities. Early notes:

> …during my research, the mosque imam remove a concrete pillar from outside the shrine of Siddi Qubba (known to cure infertility); women who had customarily circumambulated this pillar remarked that since it was un-Islamic it was best it had stopped. With no fuss and no muss, they simply searched for new pilgrimage spots. There was no sense of confrontation, but rather the baladis assimilated the alfrangi view saying "it was good the imam was there to tell us." (125)

In Medreseönü, the impact of the new style of religious education can be seen in the interaction between the elderly women of the villages and a recent graduate of an *İmam-Hatip* religious school. It was this young man's opinion that, when reading the *nazar duası* [the prayer against the evil eye] over bread in order to treat a stricken cow, the use of bakery bread *(fırın ekmeği)* was mandatory, and that the traditional use of home-baked corn bread *(mısır ekmeği)* was a sin *(gunah).* This attention to the minutiae of Muslim daily life is typical of the new Islamist "fundamentalist" movement. The elderly women were torn between conflicting feelings: they felt respect, because this young man had successfully completed his religious education; they were amused, because he was concerned with a practice which had been largely ignored but sometimes scoffed at by young men before him; and they were worried, because, although he was not condemning them for doing this practice in ignorance, they would be guilty of bad intention, and therefore of sin, if they continued to use corn bread after being told it was wrong. In this case, a young man was using a text-based education taking its strength from a national and international community, to directly challenge an orally-transmitted, local women's practice. This is just one example of the attempt by non-locals to inscribe the local individual with Islamic modernist values after decades of non-local attempts to inscribe the individual with secular modernist values.

Julie Marcus (1992) describes an attack on a women's religious visit to a shrine near Izmir (*Susuz Dede*) by young students from an *İmam-Hatip* school. "[They] came on a zealous journey to inform the women of the errors of their ways. The boys asserted that there was no-one in the grave and that the rites were pagan. When the boys tore the cotton from the tomb and kicked the candles into the fire, they were ignored. Despite their brashness, the women dealt patiently with them…" (138) The most common verbal defense used by women in such cases is the assertion that God is everywhere and only God can decide if a person's faith is pure and intentions good. In the case of these brash young men, the women may be able to excuse their rudeness on the grounds that they are young, hot-blooded (*delikanlı* : literally "crazy-blooded"), and under the influence of heady doctrines.

These examples show a gendered division of religious discourse, with women on the side of popular and traditional practice and men on the side of book-learning and orthodox practice. While disagreements of this cross-gender type are perhaps the most noticeable, it is very common for women to correct each other, give advice, instruct, and discuss proper practice. Sometimes, a woman's advanced age or acknowledged piety may give her statements authority, at other times, a young woman's schooling or training in religious practice may lend her ideas weight. A visitor with experience of other styles of practice will be respectfully listened to, and the local community will decide how much of a divergent practice to incorporate. The words of a woman back from the pilgrimage to Mecca are given careful consideration. Women may advise men, as well, but they are most likely to do so in a light-hearted manner or entirely private setting. In public places, especially in matters of religion, women are likely to defer to male authority without stirring up controversy. What they choose to do about advice they receive is worked out over time and often involves getting second and third opinions.

Eleanor Abdella Doumato (2000), in her study of religious change over time in the Arab peninsula, outlines the Wahabbi movement and its specific impact on women's religious lives. She writes:

> ...Wahabbi authority defined itself very specifically in opposition to saint worship, praying at graves, votive offerings, and Sufi *zikr* chanting and dancing, as well as fortune-telling, spell making, truth divining, and amulet wearing. In short, in asserting their own brand of orthodoxy, the Wahabbis denigrated techniques of personal and spiritual empowerment in contradiction to orthodox standards that were available to women and condemned communal rituals that appealed to women's needs. (p. 40)

By this, Doumato does not mean that Ibn Abd al-Wahhab singled out women's activities for attack, but that, while the new system offered appropriate communal rituals to men (like mosque worship), it did not provide alternate models of religious practice for women and ended up thrusting all of their practices to the margins of daily life. The Saudi example, of course, is not the only time in history in which the conjunction of nation-state power, techniques of modernism, educational reforms, and an emphasis on rationality have worked together to marginalize traditional practices and disenfranchise women. The history of the gradual medicalization of birth in the United States is a well documented example of such a shift.

Islam has always been a religion encompassing a variety of peoples and cultures. The pilgrimage to Mecca *(hac)*, Islamic education, and the transnational movement of Muslim scholars have historically been factors encouraging the integration and homogenization of Muslim practices in contrast to the adherence to the local transmission of cultural knowledge which can have pre-Islamic roots. Debates between Muslim modernists and traditionalists are not new in Islamic history, but modem technology and communication, once the weapons of modernizing secularists, have been fully integrated into the arsenal of the Muslim modernists. The "enemies" of both types of modernizers are local knowledge and traditional world-view: the "old wives' beliefs," *(kocakarı inançları)* which are "backward-minded," *(geri kafalı)*, "ludicrous," *(saçma sapan)*, "empty," *(boş)*, "superstitious beliefs," *(batıl inançlar)*, and "made-up," *(uyduruk)*.

In the current competition between a traditional Muslim world-view, which is internal and inseparable from everyday activity, and a rationalized Muslim world-view coming from institutions of Islamic education, the minute details of a person's daily life have become a symbolic battleground. When a young *hoca* tells elderly ladies that they are sinning by reading a *nazar* prayer over corn bread, he is attacking a formerly unquestioned local practice and destabilizing the basis for the traditional world-view. When a person is taught to consciously choose the right foot to step out from a toilet room, in the name of Islamic rules of conduct, the actual individual physical body is being molded by rationalized religion. The impulse in the new Islamist movement seems to be to "tidy up" (but not discard) the ritual details of the traditional lived Islamic practices.

It is crucial to stress that traditional healing practitioners whose methods are described in this work are devout Muslims who consider their practices to be based in and legitimized by Islam and who attribute any success in healing to the power and will of God, as well as to their own God-given abilities.

Types of Supernatural Phenomena in Medreseönü

The traditional belief system in this region of the Black Sea shares with other Muslim belief systems a belief in God, the Prophet, *melekler (angels)*, *evliyalar* (saints), *cin* (which is pronounced "jin," and which is translated as "genie" in English), *ecinni* (the Arabic plural pronounced "ejunnu" in the local dialect, has a purely negative connotation), *periler* (fairies), and *ruhlar* (souls or spirits of known people who have passed on). Along with these types, all of which are mentioned in the Koran, there are also *hortlaklar* (the risen dead, which are the roaming corpses of evil people), *karabasma* (literally "black pressing," the evil spirit who causes night paralysis), a mysterious green light which indicates the presence of a supernatural being, strange sounds and apparitions, and special supernatural abilities in humans, such as fortune-telling or the ability to cast *nazar* or other harmful spells. Although the word "hortlak" does not appear in the Koran (not being Arabic), there is plenty of Koranic support for the idea of the spirit of a sinner leading a troubled existence after death. Likewise, the other supernatural occurrences are integrated into Muslim religious belief and Islamic practices and prayers are used to counteract bad supernatural effects.

The image of a genie in the West is of a large, turbaned creature who pops out of a lamp to help a hero. This image is based on translated folk stories from the Middle East and is, although simplified, a fairly accurate image of the type of *cin* which can become a helpful familiar for a particular person.

They are said to be large and powerful and able to transform themselves into other forms, such as that of animals. A helpful *cin* can be passed down to another person, usually within a family. People who are assisted by *cin* should never tell about it, as they would lose the aid of the *cin*. In Medreseönü, one woman was known to have the help of *cin*. She would have fits, sometimes as long as two hours, in which she would speak about things of which she could have no knowledge. People would come to put questions to her, and she would answer. She may have stepped on a frog which was actually a *cin*, or disturbed a party of *cin* in some way, so that she became possessed. A person with spells of abnormal behavior, such as fits of craziness or fortune-telling abilities, is said to have *cin*. In common parlance, *"Cinlerimi attırma."* and *"Beni cinlendirme".* are phrases, literally meaning "Don't make my genies jump out." and "Don't cause me to be genied," which are used to mean "Don't make me mad."

Unlike the helpful *cin*, *ecunnu* are bad and can change shape to fool people and harm them. If one is attacked by *ecunnu*—for example scratched by an unfamiliar cat at night near a graveyard—one might suffer paralysis, blurred vision, or a general reduction in abilities leading to lethargy and low spirits. Only a specialist can read the necessary prayers to lift the effects of this kind of attack. People are admonished to keep their hearts clean and to resist fear, for these types of evil beings cannot harm a confident, good person.

The *hortlak* is a particularly unpleasant being—the dead body of a person who was so bad that the ground spits it out in disgust. It can be armless or legless, makes a screaming noise, can have long, vicious fingernails, and is likely to chase a victim all the way home and then howl outside the door for the rest of the night. People report seeing the long scratches from a *hortlak* on the outside walls of their homes. Dogs can attack and stop a *hortlak,* so it is good to have one along if walking at night. Guns, however, are useless against any kind of supernatural being. People have seen large shadows, strange sounds like birds singing at night, strange lights or voices, and apparitions such as coffins which they associate with the presence of a *hortlak*. A *hortlak* has the power to paralyze a person and cause illness. The corpse of a bad person turns into a *hortlak* within forty days after burial so it is fairly easy to determine whose *hortlak* has made an appearance.

Granny's Supernatural Experience

Granny, whose extensive interview about local healing practices is transcribed in Chapter 2, was prompted by her daughter to tell me the following story about her encounter with the *periler* (fairies). I was not able to record similar stories from other informants, but I am sure that there are many such stories told in the slower-paced winter days and nights. TV has taken the place of story-telling in many social gatherings, but, in the right setting, one story of supernatural experience will lead to others.

✶✶✶✶✶

When she was 20 years old, she was in the garden (field). When she was coming back from the field, she saw three lizards in a row on a blackberry branch. They were bouncing up and down. She wondered why they were doing that and she threw a clod of earth at them. It didn't hit them, it hit the twig. All of a sudden, she felt someone wringing her insides (points to chest region) as if they were laundry—her eyes went blind, and she fainted. She found out later that she had been unconscious for three days, giving no response to anything. She couldn't see or hear. For three days, the *hoca* (religious teacher and ritual expert) said prayers over her body—only at the end when he tapped her and gave her *agates* (ritual ablution), with some water on her face, and said, "If you let her go, I will never interfere with you (the *periler*) again." When the water was splashed on her face three times, she woke right up as if from sleep. When she woke up, she couldn't remember anything about the situation of her body during those three days. She had been in a dream world for the whole time, going from wedding feast to wedding feast with the *periler*. The table was full of beautiful fruits, the *periler* were in fabulous costumes. They were all dancing. Everything was beautiful. She didn't want to wake up. People saw a smile on her face while she was unconscious. When she woke up, she wasn't hungry, because she had been feasting the entire time. The *hoca* was crying. The lizards had been *periler*, and they had been doing a wedding dance when she disturbed them. If she had hit the lizards, she would have been killed.

✶✶✶✶✶

THE REDUCTION IN
SUPERNATURAL OCCURRENCES

In the old days, meaning in the childhood memories of people my age as well as in previous generations, there were many terribly frightening occurrences which took place usually at night, near graveyards, often involving a green light. This is said to have been the work of *peri* and *cin* (fairies and genies), or of *hortlak* (the risen dead). When I asked if such things still happen, most people say that they don't go on as much as they used to — with two differing explanations for this change. One woman, whose husband was one of the earliest workers to go to Germany from this village, has been with her husband on the pilgrimage to Mecca. They were able to afford the trip because of the job in Germany, and they have earned the status and respect accorded those who are *Haci* (those who have made the pilgrimage). This woman explained that they brought holy water from Mecca back to the village, some of which they distributed as gifts, and some of which they sprinkled around in special places to bring spiritual benefit to their surroundings and their family. This water is especially potent against malicious beings. She related that, as more people are going on the *Hac* and bringing back holy water, the areas where the *peri* and *cin* can do their mischief are shrinking, thus reducing the numbers of encounters with supernatural beings. This theory stands in opposition to the theory of another woman of the same age, who told me that people are becoming so bad and are harming each other so much that the *peri* and *cin* are left with nothing to do. Neither theory fits with the standard Western secularist idea that changing times bring changing world-views, and that as people assimilate scientific notions, they will see their old "superstitions" to have been false. Many of the younger generation indicated to me that they thought of some of these ideas as the silly imaginings of an uneducated village society. Most, however, have stories of supernatural events they themselves witnessed or experienced.

The "Islamist" revival movement has worked to downplay the influence on everyday life of "minor" supernatural beings such as ghosts and fairies, while encouraging the sense of the immanence of God in every detail of life. Although *peri*, *cin*, *nazar*, angels, and various magical rites are all mentioned in the Koran, considered to be an infallible and unaltered text by all Muslims, when religious experts are asked about these issues, they often opine that villagers are exaggerating something which is real but not common.

The perception of a reduced supernatural influence on daily activity has taken its toll on the respect given to someone who is familiar with the spirit world and who can tell a good story about it. Aunty Emine's husband, Uncle Ferit, has a reputation as a teller of tall tales (or as a big liar, depending on whom you ask). He can come up with a story for any occasion, and specializes in spooky stories and snake stories. His authority on the subject of snakes is unchallenged, as he is known to be immune to snakes and has caught many dangerous, poisonous snakes in the village within the remembered collective history. His authority in matters of the spirit world is increasingly challenged by his family and neighbors, however, even to the point that listeners will cut him off and show open disrespect for his "lies."

One morning, when we were gathered around the kitchen breakfast table, drinking our tea, the *gelin* from the next house appeared at the window. She had been sick with a continuous cold since I had arrived several weeks before, and had already been to the clinic because of swollen tonsils. This morning she had a severely inflamed eye which was swollen, red, and infected. Her mother-in-law had sent her over to ask Uncle Ferit to read a prayer over her as a remedy. He pushed back from the table, spread his hands out expressively, and began in a story-telling tone of voice, "Well I wasn't going to tell you this, but as I was coming home from the mosque the other night, I saw a green light near the spring by your house..." His next sentence included the word *periler* (fairies) but was drowned out by unanimous shouts of derision. One of his daughters told him to "shut up and stop being stupid." Aunty Emine exclaimed that he was "just making it up on the spot." His son-in-law, who has a reputation for being something of an Islamic expert with a rigid, text-based knowledge of religion, spoke more quietly but expressed the opinion that even his father-in-law's prayer reading might not be effective. Well, someone who asks for a prayer can't be turned away, and so Uncle Ferit was sent out into the hall to read over her as she sits on a chair. He recited under his breath and blew over her during the pauses. When they were finished, the old man and the *gelin* came back into the kitchen. Aunty Emine told Uncle Ferit that he should also read a *nazar* prayer over the *gelin*, which he proceeded to do without leaving the room.

It seems to me that Uncle Ferit still commands some respect for his ability to read prayers over sick people, but that what he enjoys most has been for the most part taken from him—the respect granted a teller of tales of the supernatural in a society with day-to-day contact with the strange and sometimes wonderful goings on in the spirit world. Because of the more modern world-view of the younger generation (with its culture of science and skepticism of old ways), he can get an audience only for his real-life stories, and mostly for his actual personal experiences with snakes. His reputation for embellishment and exaggeration continues, but the stories of the supernatural have been pushed completely off the scale of belief and can be stopped before they even begin. I am sure that he still has some listeners in some circles and in some circumstances (perhaps in the coffeehouse or on long winter nights), and I know that he tries valiantly to keep alive his reputation as a storyteller.

NAZAR: THE "EVIL EYE"

Murdock (1980) classifies the evil eye as cause of illness under "witchcraft," and calls this belief "practically universal in the Circum-Mediterranean region but surprisingly rare elsewhere in the world." (21) Other scholars, such as Alan Dundes (1992) find a wider occurrence of evil eye belief:

> The idea that a malign glance can do grievous harm to person and property is of great antiquity. it is mentioned in the Bible as well as in Sumerian and other ancient near-eastern texts, which would make it more than five thousand years old at the very least. Widely reported from India to Ireland, the evil eye seems to be common among Indo-European and Semitic cultures past and present. immigrants to the new world from circum-Mediterranean countries...brought their evil-eye belief system with them...(p. vii)

Bess Allen Donaldson (1938, in Dundes 1992), found that her religiously educated informants most often referred to Sura 68:51 to show the Koranic affirmation of the danger of the evil eye: "Almost would the infidels strike thee down with their very looks when they hear the warning of the Koran, and they say, He is certainly possessed." (p. 67 in Dundes)

In a manual of Islamic medicine, *Islamic Medical Wisdom: The Tibb al-A'imma* (A Twelver Shi'i book translated by Batool Ispahany, edited by Andrew J. Newman, and published without a date in the Islamic Republic of Iran), the prayer to counteract the evil eye suggests that revenge upon the caster of the evil eye is most effective:

> In the Name of Allah, the Lord of a frowning face and confining water and dry stone, I trust, and crushing water and searching meteor, from an envious eye and from the evil eye. I return the evil eye to him and to those most loved by him, in his liver (al-kabd) and his kidney, thin blood, heavily laden fat, delicate bone, in what he deserves. In the Name of Allah, the Merciful, the Compassionate, and therein We wrote down for them: A life for a life, an eye for an eye, a nose for a nose, an ear for an ear, a tooth for a tooth, and for wounds retaliation (5:45). Allah bless our master Muhammad and his family. (186)

The "evil eye" is a belief constellation that is found in many parts of the world. The basic underlying belief common to all evil eye beliefs is that a human glance can, in some circumstances, cause harm to people, animals, or things that are the object of the glance. The belief in the evil eye is found throughout the Mediterranean area, in widely differing cultures, expressed in different languages, material artifacts, and practices. There are studies of the evil eye which refer to pre-Christian Greek and Roman evil eye beliefs (see Dundes, ed. 1991). Because the belief can be shown to pre-date Christianity and Islam, and because it appears in a variety of contemporary cultures with various religious beliefs, the scholarship on the evil eye has generally located the belief outside of the mainstream monotheistic religions, as a "superstition," a pagan remnant, or "folk" belief. When scholars take the time to ask believers themselves about the evil eye, they find that most believers are familiar with evidence from their own major religious texts about the reality of the evil eye phenomenon. For Muslims, the reality of *nazar is* irrefutable, as it is mentioned in the Koran. There is much more religious compulsion for a Muslim to accept the evil eye as a real possibility, for example, than there is for a Christian to put up a Christmas tree in December. Most mainstream Christians would not accept that a Christmas tree was unchristian or that it was an evil or heretical practice, even if they acknowledge that the practice of bringing a pine tree inside the house in the middle of winter is a pre-Christian, Northern European tradition which is nowhere called for in the Bible. Likewise, faithful Muslims place most of their own practices and beliefs within their religious tradition and are quick to point out that belief in *nazar* cannot be classed with other "superstitions" doomed to die out as human knowledge progresses. From the outside, what may seem to be a "folk belief" is an irrefutable part of "real belief" for Muslims.

In our interview, Lale, (the same as in the transcribed interviews in Chapter 2) displayed an awareness that I, as a researcher, might be conflating religious belief with baseless superstition. Her description of *nazar* showed that she thought that I might be mistakenly classifying it as a "backwards idea." She told me that she believed in *nazar* because it is in the Koran (notice, not because she had never questioned it or because she has personally experienced it or seen its effects, but because she knows it has Koranic affirmation). In my interview with her, she explained:

Lale: I don't believe in stomach-pulling and all that stuff. I believe in *nazar* because it is in the Koran. It's read for people and animals.
Sylvia: Do you have it done?
L: Yes, because we believe in God, we do it. It is in the Koran.
S: What do you use it for?
L: For example, if you have a really nice outfit, if you don't say "Maşallah" you can get *nazar*. You believe. I mean it's not backward

superstition *(batıl inançlar)*. It's in the Koran. We read it [the prayer] and it passes.

S: How do you know you have *nazar?*

L: Like this, for example, you feel weak, you don't feel well you're depressed (literally, "your soul is squeezed"—*canın sıkılıyor]*.

S: It happens to babies a lot.

L: Yes. For example, the baby has been nursed, fed, it's diaper is changed, and still it is uncomfortable. We believe it has *nazar,* we have it [the prayer] read, the baby gets better.

S: Who do you have read it?

L: Everyone does it.

Although I had not asked particularly about *nazar,* rather only in a general way about village healing practices, Lale wants to make sure that I know the difference between *nazar* and superstitions. She lives in Samsun and has sisters-in-law living in Germany. She uses herbal teas in the traditional ways, ("We use linden when we have flu. There's quince leaf, I put in carnation, I squeeze lemon."), but rejects most village healing practices as mistaken. She considers village food to be healthier than that available in the city. She is also an experienced consumer of private clinical medicine, having had three operations because of cysts in her ovaries, traveling to Istanbul and changing doctors after the first operation in order to get a second opinion. A person like this has been in many discussions about different beliefs concerning health care, perhaps across generations, or spurred by a show on television, or due to contact with another culture, within Turkey or outside. She knows that I might have classified *nazar* as "village stuff" and works to set me straight (although she is just supposing about me, this was the first time we had met and I did not mention *nazar* before she did).

Nazar and the Health Care System

Nazar is a concept which is used in a flexible manner to explain and deal with problems of illness and strife in human society. *Nazar* is a convincing explanatory tool in the local culture, much as psychological metaphors are used in American discourse. For example, attaching importance to childhood experiences or birth order as formative of personality is a commonplace in our culture but seems strange to people from many other cultures. In the biomedical metaphor of the "body as machine," organ transplants are seen as mere replacements of broken machinery, rather than as drastic or insane measures likely to change one's personality or karma. O'Connor (1995) offers the example of a hotly contested recommendation of a liver transplant as an example of difference in ideas about the body and the self being a point of conflict between the medical establishment in Philadelphia and the Hmong immigrant community. Emily Martin (1992) has shown that culture in the United States is bound up with "key metaphors" which structure our thoughts about our selves and others. She shows, for example, that the metaphor of the "body as a machine" leads to the wide-spread cultural belief that menopause is a time when a woman's body begins to malfunction and decay. If a woman's body is compared to a machine for the reproduction of the species, then birth can be thought of as a time when a woman might break down and need the services of an expert mechanic (the doctor), and then, as well, menopause is a clear sign of the end of a woman's usefulness. The metaphor of medicine being a weapon in the war against illness has permeated our society to the extent that even treatments which try to offer alternatives to the mainstream health care culture (such as herbalism) present their goods as ways to "build up the body's defenses." It shapes the discourse of this work as well, for example, when I call women the "front line" of defense against illness (Chapter 3).

Martin (1992) discusses the difficulty of researching one's own culture. She says, "As an anthropologist, my problem was how to find a vantage point from which to see the water I had lived in all my life." (11) The explanatory models used in a culture other than one's own are much easier to notice and to describe as rhetorical devices, metaphors, or culturally-specific theories. Examining the explanatory models and "key metaphors" of another culture is a necessary project when one wants to present an idea of how that culture works. The common pitfall of examining another culture is to assume that one's own culture is "natural" and free of similar metaphors which shape thoughts and behavior. In discussing how a metaphor works (or "functions") in a culture different from one's own, it is important to realize that all humans use metaphors and beliefs as they live their lives and explain their experiences.

In the local society of Medreseönü, then, one can attempt to describe ways that the belief in *nazar* is used to manage social relations and to shape health care. Jealousy and covetousness are serious problems in a small-scale agricultural society with a subsistence economy. *Nazar* beliefs deal directly with issues of jealousy, providing a means to bring covetous feelings into the open arena of social discourse. Jealousy can be treated as intentional or inadvertent, depending on the particular issues involved in a particular diagnosis of *nazar*. The problems caused by *nazar* are serious—illness, depression, accident, the reduction of food, and the destruction of property. Because *nazar* can be cast both intentionally by enemies and inadvertently by well-meaning people, everyone is taught to be aware of its potential and quick to act if it strikes.

Part of the reduction in the impact of the supernatural in everyday life, described above, is the current de-personalized idea of *nazar*. It seems that, in the past, specific people were more likely to be singled out as the knowing or unknowing casters of *nazar*. Now, although the effects of *nazar* are recognized and treated in traditional ways, people put much less emphasis on identifying the source of *nazar*.

In terms of social relations, it seems that *nazar* beliefs are an integral part of local traditional ideas about appropriate behavior for men and women at different stages of life. Young men are less culturally restricted in their ability to look around and to make eye contact with others as compared to young women. Married men are expected to control their glances at women as a part of moral behavior, although women are often thought to be consciously attracting the attentions of men, who are thus excused for not being in control of their eyes. Older women look at people (including strangers) more directly than younger women do—they have less of a fear of being labeled improper or brazen. This might be a reason that older women are more often feared to have the power of *nazar*. In a patriarchal society, young men and women of any age are often expected to keep their eyes lowered in the presence of a powerful man. Older women, however, are often in a position of questionable relation to powerful men—for instance, a man's mother often insists that he show her deference. Barren women, who must be well into childbearing years before being conclusively labeled barren, are also problematic in a patriarchal system—and they are most often thought to be jealous of the babies of others, and so likely to cause *nazar*.

Nazar Interpreted by a Disbeliever

A man from the village agreed to share his ideas about *nazar* only with the understanding that no one from the village would be told about his disbelief. He told me that hungry children learn to milk the family cow without the knowledge of their mother. The resulting reduction in milk at regular milking time can be blamed by the worried mother on the harmful presence of *nazar* in the cow. If the actual situation were to be brought to light, the family would face the terrible shame of having hungry children who are led to steal because of their hunger. In this dire situation, where poverty is obvious, the blaming of *nazar* for additional troubles can shift and diffuse blame which would otherwise fall on family members. This same man told me that cows are often frightened when they see snakes while out grazing and their fear (rather than *nazar*) causes a loss of milk production. This would be an explanation fitting better with a scientific

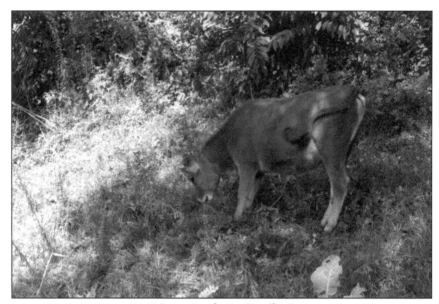

24. *Nazar* Beads on Family Cow

model of the world, but it should be noted that snakes have a special place in the folklore of the region and often replace the supernatural in frightening stories.

Women's Work

The management of *nazar* is generally women's work—if men sometimes read the *nazar* prayer or write amulets for protection, it is usually at the request of a woman who has diagnosed the problem. If men are troubled by something they think might be *nazar*, they often consult their mothers or wives for confirmation and treatment. Certain women are known for skill in treating *nazar*, but every woman has some means of taking basic precautions and providing the first line of treatment for herself and her family. In Bosnia, female healers called *bula* use their knowledge of Kornic prayers to treat a range of ailments, including those associated with the evil eye (Bringa, 1995, 178–184, and 206–216).

The Diagnosis of Nazar

People know when *nazar* is present because it manifests itself in recognizable ways. In general, *nazar* often causes depression and listlessness or a sudden onset of serious illness. During treatments, there are ways to confirm that *nazar* is actually present. If the person reciting the *nazar* prayer yawns or has watery eyes, the presence of *nazar* is confirmed. The treatments described

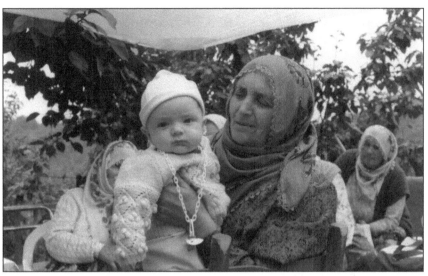

25. Aunt Emine Guards Timur from the Evil Eye when Visiting

below also have diagnostic functions. Bringa (1995) reports the combination of diagnostic and efficacious uses of a lead pouring technique (see below for the Black Sea village version) performed "at the request of women who had be bereaved by the death of a close relative, or had been upset by other events in the immediate family and were anxious and unable to sleep, though they did not know the reason why. The casting of lead and Qur'anic recitation were believed to help define the problem and thereby relieve the anxiety." (216)

The Prevention of Nazar

Nazar can be prevented through the use of amulets containing religious inscriptions (*muska*), eye-shaped blue beads, blue or red ribbon, spitting or the mimicking of spitting, the placement of an iron utensil over a milk pot, and by the simple method of hiding things from the sight of those likely to cast *nazar*. Women are largely responsible for taking preventative measures to protect themselves and their family members.

> *Durma söyle annana*
> *Başına kurşun döksün*
> *Şu gencecik uşağa da*
> *Birazcik torpil geçsun.*

> Hurry tell your mother
> She should perform "kurşun dökmek" (see below)

And she should give this fine young man
A little bit of help (to win your affections)

—Sung by Davut Güloğlu, Nurcanım

The Treatment of Nazar

The following description is of a procedure called *mum dökmek* ("pouring wax"), which is common along the Eastern Turkish Black Sea Coast and has been reported in other areas around the Black Sea and in the southern lands of the former Soviet Union. In Turkey, a more widely reported version of this technique is *kurşun dökmek* ("pouring lead"), which uses molten lead instead of wax. The woman who performed this procedure for my benefit cites the convenience and economy of wax as reasons to prefer it to lead. Wax can be melted on a simple portable gas burner, while lead may require a hotter fire. In Black Sea singer Davut Güloğlu's song above, a young man recommends the molten lead procedure for the girl he fancies, with the implication that she has too many admirers and may suffer from the evil eye. He hopes her mother will give him some *torpil*, the influence mentioned in Chapter 2, so that he can win the girl's heart. The proximity of the two wishes from the girl's mother may imply a relationship between them, as if the molten lead procedure may have some potency as a love charm.

*****

The best day to do this treatment is the first day of the lunar month. Villagers track the phases of the moon from observation as well as from their wall calendars with a page for each day and many Islamic sayings, bits of advice, puzzles, and quotations. The calendar shows the Gregorian date in large numbers and shows the Islamic month and date in small numbers. The Gregorian calendar has been in use in Turkey since it was mandated by the reform laws of 1928, but many rural people continue to rely on the traditional Islamic calendar. If the calendar is kept current, by ripping off a page each day, those who are illiterate can follow the symbols that show the phases of the moon. The Islamic calendar is lunar-based, and most traditional remedies take the lunar date into account. The best days of the week to do the treatment are Wednesday and Saturday. I have only ever heard of women performing this procedure, at least in contemporary times, while the patient can be male or female. The treatment is usually done in the toilet, because *nazar* is dirty and can be pulled out by the dirtiness of a toilet or stable. The patient squats or sits on a low stool nearly completely undressed, or wearing

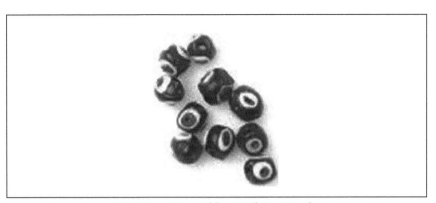

26. *Nazar Boncukları* Evil Eye Beads

old clothes that will be soiled by the dirty, waxy water poured over the patient at the end of the treatment. As with every traditional remedy, the practitioner starts by saying *"Bismillahirahmanirahim"* the Islamic prayer for beginnings. The main ingredient for this treatment is a block of beeswax, which is melted in a small frying pan used just for this procedure. The block of wax is first passed around the patient's head in a counterclockwise direction while a prayer is recited by the practitioner under her breath (about three times). The block of wax is then melted and poured into a bowl of water resting on the patient's head. This process creates a crackling, hissing, spitting sound, and the louder the sound is, the stronger the *nazar* is said to be. The practitioner then removes the wax from the surface of the water, where it has formed a pancake-like shape. The underside of the wax is studied for bubbles, which indicate *nazar,* and for the shapes of bird heads, which indicate enemies. The bubbly parts are ripped off of the pancake of wax and set aside. The remaining wax is squeezed into a solid ball then passed three times around the neck with another prayer. It is re-melted and the hot wax is poured into the bowl of water, which is now held over the patient's bent neck. Again the wax pancake is examined and the parts indicating *nazar* are removed and separated into two distinct balls of wax. The next step is to pass the squeezed wax around the right arm and then the left arm, melt the wax, and pour it into the bowl held over the patient's arms, which are held straight out together in front of the body. The procedure is repeated for the waist and for the legs, for a total of five successive meltings and pourings. It is possible for the practitioner to differentiate between areas of the body strongly affected by *nazar* and those not affected. A patient's physical or mental complaints can be traced to the effects of *nazar* in different parts of the body. After the final examination of the wax and removal of the *nazar*-affected parts, the remaining wax becomes the third ball of wax. The disposal of these three balls of wax is a crucial part of the procedure. The first ball is to be buried under a tree, the second is to be thrown into flowing water, and the third is to be tossed onto a busy intersection to be trampled and run over by passing traffic. Some of the water in the bowl is poured over the head of the patient as the patient straightens up into a standing position. This is repeated three times and the water must dry on the patient. The patient is now considered dirty, and should not touch a baby or perform any ritual requiring cleanliness (such as prayer) before getting rid of the dirtiness by entering a stable (which is dirty and draws dirt to itself) three times. A patient can also enter someone else's house three times, but the implication is that the dirt will then stay there, and so this would only be used against an enemy. If the patient needs to pick up a baby, the baby can be first passed over the head of the patient to neutralize the power of the dirt. The person doing the passing over must then go three times in and out of a stable to get rid of the dirt thus acquired.

*****

Aside from this complex and time-consuming procedure, and aside from the most common treatment of *nazar* through prayer and blowing, there are a few quick methods for averting the evil eye. One is to say '*Maşallah*' mimicking a spitting sound three times in the direction of a person or object considered especially beautiful. This can even be done in a conversation, usually in a light-hearteded manner, after a person or thing is highly praised. A person who is thought to be afflicted by *nazar* can have someone take a small pinch of salt in their fingers, circle the person's head three times, and then throw the salt into a flame. The sparkling of the salt is taken as a sign that *nazar* had been present. Dundes' (1992) book gives examples of the widespread uses of salt, spitting, and diagnosis through the use of a bowl of water and a hot substance (molten lead or live coals used in many regions).

Breastfeeding and Nazar

Mother's milk, like cow's milk, is susceptible to the bad effects of *nazar*. Mothers are admonished by older women not to talk about nursing and not to nurse in front of others. An abundance of milk is a good thing which might easily attract *nazar*. This worry about *nazar* made it difficult for me to collect information about breast-feeding in the village. When I spoke to mothers of young children about my own breast-feeding (which I learned to do only in select company), they seemed more willing to talk about it. The nurses at the clinic strongly encourage breast-feeding, but realize that it is a difficult subject to discuss because of the possibility of *nazar*. I saw many women "putting their babies to sleep" in a position which I later realized from my own experience was probably nursing—reclined on a bed next to the baby, supported on one elbow, usually with the mother's back to the door. Even though people often glance in the room where a mother is with her baby, to make sure everything is fine, there would be no chance of inadvertent *nazar* because of the mother's position. My first idea about how I should breast-feed in the village setting was that I only needed to be sure not to indecently expose myself (this being the major concern expressed in American debates about public breast-feeding). Even in all-women gatherings, however, I became aware that I should be very discreet about nursing so as not to attract attention and possible *nazar*. My mother-in-law would often tell other women that the baby was sleeping in my lap, when he was actually nursing, covered with a blanket. Turning one's back to the room is another way to shield the baby and the nursing mother from unwanted glances.

Life Transitions and Nazar

Nazar seems especially likely to occur during transitional times in an individual's life. Weddings are a time when *nazar* may be present and preventative actions are taken. It is possible that the red color of the henna used to stain the bride's hands is an "eye-catching" preventative technique. The sacrifice of a rooster on the doorstep of the groom's house as the couple enters is meant to purify the couple of any negative influences. In some regions of Turkey a drinking glass is broken on the doorstep for the same reason. The period of forty days after a woman gives birth (*lohusa zamanı*) is also considered to be especially dangerous for both mother and baby. They are both prevented from going outside the house. The woman's hair is tied with a red ribbon, and the baby is pinned with amulets or beads against *nazar*. All visitors exclaim "*Maşallah*" on first sight of the new baby to deflect the possible ill-effects of their admiration. In important times during an individual woman's life, especially in times of transition, *nazar* is a force with which to reckon.

CLINICAL PRACTITIONERS AND BELIEF

Clinical practitioners have an ambivalent relationship to the beliefs held by their patients. On the one hand, they are from the same general culture, although they may differ in terms of regional affiliation and class. On the other hand, they have been trained in a belief system based on the microbiological model, which is often radically distinct from the explanatory models which make sense to their patients. Patients quickly realize in discussions with health professionals in a clinic or hospital that this difference exists. According to Snow (1977):

> Magic and religion do entertwine in the attempt to solve the problems of everyday living and such attempts are too often seen as ignorance, as superstition, as evidence of subnormal mentality when they come to the attention of the health professional.... [The informants among whom I work] know that many of their most valued and deeply held beliefs are different from those of the mainstream middle-class citizen, and these same beliefs are seen as laughable and ridiculous. They are quite aware that their medical beliefs and practices are not shared by mainstream medicine and they largely know which beliefs these are: this does not result in their being dropped, it results in their being hidden. Too many poor patients are also quite aware that many physicians and ancillary health workers see them as shiftless, dirty, ignorant, lazy and inferior and would prefer not to have to deal with them. (44–45)

She makes clear that class differences play a big part in the perceptions of one group toward the other. In Turkish culture, villagers are at once praised as the "salt of the earth" and damned for being poor and uneducated.

It seems to be a human tendency to scoff at the health care beliefs held by others. The current trend in academia, however, is for scholars of health care systems to see the mainstream biomedical model to be itself a culturally constructed and constructing metaphor and to attempt an even-handed examination of the salient health-related metaphors in other cultures. According to Gevitz (1988):

> As in the case of sectarian medicine, folk and religious healing have also been the subjects of scholarly studies recently which have been less concerned with normative issues than with placing these phenomena within social cultural and historical context. Rather than dismissing the adherents of folk and religious healers as a weird fringe element or approaching them from the standpoint of psychopathology, such works examine the intellectual origins and logical coherence of these systems and what functions they serve to participants. While many scholars continue to focus on folk and religious healing

among marginal groups, greater attention is being given to unorthodox beliefs and practices accepted by people generally considered to
be in the mainstream of social life. (27)

Turkish clinical professionals are committed to the truth of the biological
method to varying degrees. They may make a distinction between personal
beliefs and professional discourse. They may wear evil-eye protection beads
around their necks at the same time as they express skepticism about the va-
lidity of the *nazar* belief system. If they are practicing Muslims, or at least respectful of Muslim beliefs, they must acknowledge *nazar* as a real phenomenon. They may, however, find *nazar* illness to be an overused category of
ailment. Pierce (1964) concerned himself with describing the culture of a
Turkish village, but he could not resist giving the following example of the
nazar theory of a doctor in the capital:

> …in addition to the formal religion, all Turkish villages have many
> folk-beliefs. I do not have detailed data for Demirciler on this sub-
> ject, but belief in the evil-eye is common, and the villagers in Demir-
> ciler displayed the ever-present blue beads that are thought to be a
> protection against this menace. A well-known physician (an eye spe-
> cialist, incidentally) in Ankara told me quite seriously one day that
> the evil-eye was not a supernatural phenomenon at all. He theorized
> that certain wave lengths in light were harmful to human beings and
> that certain people had the ability to store up these harmful wave
> lengths and release them at will. These frequencies when directed to-
> ward an individual (children were supposed to be most susceptible to
> these), cause poor health and can result in a general deterioration
> ending in death. He did not explain how the blue beads served to pro-
> tect one from this. (89)

In ethnography, the ideal informant (whose very existence has been rightly
called into question) has been untouched by the outside and has thus never
learned to hide his or her beliefs in the company of those who may not share
them. What is striking about the Pierce example is not so much that the doctor in Ankara wants to have a scientific explanation of *nazar*, but that he did
not realize that Pierce would think his idea ridiculous.

Another example of the complexity of the clinical professional's relationship
to his cultural environment is the combination of secular and Islamic symbols
displayed in the private office of Dr. Deniz in Ordu. The objects on display can
be read as a text meant to inspire confidence in the doctor. In his waiting room,
there are bookshelves filled with a several encyclopedia-like series on the lives

of saints. A plaque which reads: *"Hastanın ilaç kullanması bir sebeptir. Şifayı verecek olan ise Allahü tealadır."* *Hadis-I-Şerif* ("A patient's use of medicine is a means. If anyone gives a cure, it is Exalted God." Sacred Hadith). The waiting room, then, is set up to be "read" and understood as a proper display of piety. This is mainly a post-1990's type of display. The encyclopedias are made available through newspaper subscriptions, and often remain unopened on the shelves, used as a sign more than as a informational resource.

In contrast to the religious markers in the waiting room, the doctor's inner office displays a large picture of Atatürk above the desk and a wall-sized mural of one of Atatürk's sayings about doctors: *"Beni Türk Hekimlerine Emanet Ediniz."* ("Entrust me to Turkish doctors."). This is both a nationalistic request ("I don't want foreign doctors—either in the Ottoman sense of using Armenian, Jewish or Greek specialists, or in the more recent fad of preferring European specialists—Turkish doctors are the best, or should be trained to be the best") and a secular request (not "Entrust me to God."), a pithy formula which combines two of Atatürk's most famous political projects. The set-up of the doctor's inner office is more like the officially-sanctioned, secular displays of a public clinic. The waiting room, however, is more like a private living room, with religious books seeming to make a statement about the doctor's personal tastes. Once again, the boundaries between traditional and clinical, religious and secular, personal and private are seen to be blurry and shifting, in constant interaction and negotiation.

"Faith," then, is a tricky subject, whether the beliefs under examination are one's own or those of others. In academic circles, there has long been the idea, recently challenged from all sides, that scholarly neutrality is possible and ideal, that one's own beliefs can be separated from one's analysis of a subject matter. When one's subject is human behavior and culture, careful attention to what people actually say can lead both to an awareness of the often insurmountable difference between the specific details of people's beliefs and to a new understanding of how all humans use their beliefs to structure and make sense of their lives. The focus of the next chapter is an individual healer, an elderly bone-setter who learned her techniques in the traditional manner. While an outsider might expect that this woman would be a fount of outlandish traditional beliefs who expects her patients to accept her bizarre treatments on faith, she is living proof that an illiterate healer can be a down-to-earth paragon of empirical knowledge based on a lifetime of experience.

CHAPTER 6

A Traditional Healer

She could cure a bullet wound in a mere couple of days. The broken wing of
a little bird would be child's play for her. She was famous in this small town,
and for miles around too, for her healing arts. Even the smugglers, even the
armed pirates along these coasts knew that her medicines could restore the
dead to life.

—Yashar Kemal, *Seagull*, 1981 (p. 7)

A happy, noisy group of women and children from the village below are
visiting a family in the village up the hill. I have asked to visit with Aunty
Zeynep and to see her at work, and the expedition has turned into a boisterous get-together for women who can't always find the time to sit and chat with
each other. My tape-recorder (with its sound-activated red power light) is an
object of great interest to the children. The women make a joke of my recording their conversation—"She's going to write it all down in a book! We'll be
famous in America!" Back in the U.S., I will listen to the tape, remembering
the festive atmosphere of a women's mid-day social visit, trying hard to deci-
pher the voices and sounds which pile up on top of each other (including the
South American soap-opera on TV), the overlapping and the interrupting,
the laughing short-hand conversation about familiar people and events, the
comfortable use of local phrases and pronunciation.

Aunty Emine and Aunty Zeynep have known each other for almost all of
their lives, and are both accomplished healers who can compare notes about
bone-setting experiences. As the initial chit-chat flows into talk about health,
Aunty Emine and Aunty Zeynep try to accommodate my interests by discussing people they have known and treated. Aunty Zeynep is asked to take a
look at the new infant in the household, since he has been fussing and not
sleeping well. Aunty Zeynep holds the baby and begins to recite the *nazar*
prayer. Conversation flows on around them, and the prayer is over in a few
minutes. After tea and cookies, our visit draws to a close. Most of our group

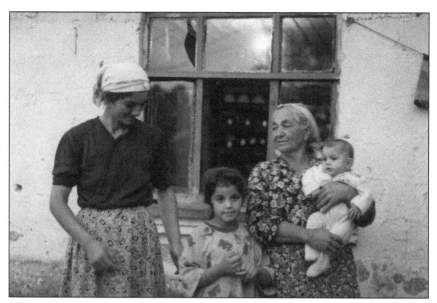

27. Aunty Zeynep with her Other Gelin and Grandchildren

heads home to work in the gardens, but Aunty Emine and I go with Aunty Zeynep as she goes on what resembles a doctor's rounds.

The next woman we see has a severely sprained ankle, which has swollen up to the knee until she can hardly walk. The woman is from the same generation as Aunty Zeynep and Aunty Emine, and has limped over to her daughter's house with great difficulty, using a walking stick. Making sympathetic sounds, Aunty Zeynep begins by softening the woman's ankle by wrapping it in hot towels. She gets the woman to sit on the carpet with her feet in front of her. Aunty Zeynep asks for olive oil and begins to massage the oil into the swollen limb with her thumbs. As she works, she tells the woman that she will have to massage her own leg for it to heal properly. The woman protests that she can't touch it herself, because of the pain. As Aunty Zeynep's hands move down the leg to the ankle, the woman lets out a scream of pain. Aunty Zeynep soothes her, asking her to not be afraid. She recommends that the woman wrap her leg every night in hot towels and stay off her leg for as long as possible. After the leg is softened and the swelling is slightly loosened, Aunty Zeynep holds the woman's foot in both of her hands and slowly turns it to check if the joint and bones are dislocated. She listens for sounds coming from the joint, which would indicate dislocation. She scolds the woman for waiting before asking for help, telling her that there is only so much she can help when the swelling is so severe and the problem has been left without treatment for so long (about a week has gone by since the woman fell and twisted her ankle). Her tone of authority, her diagnosis and instructions for care, and her frustration with the "non-compliance" of her patients reminds me of a clinical doctor.

When the massaging is finished, Aunty Zeynep has our hostess, the patient's daughter, bring cloths soaked in softened beeswax to wrap up the leg. The women agree that pine sap works as well as beeswax for this purpose. The wax hardens as it cools, creating a protective casing around the injured limb and keeping it from moving out of place. Aunty Zeynep admonishes the woman to stay off her leg, threatening permanent disability if she continues to use it.

The treatment over, we sit around and chat over tea. Aunty Zeynep demonstrates various techniques of bone-setting, joint adjustments, and replacing dislocated veins, tendons, and muscles. She gets a young girl, about eight years old, to submit to her various demonstrations, which she does with alternating giggles and yelps. Aunty Zeynep has a specialist's vocabulary, with particular words for body parts and conditions. She stresses the importance of the particular sound "*Kart!*" which indicates a joint returning successfully to its place. After a while, the conversation becomes more general, with talk about good *gelins* and bad ones, a sensational shooting incident of the night before, and the current state of a local woman with mental health problems.

The elderly ladies turn to one of their daily concerns, and favorite topics of conversation, the health of their milk cows. Aside from treating human patients, Aunty Zeynep is an expert in the care of cows. She knows causes of infertility, she can diagnose illnesses in the animals, and she is often asked to help out when a cow seems to be afflicted with *nazar*. During this visit, in fact, she is asked to read a prayer over a piece of bread, which will then be fed to the troubled family cow. As a traditional specialist, this is just one part of Aunty Zeynep's daily routine. She begins the prayer and blowing, but can't resist participating in the conversation, which continues. She apologizes for interrupting the prayer, says what she wants to, and then starts again at the beginning. As she recites, she is overcome by yawns, a sure sign of the presence of *nazar*.

Other topics of conversation include wedding invitations, traditionally given in the form of new colorful head scarves but now increasingly in printed card form, wedding gifts, and the care of babies. Aunty Zeynep warns the young mother in the room not to kiss the baby excessively on its face, as it can develop a rash. Later I learn that kissing a baby too much is thought to hinder its development or cause illness. Our tea glasses are continually refilled on the small tables pulled out for our visit. We snack on cakes and biscuits until the conversation reaches a natural lull. Then our upturned palms are splashed with lemon cologne, and we gather our things and stand.

Before leaving this house, we stop in another room to visit a woman on her deathbed. Our hostess has been taking care of her invalid mother-in-law for four-and-a-half months. The room smells sharply of ammonia and antiseptic. The woman is painfully thin with a gray skin-tone. When we come in, she turns her head slowly away from the wall to face us. She recognizes Aunty Emine and is introduced to me. Holding the woman's bony hand, Aunty Emine says some consoling words about the power of God, wishes the woman relief from pain, and we leave.

*****

Meeting Aunty Zeynep

Aunty Zeynep is a woman in her sixties, who lives in Çandır, the village far up the road from Gebeşli, where Aunty Emine lives, and more than twice as far from the shore road and town center. Aunty Emine was born in Çandır, and visits her relatives and friends there with some frequency. Çandır was only recently incorporated into Medreseönü and retains a feeling of more independence from the goings on in the town center. Unlike the other villages associated with Medreseönü, Çandır is known for having horses as well as cows. Many families use horses in their daily trips to fields and for bringing the cows to and from grazing. Elderly people relate that, in the past, horses were common in all of the villages, and people got to nearby towns by going across the hills on horse trails rather than along the coast as they do now in vehicles. When Aunty Emine was asked about traditional healers for me to interview, she immediately thought of Aunty Zeynep, who is known by all in the region to be a bone-setter (*kırıkçıkıkçı*), the one who deals with breaks and dislocations).

In 1993, I was taken up to Çandır by Aunty Emine for the express purpose of meeting Aunty Zeynep. I first met her during the social visiting described in the previous section, which can be called "going on rounds." The two Aunties then decided that we should come at another time to videotape some of her demonstrations. Because her techniques are based on the physical touching and manipulation of injured body parts, video is an excellent medium for recording them. I cannot do justice in print to the level of detail in her demonstrations, for which she would often grab her own arm or leg, or that of a nearby child or of one of us. A lengthy translation of the verbal portion of her explanations would be futile: "This comes out, see, so I take this, and rub like this, then *kart!* I push it back in."

So, on another afternoon, Aunty Emine, my husband, and I went up to Aunty Zeynep's house in Çandır. After walking up the winding dirt road through hazelnut groves, we came to the flat section of road above which sits the Çandır graveyard. Aunty Emine recited some prayers for the souls of her parents as we passed. A couple of times a year she will come up to this grave-yard, cut back the grass and weeds from their graves, and recite prayers, but today she is just praying in passing, as a sign of respect and piety. As we came into Çandır, Aunty Emine began to greet people in their yards alongside the road. We came up to a group of houses arranged up a steep slope along a ce-ment set of stairs. This was a family compound, which had grown up the hill as sons built additional rooms onto their parents' house on the road. Aunty Zeynep's house seems to me to be desperately poor. There is a broken pane of glass in the single window of the kitchen, which also serves as a room to re-ceive guests. We sit on a lumpy mattress atop a rusty bedspring. The pans and bowls arranged on shelves above the sink are the old tinned copper ones, and their surfaces look ready for re-tinning. Aunty Zeynep is wearing a homemade skirt over a homemade house dress. Her grandchildren run about without shoes, their clothes patched and dirty. We are only later to hear about her hus-band's mental/spiritual illness (described in his story in Chapter 2), and the devastating boat accident that will handicap both her grown son and her son-in-law has yet to occur. The house's condition is enough to make us aware that this is a family with little economic security.

Despite her poverty, or in defiance of it, Aunty Zeynep has a confident air. Her arms are thick and her hands obviously capable. She is a busy woman with housework, garden work, cows and grandchildren to watch after, and a busy circuit of patients who value her expertise and depend on her to allevi-ate their suffering.

Her techniques include the adjustment of joints which have been wrenched out of place, the diagnosis of breaks, fractures, and dislocated ten-dons, the alignment of broken parts of a bone, the wrapping and setting of broken or sprained limbs, the reduction of swelling through the use of heat and massage, the diagnosis of gangrene and infection, the manipulation of the skin near the spine for the relief of aches, the prescription of herbal reme-dies, the reading of *nazar* prayers, the application of heated leaves on the throat or chest for coughs and sore throats, the application of various poul-tices for the reduction pain and swelling, the procurement of pain-killers from the local pharmacist for her patients, and the application of heated drinking glasses to create vacuum pressure on special points on the back for the treatment of various inner ailments. The setting of bones, joints, and ten-dons, as well as the treatment for *nazar* are techniques she performs on animals as well as humans. Locals, in general, know many techniques for cracking various aching joints and the spine, which usually involve another person who lifts or pulls. Aunty Zeynep's knowledge goes beyond these everyday techniques. She is an expert.

On this visit to her home, Aunty Zeynep told us a story, which she repeated on another visit two years later, and is clearly very important to her. The story can be translated as follows:

> Aunty Zeynep:...Once I went to Doctor Gündüz. The wife of Hace's Yılmaz fell out of a tree. I healed that leg. The leg was fine. She went to the doctor. When she got there, my girl [to another lady her age in the room] Doctor Gündüz said to her "My girl, who fixed (pulled) this leg?" "So-and-so fixed it." I thought I was going to be jailed. First. I went. The doctor said, "How did you fix this?" First, I said, "I left it in boiled water, I softened it really well in the boiled water. [demonstrating on her own leg] After that, I searched with my hand to see where there was broken bone. After that, this leg, this heel." I said "I gathered it together from this side and that," I said. "I pulled the leg down, I pulled it upwards. These pieces right here, I sought them with my hand." I said. "Before it swelled." I said. "With only beeswax." I said. "And so I wrapped it this way." I said. [to us, as explanation] With heavy wax paper, thick paper. I wrapped the paper around here like a bracelet. "I wrapped it." I said. He asked me, "How many days [did it take] Exactly how many days did you leave it?" He asked me. "I left it exactly five days," I said, "On the fifth day I opened it." "Then what did you do again after that?" he asked me. "Then again I massaged it well with olive oil. I made a dressing. Once every three or four nights," I said. "Then I wrapped it up again," I said. "I didn't let her step down on it," I said. At that time, he said to me "I'm going to bring you here," he said to me, "I'll make a place [for her in his practice], I'll bring you here." "No," I said, "I've got small children." "Well then, you're going to give up this practice," he said to me. "My grandmother taught me this," I said. He brought me a basket of bones. [to us] Do you know what kind of bones? [M. asks, "This is Doctor Gündüz?"] Yeaa. He brought me those bones, cows' bones. He said, "Let me see you straighten out these bones and muscles." They were separated from each other. Look, there were some muscles in place and some were out. "How are these muscles? How are you going to bind these?" he said. How was it? They were all muscle, muscle

[separated] like this. "This," I said, "I would do this way." There is only one muscle here, one is missing [showing us on her own finger], isn't it so? "This muscle has cooked [merged] into the flesh," I said, "it is knitted in the flesh. There is flesh inside it [the bone]. With just one muscle, it won't come out right. So," I said, "if this same thing comes here to a doctor, could he attach the muscle? He can't attach it. It would be knitted with only one muscle. Just the same way it would knit in the flesh. There are some wrenched bobbins [local word for wrist bones]," I said. He said, "What are those wrenched bobbins?" [he doesn't understand her terminology] "Eeeh, those wrenched ones," [she demonstrates] I said, "they put a platinum bone in, they put in iron," I said. "When I don't do it, I send them [to a doctor]," I said. I'm telling them this [to the injured people]," I said. "When the bone won't take here, right? Then they put in a bone or stitch them together. Then it gets straightened," I said. "But with that kind of other dangerous stuff, I send them [to the doctor]," I said…"

I find this story particularly fascinating because it shows the interaction between a traditional healer and her modern medical counterpart. This story disproved my original hypothesis that traditional and modern experts had no contact and no respect for each other. In this story, Aunty Zeynep shows that she had been afraid of the legal consequences of practicing bone-setting, a form of traditional medicine. She discovers that the doctor was impressed with her work, but that he wants her either to practice in a formal clinic situation or to give up her art. She also tells the doctor that she is aware of her own limitations and that she does not hesitate to send a patient to a hospital or doctor if she cannot perform the necessary operations. The story shows two types of experts negotiating their roles in relationship to each other.

The traditional healer cites having small children as the reason she cannot join the doctor in his domain. This suggests to me that the traditional healing practices, performed by a woman with special skills and training, are considered to be inseparable from her normal life, and not an isolated profession which takes the place of other duties. The mention of her small children could also be seen as a strategy to dissuade the doctor from any punishment he might have been contemplating. Although the Doctor has the power of the law and of the medical profession behind him, Aunty Zeynep has the power of her knowledge and of her respected status of mother in her favor. When the Doctor tells her she must give up her practice, she challenges his right to make this demand, saying that her grandmother had taught her. Her art, she seems to imply, should be respected because of its lineage. The doctor then proceeds to test this knowledge with the cows' bones, and Aunty Zeynep never mentions if he said anything more about giving up the practice. The outcome of the exchange being that the two experts know each other's skills and power a bit better, and both continue to practice in their accustomed manner.

Throughout our initial interview, Aunty Zeynep checked in various ways to see if we were earnest in our interest in her art. Her story about the doctor impressed with her work could be seen as a rhetorical strategy to provide evidence from a biomedical expert of her skill. She needed to know that we were not dangerous for her, perhaps outsiders who would report her illegal practice. She wanted to show us her abilities and impress us with the extent of her experience and her commitment to her practice. I imagine that she had these things in mind as she demonstrated a technique on Muammer's wrist for the video camera. When I asked her to demonstrate on my wrist as well, she deftly dislocated my wrist and then popped it back into place. In an excruciatingly real way, I learned the power of her grasp and the confidence of her technique. My scream and then my laughing relief after the demonstration were proof of my temporary powerlessness in her hands. I was impressed, convinced in a visceral way of the woman's abilities.

One thing that stood out very clearly on the cassette recording with Aunty Zeynep was how quickly she understood what I was interested in and how easily she stepped into the role of an expert providing information. She needed no coaxing to start, and expected some kind of financial reward at the end of the video taping session. As far as I know, she has never been interviewed by a professional researcher, but she fields questions from her family and neighbors all the time. She may have considered me to be a kind of student who would pay for my lessons. Confused about her hints at the scene, my husband and I were set straight by Aunty Emine, who recommended that we send her some money as we were leaving the area. As a known traditional expert, Aunty Zeynep is used to being asked about healing techniques. She did make a perhaps-pointed reference to the lack of respect city people show to villagers. Many elements in the interview suggest ambivalence about sharing information with an outsider. The story about the Doctor, after all, was a story of a powerful and potentially dangerous outsider. Aunty Zeynep was careful to check our intentions and respect for traditional medicine. Points in our favor included our local family connections, our fame in the area as the first American bride and the first local boy to go to America, and the fact that we had come from another village just for the sake of meeting and interviewing her about her healing practices.

A Specialist's Language

"Aunty Zeynep uses a specialist's language when she talks about her art. She has words for each part of the body, including words which are not part of everyday speech in the area. I had to clarify many terms when translating interviews and video tape, and even local helpers had to be shown the body parts in question to venture a guess as to the correct translation of Aunty Zeynep's terms. Institutionally trained doctors have Latin terms for body parts, as well as common terms (not the terms Aunty Zeynep uses) to explain things to their patients. Like a doctor, Aunty Zeynep has phrases to describe particular conditions, such as *"kemiğin arasına et girmiş"* (tissue has gotten in the break in the bone) to describe a situation which she considers to be beyond her abilities to heal, a situation in which a person has waited too long to come to her, when there is a high risk of infection, and in which case she sends the patient to a doctor. This special language is a part of Aunty Zeynep's training and sets her apart from the general population—it makes her an expert.

Although she makes use of a specialist's language, Aunty Zeynep also faces difficult in describing certain things that she can feel in the body of a patient. When describing physical problems and their treatment, she often resorts to reproducing the sounds of the re-locations and needs to touch actual limbs to demonstrate the physical procedures. Hinojosa (2001) reports on contemporary Mayan bone-setters:

> The contact rendered through the bonesetter's hands enables him to directly assess the problem in the client's body. His hands serve as his primary vehicle for diagnosis and treatment, but in a nonmechanistic way. Bonesetters stress that their hands "know" the body and can directly determine what is wrong with it. The source of this intuition is indeterminate, but bonesetters locate the knowledge for bodywork quite explicitly in the hands.... When a bonesetter places his hands on a body, therefore, his hands guide him, and not the other way around. (p. 5)

Aunty Zeynep's use of beeswax-soaked cloth resembles the methods of the Mayan bonesetters who treat fractures, who "wrap the area with a gauze or cloth, or...immobilize the limb using available materials, such as cardboard or sticks.... most bonesetters prefer immobilizing arrangements that can be easily removed. This is because bonesetters generally check the injury site several days after the initial reduction to examine its alignment and progress." One of Hinojosa's bonesetter informants says:

[The fracture] *has* to be checked. If the bone hasn't moved out of place, it's because the site is knitting together, binding together. This has to be confirmed, though, because if it isn't, the bone might move out of place again, leaving the person crippled." (p. 5)

Aunty Zeynep's equivalent of the knitting of bones is the verb *tutmak*, which can be translated as "holding," "taking," or "sticking."

Again, in a point of similarity between Aunty Zeynep and the Mayan bone-setters studied by Hinojosa, the work of bone-setting is connected to the spiritual world only so much as the talent to be a bone-setter is taken to be a God-given one and all curing is ultimately in the hands of God. Aunty Zeynep uses only prayers which any woman can use to aid healing or to ask for blessing or assistance, she is not considered a specialist in spiritual matters. Unlike the Mayan bone-setters who do not seem to learn their art from family members, Aunty Zeynep specifically credits her training by her grandmother. Like the Mayan bone-setters, however, she links the story of her own severe injury to the start of her apprenticeship. Hinojosa speculates:

> In persons in whom a bodily grounding is heightened, through pain, for instance, a heightened bodily attention can emerge as a consequence, something especially evident in a vocational context. Injury, especially, may enable the bonesetter's body to better respond to and coexperience the suffering of other bodies, while at the same time legitimizing for locals the bonesetter's authority to utilize his body for healing. The health problems experienced by bonesetters authenticate their bodies as sources of knowledge and constitute a vector through which healing knowledge is revealed. (p. 8)

RETURNING TO AUNTY ZEYNEP

In July of 1996, I have my second formal interview with Aunty Zeynep, accompanied by Aunty Emine, Muammer, and our four-month-old son, Timur. We take her a gift of cloth for making a skirt, to show appreciation for her previous information. Aunty Emine had sent her some money the previous year to show gratitude for our first interview. The two women have known each other for a long time, since Aunty Emine comes from the village where Aunty Zeynep has lived all of her married life. As we sit down, the two women start to chat about a very important part of the life of village women, taking care of cows. Aunty Zeynep's husband is sitting in the room, but does not participate in this initial conversation. The women complain about the heat and the fact that no one is buying meat because of the mad cow disease scare from England. Because of this they can't even sell their cows and be saved from the work of keeping them. They agree that husbands are no help when it comes to cows. Aunty Zeynep tells how her cow's hip became dislocated when it turned a corner. She immediately put it right, but now she worries that if she tries to sell the cow, people will wonder why she has picked this particular time to sell it, and might guess that it had been injured.

We turn to the topic of feeding babies and it comes out that both women agree that yogurt and *pekmez* (condensed mulberry syrup) is better for babies than formula. Aunty Zeynep says that a doctor had come to the village and recommended that babies eat yogurt and *pekmez* instead of store-bought baby formula. Aunty Emine responds to Aunty Zeynep's inquiry about her health by telling her about her high blood pressure (*tansiyon*). The doctor told her that yogurt water is good for lowering high blood pressure. When Aunty Emine asks her how she is, Aunty Zeynep tells us about her attempts to heal her son and son-in-law after their very serious fishing-boat accident. For the son's multiple fracture in his arm, she put egg-sized wads of cotton under his arm to hold it in position. A doctor in Istanbul recommended various exercises to strengthen their injured limbs. The husband explains that all this misfortune came from *nazar*, which caused their accident.

I ask Aunty Zeynep to check baby Timur's limbs, telling her that his shoulder joints make noises sometimes when he moves. She said that his bones were thin/weak (*zayıf*), which is normal for a baby, and that they will fill out as he gets older. She said the noises are normal for babies.

Turning to general talk about health, we discuss the impact of diet on health. Everyone agrees that everyone should drink a lot of water to be healthy. Aunty Zeynep's husband says that fat, oil, and butter are good for people. Aunty Emine tells him that her doctor told her not to eat them because of her *tansiyon* (high blood pressure). He doesn't reply, but he obviously doesn't agree with the doctor. He proceeds to tell a story (summarized in Chapter 3) in which even a professor doctor in Istanbul was unable to help him, whereas a local religious healer (*hoca*) was able to cure him after seven years of illness. Aunty Zeynep's husband chooses to tell us the complete story of an important illness in his own life, realizing that the session is being recorded. Perhaps he is inspired by our questions about health, or by Aunty Emine's doctor's opinions, or even by a sense of competition with his wife, who is the expert we have come to interview.

Then Aunty Emine asks Aunty Zeynep for more specific information for me about bone-setting, and she begins to tell about a woman who fell out of a tree and broke her leg. While she describes a break or a technique, Aunty Zeynep demonstrates using my leg. In this case, she wrapped the leg and waited three days with it well wrapped, then checked it for any signs of blackness, which indicates gangrene. If she ever sees blackness, she immediately sends the person to a doctor. In this case, there wasn't any blackness, so she had the patient wait two more days and then sent them to get an x-ray. The patient was afraid to tell the doctor that she had been to a *kırıkçıkıkçı*, but the doctor and his associates were amazed at how well the job had been done. This was Dr. Gündüz, who had wanted to put her to work at his clinic (this is an important story for Aunty Zeynep, who told a full version of the interaction with Dr. Gündüz, translated above, when I first interviewed her). Ironically and sadly, the same woman who had been successfully healed of a broken leg died of breast cancer from a lump that was "no bigger than a hazelnut." Aunty Zeynep had sent her to a doctor in Ordu because of the lump, then she went to Ankara, but she still died. And she had been pregnant, too. The women sigh and shake their heads.

Conversation turns to a recent car accident and how badly injured a man was. Then the women discuss young people, scheming to arrange the best possible matches for them. As the visit ends, the women agree that people should teach their daughters by giving them examples of the bad things that happen to others, rather than by beating them.

A Story about Bone-Setting

Uncle Ferit told me the story about a bone-setter summarized below: (July 5, 1996)

*Kırıkçıkıkçı*s don't use plaster for breaks—plaster can break the bone into pieces. Once a guy went to a doctor for an operation on his heart. He paid his money to the doctor and the nurse. A woman came in behind him with a broken shoulder. The guy turns out to be a *kırıkçıkıkçı*. He fixed the woman's shoulder right there in the waiting room. Then he tells the nurse to give him back his money because he has given up on having the operation. He says, "This isn't a hospital, it's a house of torture!" Later, the guy is sitting on his balcony with a friend and sees two women coming towards them. He says to his friend, "That's the nurse I got my money back from!" His friend says, "You made her sorry/wretched (*perişan*), she won't come to you." The guy says, "Yes she will, she needs me." The woman approaching with

the nurse had fallen down the stairs and broken her tailbone. Our guy
fixes it. They offer him a lot of money—he says, "No, all I deserve is
this," and he takes a small amount of money.

This story shows that the traditional healer doesn't really need the doctor
because he can do without the operation and save the money. The nurse
comes around to respect the traditional healer more than the medicine she
was trained in. The story is amusing to listeners because it shows the traditional healer, on his own, besting the powerful and expensive clinical medical
system and still not taking advantage of people by taking too much of their
money. The traditional healer is shown to be more expert in fixing breaks and
more righteous than the doctors. For a different audience (men in a coffeehouse, for example) Uncle Ferit, talented storyteller that he is, would probably exaggerate the sexual innuendoes of a man being petitioned to fix a
woman's broken tailbone.

In many accounts of healing by bone-setters, the traditional healer is set up
in opposition to a doctor. Both are specialists who have acquired local regard
because of successful treatments (in the general Turkish media, there has long
been an interest in presenting stories of people who have remained crippled
for life because they went to a traditional bone-setter). They meet each other's
patients and check each other's work. A bone-setter can refer a person to a
doctor if there is a chance of being blamed for faulty treatment later—a doctor, however, is not meant to refer anyone to a traditional healer, although
they can admire a good traditional treatment. People argue the merits of the
two styles of treatment, with no clear majority supporting one side or the
other. Some families take children to bone-setter (because children's breaks
and sprains are common and can heal faster), whereas they recommend a doctor and x-rays for an adult. Some people, especially those who live in big cities
where they mainly know about bone-setters from alarmist newspaper accounts, fear bone-setters and only resort to using their services if the clinical
medical approach has been fully utilized but has been unable to solve their
problem.

What Makes a Person an Expert?

In Medreseönü, when the topic of bone-setting comes up, the name of
Aunty Zeynep almost invariably comes up. She has practiced for years, with
great success. Most people know someone who has been treated personally by
her at some time in their lives. She lives in extremely poor conditions, her hus-

band and sons having had consistent bad luck. Her bone-setting is a profession for her—it gives her an important identity in the area, it gives her a reason to be socially active without incurring a reputation as someone who takes advantage of other's hospitality without being able to return it, and it gives her a source of necessities and even of cash income. Although she does not state a fee for her services, she knows that people value her expertise and will give her either goods such as dry foods or cloth for clothing, or money.

Although Aunty Emine knows many bone-setting techniques, she has never considered bone-setting as her vocation in the way that Aunty Zeynep does. Once, another well-known bone-setter in the area, who had passed away before I came to the area, came to Aunty Emine with broken ribs. She described the proper procedure to Aunty Emine, who then fixed her. In these kinds of circumstances, which mainly occurred before it was easy to transport an injured person to a medical doctor, Aunty Emine would gladly help a needy person. These days, she would rather send someone to a doctor than worry about being blamed later for a faulty diagnosis or treatment. She does not look for patients and does not consider bone-setting to be a livelihood. She was well-known for midwifery in her younger days, and she is still asked to perform the ritual preparation of a corpse by the families who do not have anyone among them who can perform this special ritual. She is often asked health-related questions by family and neighbors, among whom she is known to have a knack for such things. She could certainly be called an expert, especially because of her ability to safely deliver breech births, but she is not as much of a professional as Aunty Zeynep.

THE EDUCATION OF A TRADITIONAL HEALER

Aunty Zeynep was taught by her grandmother, when she was a teenager, before she was married. She had fallen and injured her ribs. When her grandmother fixed the problem, she asked to be taught the art of bone-setting. One of the ways that her grandmother trained her granddaughter's sensitivity to the invisible problems under the skin was to break a pottery jar inside a bag and ask her to put the pieces back together through the bag, without opening it or looking inside. She would also have her granddaughter feel the limbs of people who had come for help, so that she would get used to what was normal and what was broken, fractured, or out of place. There was also plenty of opportunity to practice by ministering to animals, mostly cows. With the agricultural life on the steep hills of the region and with the difficult life on the sea, people seem to be constantly wrenching their limbs, falling out of trees or off roofs and breaking bones, spraining their ankles, and having their shoulders dislocated.

Both the traditional bone-setter and the clinic staff agree that the best thing a person can do to speed recovery is to get help immediately, before the problem sets and swelling makes relocation difficult. Both types of practitioners scolded their patients for delaying treatment, warning them about the risks of slow and imperfect recovery and the danger of infection.

AUNTY EMINE ON BONE-SETTING

I asked Aunty Emine about bone-setting in an interview (1993):

Aunty Emine: I don't fix broken bones now, I'm afraid. When they scream, I can't stand it. Now, say your wrist comes out. I hold it here, and I squeeze hard here, I press here. It clicks right into place. I don't get involved with surgery. If there is a fracture, if you just touch here, the person faints. If there is a fracture in the bone. Then I leave it; I send them to a doctor. They do an x-ray, they look, and there's a fracture. They say, "Are you a doctor?" I don't move it. If I mess with it could open up the fractured bone. Then tissue can get in and it is harmful. When I squeeze like this, I see the person's screaming, about to faint, then I say, "There's a fracture."
Sylvia: If there isn't one?
A. E.: If there isn't, then it pops back into place. If this shoulder gets dislocated, this shoulder. I pull slowly, and I press with my other hand here, I press here. I put my hand behind the shoulder, push, and then it goes back in place. However, I've never treated here, I've never adjusted a hip. [indicates her own shoulder] For this there was a woman, I learned from her, she's from Orta Köy. My shoulder got dislocated...
S: How did you learn?
A. E.: When I fell, my shoulder...My foot slipped, I fell, and this came out of place. Oh God! This got all swollen. It was right before my daughter's wedding. It [the shoulder] had gone backwards. It was like this, I mean, I took hold of it right away, with this hand, I let out an "Aiii!" I pulled it, "Pop!" it went right into place. My arm was useless, when my girl was going to her husband. But it got back [to normal] fast.
S: How old were you then?
A. E.: I was 39 years old then.

Describing the Difference between a Doctor and a Bone-Setter

When discussing bone-setting, Uncle Ferit made the analogy that because a doctor is educated, he is like an architect, but a *kırıkçıkıkçı* is like a construction worker, experienced in putting one brick on top of another. He said, "In our Turkey, not like Europe, our people go to the doctor with a broken bone. The doctor takes an x-ray and puts a plaster cast on them. Then they come home, take off the cast, and go to a *kırıkçıkıkçı* to get it fixed." (Interview, 1993)

Payment for Services

In a discussion about bone-setting, Aunty Emine explains that she used to fix babies and children when they were brought to her with broken or dislocated bones. She never asked for money, although, if the parents felt like giving her something, that was fine with her. In contrast, some women charge for helping others. She gives an example of a woman who charges up front, even to read the evil eye protection prayer, which is very shameful. Traditionally, a prayer that is in exchange for money would be considered bad-intentioned. If the person is asking for money instead of for God's help in alleviating someone's problem, then the prayers are useless—a person may be able to fool other people, but no one can fool God. (Interview, 1993)

The efficacy of a prayer depends on its correct recital, which is not difficult for most people who have memorized the basic prayers. The person reciting the prayer must also be well-intentioned (*iyi niyetli*) and clean hearted (*temiz kalpli*). The work of a bone-setter, in contrast, is recognized as a personal gift which is strengthened by experience.

The Traditional Healer

In Medreseönü, there are a few recognized healing specialists and many individuals who are thought of as practical or helpful in the treatment of everyday problems. In the course of her lifetime, a woman learns various healing techniques, which she will use to benefit her own family members. When she starts to acquire social status, because of age and family connections, she may be asked for advice by those outside her immediate family. Like Aunty Emine, she might have a period of very active service as a midwife and healer in the community, followed by a gradual lessening of interest or willingness to treat. In contrast, she may become more like Aunty Zeynep, who continues to develop her role as an expert as she ages, in part because she and her family need the social security that her practice brings. The formation of an expert, in traditional village culture, occurs not through an institutional training along formal lines, but through a negotiation between the changing needs of the community and the skills and interests of certain individuals.

THE STATUS OF A TRADITIONAL HEALER

Hinojosa (2001) suspects that the relatively low status of the Mayan bone-setters he studied may have to do in part with the perception that they are not spiritual experts. He also notes that their willingness to treat breaks and fractures in animals can reduce their status, especially in the eyes of clinical physicians. (p.12) This is almost certainly the case in the Black Sea village setting, in which the traditional midwife who can assist in animal birth and the bone-setter who can treat animal fractures are accorded only local status and are denigrated on a national scale by clinical professionals as dirty, dangerous, and ignorant.

As long as people make their living in the physically punishing world of agriculture, it is likely that the services of a local bone-setter will continue to be needed. The clinical methods for treating these common injuries, associated as they are with great expense, inconvenience, long periods of immobility, and even malpractice, have not been able to win the loyalties of most villagers. As villagers move to cities and enter new professions, new types of physical treatments and experts develop. The knowledge of the internal body which can be obtained through experienced touch and the ability to manipulate the body without breaking the skin are, after all, growing in popularity among the world's urban elite in the fields of massage, chiropractic, acupressure, reiki, and the like.

A TRADITIONAL HEALER IN A
NOVEL BY YASHAR KEMAL

In Yashar Kemal's novel *Seagull*, the young boy Salih, whose Black Sea family now lives on an island near Istanbul, comes home with an injured seagull, hoping his grandmother will help it. The interaction between them reveals much about the traditonal role of elderly women in the healing arts:

'Granny,' he blurted out, 'you've got an ointment...' he was surprised
at his own daring.

'Indeed I have,' she said, 'but it's only for people.'

'Won't it do for birds too?'

'Certainly not,' she said turning up her wrinkled nose distainfully. Her
head was bound tightly in a white kerchief. The lines on her furrowed
face were deep-set. 'My ointments are for human beings.'

If there was one thing his grandmother prided herself on it was her
healing art. People paid her a lot of money for her ointments. Salih
resorted to cunning. 'I know, granny,' he said. 'Who would know better than me that your ointments are the best ever. Why, if you gave
them to the doctors, who knows what a fortune you'd get...We'd become rich in a day.'

'I'd never give those heathens anything,' she said mulishly.

'Don't, granny. How right you are!'

'Never!' she repeated. 'My ointments will die with me.'

'But isn't that a pity, granny? Look how many people they've saved.
If they could save my seagull too now...'

'Never!' his grandmother shouted. 'My ointments aren't for birds and
beasts. They're hardly enough for human beings as it is.'

Salih fixed his eyes, huge and tearful, on her, trying to put all the love
and pleading he could into his gaze. 'Remember, granny, when Fethi
broke his arm? In two it was, but you tended it with your ointments
and bound it up, and when he came back only a fotnight later his arm
was as good as new...'

'And so it should be,' she said, pleased. 'My ointments are distilled
from the most wholesome plants and flowers that grow in these hills.'
(p. 20–21)

In another section, Kemal uses the passage quoted at the head of this chapter to describe granny as one who has the respect of all, even the pirates. In
this novel, the figure of granny is both important to the main character Salih
and feared by him because of her power and ill-temper. This characterization
of an elderly woman who is respected and holds power over others because of
her knowledge of healing fits the Turkish cultural model of a woman who has
gathered social leverage through years of experience and learning. Over the
years, she has become recognized as a traditional healer, like Aunty Zeynep,
bone-setter from Çandır.

This chapter addressed the setting of bones, a common concern for villagers, both male and female, because of their hard physical labor. The next

chapter takes up another issue of general concern for all villagers, which, however, is understood to be a health concern particuarly of women—the issue of reproductive health.

CHAPTER 7

REPRODUCTION AND REPRODUCTIVE HEALTH

Müjde Amine sana,
Nur getirdin cihana.
İşte doğdu son Nebi
Yüce nurlar sahibi…

Glad tidings, Amine, to you
You brought light to the world.
Lo! he is born, the last Prophet
The Master of exalted brilliance

—Bursalı from *Mübarek Hanımlar* 1990, p. 9
a poem on the Mother of Prophet Muhammed

On a sweltering summer afternoon, I head up to the house of Aunty Emine's daughter, Nazmiye. I am trying to find a breeze and hoping to get some tea. From Nazmiye's front yard, you can see all the way down to the sea, which today is shimmering and hazy with heat. There is a breeze here, and the curtains are blowing out of each window. Nazmiye's middle daughter sees me coming from the kitchen window. "Greetings, *yenge!*" (What younger family members call a woman married into the family) I love visiting this house, because the girls always greet me with a smile. Even Nazmiye's husband, who is extremely shy, is amused by the very fact of an American *gelin* and sometimes recites his one memorized English lesson to me. I always find a good welcome here. Today, something unusual is going on when I arrive. An older woman and her daughter-in-law are here, but they are not merely visiting. A white-haired traditional expert, Aunty Pakize, is also here, and it turns out that she is going to treat the daughter-in-law, Hatice, for a "fallen stomach" (*mide düşmesi*). This is the first time I am really meeting Hatice, who is eighteen and has been married less than a year, and she is very shy. Nazmiye's

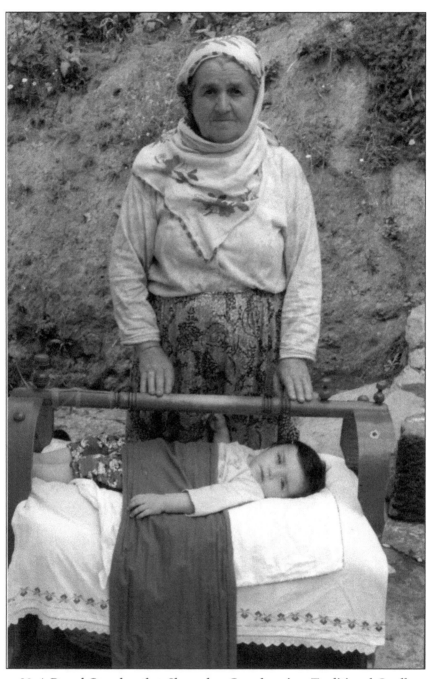

28. A Proud Grandmother Shows her Grandson in a Traditional Cradle

daughters know my research interests, and arrange for me to be in the bedroom while the treatment is being performed. Aunty Pakize lives with her husband in Germany, but her grown children remain in the village house and keep up the farm. Every time she comes back from Germany, women come to ask her to pull their stomachs (*mide çekmek*), because she is known for being good at it. The treatment is to reposition the stomach (*karın* or *mide*) and intestines (*barsak*) so that they do not press on the womb (*rahime*) and prevent conception. The procedure is also used when a person, man or woman, feels extreme abdominal pressure and cramping, as if someone is squeezing one's gut very hard.

Hatice is worried that her fallen stomach is preventing conception, so she is hoping that this procedure will help her have a baby. In the small, brightly-lit bedroom, two of Nazmiye's unmarried daughters and I watch the procedure and chat with Hatice and Aunty Pakize. She pulls up Hatice's undershirt, lowers the waistband on her skirt, and begins to massage her stomach. She kneads and probes, finding that, indeed, the stomach is too low and presses on the womb. After a few minutes of massage, she grasps Hatice's stomach with both hands and gently pulls it up toward her chest. She holds the stomach in that way for about fifteen minutes, as we chat and giggle about methods for increasing the chances of conception, including paying attention to the best time in the cycle to try, the most efficacious positions in intercourse, and the need to delay the post-coital ritual ablutions until enough time has been allowed for conception to take place. I noted during this particular procedure that unmarried women close to the patient were not only present but also took part in the conversation about sex, storing away information for future use. We all tell Hatice that she is worrying too early, that there is plenty of time to conceive, that she is young and working too hard. Aunty Pakize tells me that the signs of a fallen stomach, besides failure to conceive, are bad menstrual cramps and abdominal pain. Hatice warms up to me after a while and is able to talk more openly about her fears.

After she has pulled the stomach for long enough, Aunty Pakize presses a roll of white cloth into the space below Hatice's navel and binds it into place with a waist scarf (*peştemal*) around her waist. She tells her to lie down for as long as possible in the same prone position, until night, if possible. This is not possible, because Hatice's mother-in-law, who has been visiting with Nazmiye in the living room, comes to get her after about an hour.

Later that summer, when it becomes clear that Hatice has not conceived, she asks Aunty Pakize to repeat the procedure. Everyone agrees that she did not rest long enough the first time to let the treatment take effect. Hatice also admitted to having lifted heavy things and having jumped down from a cherry tree, both considered ruinous to the beneficial effects of stomach-pulling. The procedure was again done at Nazmiye's house. Aunty Pakize doesn't take any money for doing the procedure, but if the woman successfully has a baby after being treated by her, the woman usually gives her a gift such as a scarf. Aunty Pakize also treats women with this technique after birth to solve problems coming from childbirth. At this time, I asked Hatice if she had been to a doctor about her infertility, and she shot me an alarmed look and said "No!" as if the very idea was crazy and terrifying.

In conversation with Hatice and an unmarried friend of hers, I was told that some women who do procedures to aid conception actually look or feel inside the woman's uterus, but these young women agreed that that was going too far.

*****

The following year, on another summer evening, this one quite chilly, my husband and I walked up the dirt road to the crest of the hill and then down the other side to the newly built house of Mehmet and Hatice. Mehmet, who works as a fisherman, is a school friend of my husband's brother. The new house is across a small yard from his parents' house which I had visited a few years previously. The young couple seemed well established in their new home and integrated into the family and community. They had one growing concern, however, which has consumed their thoughts and resources since early in their marriage—they have not been able to conceive a child.

Despite the ministrations of Aunty Pakize the previous summer, Hatice had still not conceived. The couple had both been tested by a doctor in Fatsa, the nearest town with a hospital, and Hatice had been confirmed as the infertile one. The doctor in Fatsa told them that their only chance to conceive was a test-tube conception. At the time, this procedure would cost them 500 million Turkish Lira (about $4,200), which was much too high for them to consider. Their next step was to consult a doctor in Ordu, a bigger city nearby. She told them that Hatice's fallopian tubes were closed and that she would therefore never conceive. She expressed contempt for the Fatsa doctor's idea of a test-tube conception: "What does he know?"

At this point, the couple was driven to further measures, going as far as Istanbul, where Hatice's sister had been aided by a doctor there when she had had problems in pregnancy due to her very young age. The Istanbul doctor offered two choices, an operation on the fallopian tubes for TL 60 million (about $430), or a test-tube conception for TL 400 million (about $2,860). They chose the operation. The doctor guaranteed that Hatice would conceive within a few months of the operation. He recommended that she stay as long as she could in the hospital, since the charge would be the same for any time under three days. The couple left the hospital eight hours after

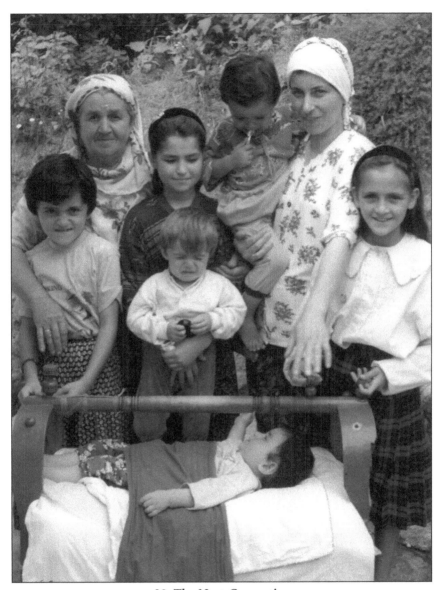

29. The Next Generation

the operation to catch their bus back home to the Black Sea. By the middle of the trip back, Hatice was doubled over in pain, Mehmet was frightened for her, and they were both mortified by the idea that they were making a spectacle of themselves. They reached home, where Hatice recovered before too long.

As we sat in the kitchen, having finished the business of collecting the tea glasses, washing, drying, and putting them away, Hatice and I talked about their traumatic trip to Istanbul and her hopes and fears since the operation. Muammer and Mehmet talked about the same things outside over their cigarettes. Later Muammer told me that Mehmet was staying home from fishing in order to be available when Hatice's cycle reached its optimum time for conception. This means that the couple is willing to sacrifice his income as well as all of the savings they had put into the trip and the operation in order to maximize their chance to become parents. In a telephone conversation with Nazmiye (January, 2004), I learned that Mehmet and Hatice now have two sons, a year-and-a-half apart in age. The operation in Istanbul is credited for Hatice's fertility. In July of 2004, my trip to Medreseönü coincided with the two brothers' circumcision celebration (*sünnet düğünü*—the term *düğün* being used equally for circumcision and for wedding celebrations).

The Fallen Stomach

As mentioned in Chapter 2, concepts of the body and its functions and problems can be distinctly linked to gender. For example, women are considered to be more likely to suffer from "stomach-falling" (*mide düşüklüğü*), which can have effects ranging from a temporary discomfort to infertility. The particular vulnerability of women to this problem seems to be founded on the idea that women's bodies are more open below, so that women can more easily lose something through "falling" or have something slip downward. Women are advised to remain prone for a while after intercourse to prevent the falling of sperm and thus to increase the chance of impregnation. Pregnant women must be careful about jumping and lifting because a miscarriage is a kind of "falling" (*düşük*). A common problem for birth control methods reported by the Health Clinic nurse was the slipping or falling of the spiral or I.U.D. Women who have been treated for a fallen stomach can destroy the efficacy of the treatment in the same ways that a miscarriage can be caused, by jumping down from a high place or by lifting heavy objects.

In the lengthy interview with Granny about health and illness, the concept of a "fallen stomach" was not specifically tied to women or to reproductive problems. Her addition of a "fallen heart" illness is not something that came up in any other interviews.

S: This "fallen stomach"…

G: Some used to do it, like this, with wild bee honey, they'd pull it like this, those who knew, those who were used to it. Like this, like this, with honey, with syrup, they'd pull it well, they'd put it back in place. An expert would get it back. In the old days, those with a fallen stomach, those with a fallen heart, whatever they had, like this, with pulling, they'd put it back in place. They'd pull, like this. They'd wrap your waist lightly with a scarf, that would hold it, and it would pass. Thank God, it is God's will…

In my observations of actual contemporary practices, however, this affliction seems to have become a "female problem"—perhaps because it offers a local and inexpensive treatment for the much-feared problem of infertility, administered along with the friendly advice of an experienced female elder. When stomach-pulling does not solve the problem, as in the case of Hatice and Mehmet narrated above, the importance of fertility can come to outweigh the shame of visiting unfamiliar male doctors, the rigors of a long journey, and the heavy financial burdens of clinical fertility treatments.

Comparison with Mayan Manual Medicine

Hinojosa (2001) in his study of Mayan traditional healers, reveals that a technique such as the vigorous massage of the abdomen can be performed in similar ways according to very different concepts of the body. He writes:

Most Comalapans practicing manual medicine also concentrate on stomach or body massage and underwrite their work with non-Western views of the body. For example, they view the stomach as containing a pouch-home to very active naturally occurring worms. The task of the massagers in the case of severe stomach pain, then, is to massage wayward worms back into their pouch, thus easing the upset." (p.3)

The concept of the worms is quite distinct from any concepts of the internal abdomen which are present in the region I studied, but the idea that massage by an expert can relieve extreme pain is similar. The Mayan practitioners (who practice bone-setting as well as abdominal massage) are mostly male, but, while men and women in Medreseönü may know the art of stomach-pulling, I only observed women perform it for the specific treatment of infertility.

The inhabitants of Medreseönü know about parasites, including intestinal tapeworms and roundworms (called *tenya*, *kurt*, or *solucan*), in stock animals and humans, which they treat with remedies which cause constipation (like quince *ayva* or pommegranate skin *nar kabuğu*). After a period of constipation the worm passes with the stool. (*kurt dökmek* literally 'to drop a worm') Another common remedy is *pelin otu* (wormwood, absinthe) for killing worms. Collard green seeds (*lahana* in standard Turkish, *pancar* in Black Sea Turkish) in a glass of broth of tonka bean (*acı bakla suyu*) on an empty stomach can rid the system of parasites.

REPRODUCTION AND REPRODUCTIVE HEALTH

Issues of reproduction and reproductive health are of central concern to women in Medreseönü. As we have seen, women are the primary care-takers in their families and villages. Women are held responsible for the health of family members, and particularly for the health of their infants and children. Reproduction is considered to be a woman's area of concern and knowledge. In general, people have a practical knowledge about the factors involved in reproduction. Children grow up hearing conversations about sex, pregnancies, and birth. They witness the reproductive cycles of animals and know that both male and female pass characteristics on to their offspring. Birth, growth, and death are all integrated into the life of the community. When a problem occurs, such as Hatice and Mehmet being unable to conceive, it is discussed in groups of women and children of varying ages. The unmarried women I spoke to knew about various kinds of birth control and techniques to facilitate conception.

One metaphor of reproduction found in traditional Turkish communities is expressed by the analogy of the man's contribution to reproduction as the seed, and the woman's as the field. This cosmology was found by Carol Delaney (1991) to be the major determinant of gender relations in an Anatolian village setting. On the Black Sea Coast, the inhabitants consider Anatolian villagers to be extreme in gender segregation, veiling, and patriarchal family relations. Many women expressed the idea that Anatolian women did not stand up for themselves the way that Black Sea women do, perhaps out of ignorance, and are therefore to blame in part for their oppression. In my research, I found that people framed their basic concepts of reproduction with their knowledge of the animal world, mainly the closely observable world of domestic animals. Rash male behavior is often compared to the behavior of bulls or roosters—they are important for reproduction but difficult to deal with and less useful than the females who provide milk and eggs. In the agricultural setting, male domestic animals are the first to be killed for meat, and people are wary of becoming fond of them. This is in contrast to the loss of a family cow, which, as shown in Chapter 3, can be a financial and emotional blow for a household.

During their Black Sea research, Beller-Hann and Hann (2001) were told "A woman is a basket. You empty it and then fill it again." (*'Kadın sepettir. Boşaltıyorsun, sonra yine dolduruyorsun.'*) and 'A woman is like a field. Whatever you sow will grow.' (*'Kadın tarlaya benzer. Ne ekersin o biter.'*). These researchers are sensitive to the fact that partiarchal metaphors may be subtly used even as they are presented as the proper ways to think about the world. If a woman is thought of as a field, for example, a mother cannot be blamed for faulty seed which produces a handicapped child, although Beller-Hann and Hann find that blame for a handicapped or weak child can be put upon the mother's brother (134). As discussed in Chapter 3 in the section on metaphors, a basket can be claimed as a sign of women's independent work and mobility, as well as a symbol of the patriarchal oppression of women.[1]

The young women I interviewed about reproductive issues have learned the clinical/biomedical model of reproduction, and speak about their ova ("my eggs" *yumurtalarım*). They also spoke about the causes of both female and male infertility, such as blocked fallopian tubes ("my eggs are not falling" "*yumurtalarım düşmüyor*) or the possible effects on a man of a bout of childhood mumps. One traditional idea in current circulation, which does not conform to the biomedical model, is that some women are said to only bear sons, or only bear daughters. Evidence for this idea is found in the animal world, in which some cows are known to bear only offspring of one sex.

Among the previous generation, infertility was considered to be the woman's fault and was sometimes a cause for divorce. Barren women were often associated with the power to cast *nazar* (even now, one of the most common sources of *nazar* is the longing glance a woman with no children may cast on a baby), or with various kinds of magic or fortune-telling powers. People now believe that either partner could be the cause for infertility, but the women concern themselves more with remedies for infertility. For example, Hatice took it upon herself to try the traditional measures to increase fertility, such as having her stomach pulled by the local experts, and

---

1. Metaphors about reproduction often involve ideas about common human body elements, such as blood, semen, and milk. Care must be taken, however, to distinguish how these elements are conceptualized, for this can vary widely in different cultures. For example, in Sri Lanka, McGilvray (1982) finds a concept of "two semens" male and female which combine in a fetus (52). This shapes ideas about milk, which is connected to a female type of transformation of blood (61) and shapes explanations of infertility (63).

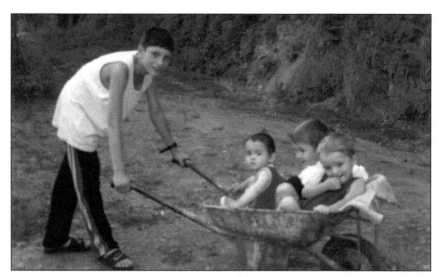

30. Maşallah

only required the increasing involvement of her husband as the local measures failed and more expensive, distant remedies were sought. This is the
traditional division of labor—women are to see to the daily needs of their
families, tend the gardens and fields, and to provide care for their families
and neighbors, while men are to supply money and labor for the physical
structures and necessities of the home, do the heaviest seasonal agricultural
work, and provide links between their own families and the world beyond
the village.

    As clinical medicine becomes more readily available and gains a following,
doctors, who are unrelated male experts trained in distant institutions, become more involved in the realm of health care. Currently, most women in
the villages deliver their babies at home, attended by a trained midwife in the
employ of the Health Clinic. Women are increasingly making use of new technologies such as ultrasound devices, which require visits to doctors in Fatsa or
Ordu. Women combine techniques as they see fit and as their family income
allows—for example, some women want to have regular ultrasound scans but
then have their birth at home with a clinic midwife in attendance. As cash income increases, more women are choosing to have their babies delivered by a
private doctor in one of the nearby hospitals. Hospital births are very likely to
be cesareans, for reasons discussed in the section "Hospital Births" below, with
a cesarean rate of up to 80% in the Fatsa Hospital. Most of the pre-natal care
and the assistance to the mother and baby in the weeks after birth is still provided through the traditional channels of female relatives and friends.

I collected most of the following information about pregnancy, birth, and the care of babies during the visits I made after the birth of my own child. The topic was of interest to me, and came up regularly in conversation with women of all ages. This chapter will present information I collected when asking about birth control and family planning, traditional births, then stories about particular experiences with hospital births. I will examine some of the factors that shape women's choices about where to deliver their babies. Then I will look at two cases of problems with reproductive health which serve as examples of the ways in which women move through levels of health care options, from most familiar and inexpensive to farthest away and most expensive, until a satisfactory outcome is reached.

Birth Control and Family Planning

According to Nurse Rahime, the Health Clinic provides birth control pills and condoms for free, but sends women to the city hospital if they want to have a spiral (I.U.D.) inserted. She relates that women usually don't get a spiral until after their first child, because they fear that harm can come to their uterus which would be irreversible. Nurse Rahime told me that it is hard to get women to stop working for the required 15 days after a spiral is put in, so there are cases of spirals slipping soon after insertion. Notice that the failure of a birth control device is blamed on the over activity and heavy work of village women, just like the failure of stomach pulling to result in conception, or the failure of Hatice's Istanbul operation to work.

The side effects of birth control pills that concern the local women are diabetes and heart irregularities. There is no common perception of a link to cancer, according to Nurse Rahime. When I asked an unmarried woman about the free birth control provided by the Clinic, she let out a laugh, "That's only the first pack of pills! If it were all free, they'd have a long line outside the Clinic door!" The women who are so anxious for birth control are married women who want to space their children and limit their family size, in recognition of the economic and health benefits of smaller families. The subject of female sexual activity before marriage never came up within my hearing, so the interest in birth control of a woman who has never been married is meant to be purely theoretical.

Family size is often cited as a problem in Black Sea communities. Although large families are the norm in the previous generation, most families with small children use birth control to limit their family size to two or three children. In the previous generation, there was little birth control available, there was a higher risk of infant and childhood mortality, and agricultural labor was needed. The family lands in the area have been subdivided among siblings to an extent that everyone agrees has gone too far and is hard to sustain. Part of the push to jobs in big cities and Europe was the sudden ill-fit between traditional family size and local economic potential.

Older women speak about various traditional practices used in the attempt to induce an abortion. Some substances, such as soap or caustic agents, were inserted into the uterus, but often had dire side-effects. A miscarriage is called a *düşük*, which is associated with the baby falling (the same term is used when a stomach presses down out of place and causes cramping and infertility), and the most commonly cited reason for a miscarriage is a pregnant woman's fall to the ground. I was told that, before medical abortions, women would jump from high places to try to start a miscarriage. Now, medical abortion is legal and free, although many women don't have an abortion before their first child for fear it will ruin their chances of having children in the future. In other words, it is a technology used by married couples for spacing children. The pregnancy of an unmarried woman is something that was never discussed in my presence, and I thought it an inappropriate subject for an interview.

While the limiting of family size is of great importance for women who have had children, the conception of the first child is perhaps the most consuming concern for a newly married woman. On one of my visits to the Health Clinic, I witnessed the following scene. A red-faced young man of twenty-seven came in, asked a hurried question to one of the nurses, and hurried out. When he returned, he had been to the pharmacy next door, and was carrying a pregnancy test kit (which costs about $3.50). His new bride, in her early twenties, came with him the second time. The nurses told me to come along as they were taken into one of the observation rooms. The young woman was ten days late for her menstrual period, and wanted to find out if she was pregnant. The groom was leaving the next day for his compulsory military service, which would last almost two years, so they were really hoping that she was pregnant. The nurses sent the woman into the bathroom with a glass. She complained that the glass was filthy, but came back with the requisite sample. One of the midwives (several nurses had also come to see the results) opened the package from the pharmacy and did the test. After a minute or so, the nurse congratulated the woman and showed her the positive marker. Everyone embraced, and the woman kissed the midwife. The appropriate phrase "*Gözünüz aydın!*" (May your eyes light up!) was called from all of the staff as the beaming couple left the clinic. The happy news, the perfect example of how life should be, was fast on its way to all ears.

The Village Midwife

The word for midwife is *ebe*. This term now denotes the institutionally-trained midwives who are associated with the government Health Clinic. To speak of the traditional midwife, women use the term *köy ebesi* (village midwife). Traditional midwifery is now completely outlawed, and the Turkish media frequently relates formulaic horror-stories about the mistakes of village midwives in the effort to eradicate their practice. It seems to me, although I can have no solid proof to support this conjecture, that young women who might have been drawn to traditional healing practices or midwifery are the same ones who are now sent to nursing and midwifery schools. The young clinic midwife whose dress symbolizes her adherence to modern Islamist conceptions of Muslim propriety, for example, was the daughter of an institutionally-trained nurse and the granddaughter of a village midwife. Village women who used to be practicing midwives, such as Aunty Emine, are still asked for information on pregnancy and birth-related issues, and may still be called upon in an emergency.

Aunty Emine on Breech Births

I ask Aunty Emine about delivering a breech baby. Typically, she uses specific cases of individuals known to me to illustrate her descriptions. During all of her explanations, she shows me what she means with hand gestures, pointing to parts of her body or moving her hands as if she were performing the procedure. (1993)

> Aunty Emine: İrfan, and the blond one who's coming, Temel, those I delivered, they're mine [i.e. she delivered them].
> Sylvia: Was it easy?
> A: It was easy. Now you know the woman who came with her son, who brought iron? Well, that woman's baby always came out backwards, came bottom first. I delivered her three children. The kid is coming like this, I feel around, moving my hands around and around, when the contraction comes, I move my finger around, I put olive oil on my fingers, and massage like this [shows circular motion with her right hand], before that I put *kolonya* [on her hands, *kolonya* is an alcohol-based cologne used in every Turkish household for its fresh smell and sterilizing properties]. I take hold of the feet, with my fingers. This hand [her left] stays on top, holding the baby's head [which

she feels through the mother's belly], so I can feel the head. The legs pop out with the fluid. I put my [right hand] fingers in and pull the baby's legs out. I hold the head and press down [with left hand]. My brother's wife is a trained midwife. She was amazed. She asked, "How do you deliver them [breech babies]?" She was scared. [I said] "I can't do it alone. It's God's doing. The Good Lord pushes and I catch."
A midwife said "The woman's breech!" She let out a scream and said "Straight to the hospital!" I said, "Wait, forget the hospital." I said. That was a village woman [the midwife] "You hold the woman, I'll deliver her." I delivered her. My hands are small, her hands were big. Look, your hands [she says to me] are small, you could do any delivery. Your hands are narrow, they'd be soft, it'd work. And my hands are small, I just pop them out.
She said, you know that Pakize Yenge [the neighbor who does stomach-pulling], she came here? "Yenge, save me! I'll withstand it, just save me!" That's why she really loves me. I delivered her three girls. One was breech. Now, here's how I do it. The woman gets soft, right? [the cervix] Well, you don't force it, you go with the contractions, you help the baby. I rub and rub like this, and I put pressure [on the belly]. Like this, like this [she shows a circular motion as if feeling the woman's belly]. Wherever the baby has settled, I put my hand there, and the baby comes with the contractions. He/she makes a place in the lower groin. If you press him/her there, birth is easy. Let Nurcan Yenge tell you and you'll see. Nurcan Yenge says, "Where were you before?" [meaning she wishes Aunty Emine could have helped with her first birth] You know her daughter Rabiye? "Where were you for her?" she says.
[There is a pause and then we start to discuss bone-setting, excerpts in Chapter 6]
S: Do cows' births resemble humans' births?
A: I do cow deliveries too. Now with a cow, when the calf's coming, the leg comes first, if you pull one leg, then the delivery is hard. You don't pull it, you get both legs together and then pull. You've got to get both legs. Then you push down. In a woman's delivery, you pull towards the back, not over here, but to the back. Same with a cow, in the delivery, you don't pull forward, you push down. With a woman, you pull like this, pull toward the back. With a cow, the cord can come to the calf's throat. For that, I oil my hand and I take out the calf's head by turning it. Either the head or a leg [can get caught in the cord].

My mother's cow was dying. I went, to my mother, may she rest in peace, I had gone just by chance from here. They were lamenting "OOOhh, the cow is dying!" "You stop," I said, "Don't come." I went over there, my girl Fatma was small then. I went beside the cow. Its legs were in the air, like this, they were ready to kill it, they had a knife in their hands. "Stop!" I said. They stopped. I turned the cow over. She let out a big sigh. "Take hold of the cow right away." I said. They held her. I put one hand in, saying "Once more, once more." I put my other hand here on the cow. The cow had a big contraction, I pushed down, I pulled the calf. My gosh, my arms were about to drop off! It was so hard, but I delivered it. Then my father came over, and he kissed me. "You're unbelievable!" he said. "You didn't let me go to school." I said. "I would have made you an engineer!" he said. [she laughs].

Aunty Emine has always been known for her sharp intelligence, and has always resented her father for keeping her out of school so that she would help with chores and the younger children at home. Her brothers were educated and have been fairly successful. Aunty Emine travels widely, keeps a bank account, and deals swiftly with bureaucratic tangles, all without being able to read. Her accounts of successful deliveries in adverse circumstances highlight her skills and perseverance, showing that a village midwife is neither ignorant nor helpless.

Granny on Childbirth

In the interview with Granny, given in Chapter 2, the issue of childbirth was not a particularly notable topic, perhaps because it went easily for her.

S: How did they do childbirth in the old days?
G: I didn't have any trouble in childbirth. Those who couldn't birth the baby, they'd pick them up as they were and take them straight to the doctor. *Ya upala!* (Sound indicting fast departure) If her fate was to die because of this, if her luck had run out, she'd go (die) because of it. (The baby had) one hand in, one hand out, they couldn't take the baby out. I didn't have that kind of birth. Well, it was difficult, excuse me for saying it, but I never suffered. I never saw any doctor business (*doktor işi görmedim.*).
S: Normal, at home...
G: Normal, at home. No one was home, at my house, dear. I had no one next to me. Struggle and struggle, I came back from the quarry, got in birth position, screaming and crying, it happens! (She giggles)

S: Wasn't there a midwife?

G: A village midwife, old woman's stuff, old, old wives…Now *they* would really take care of you.

Granny seems slightly embarrassed about the topic and also proud that she could manage on her own. Her nostalgia for the old wives' care and concern contrasts with her dismissal of "doctor business" which she has managed without for most of her life. In this, she resembles the first generation of Ransel's (2000) Russia and Tatar informants, those born before the First World War.

Home Birth

I asked Yıldız's mother about her births. She is a woman from the older generation who had home births with a village midwife. She lives in Afırlı and is 68 years old. She had nine babies born at home, all normal, no breech births,—and one baby who died "because the water broke." She said, "In those days, there were no hospitals!" ("*O zaman, hastane, mastane yok, ya!*") More recently, her *gelin* had to go to the hospital for serum (given with an I.V.) while pregnant, but then had a normal delivery at home. (1996) For most women until the 1990s, normal birth meant home birth, attended by either a village midwife or a clinic midwife. Hospital births are becoming increasingly common.

Nurse Rahime Talks about the Old Ways

While on a visit to the home of Nurse Rahime, she, along with her mother-in-law and her sister-in-law, gave me a lot of information about birthing, birth-control, local traditions, and traditions from other parts of Turkey that they had heard about. Because of the mother-in-law's presence, I could get a sense of how things had changed over time. For example, she had given birth five times at home before there was even a local doctor, and proudly reported that four of her children (including the current mayor) are teachers and one a policeman. I take this to be a counter-claim against those who might say that the old ways had no value and were foolish or dangerous. Nurse Rahime told me about some traditional practices which horrified her and serve as proof that progress has been made because of clinical medicine. She told me, for example, that, in the old days, they used to put a sack of cow dung under the woman after she gave birth, so that she would stay warm. She called this practice "very dirty," and said that many women died of tetanus because of this practice.[2] Nurse Rahime's knowledge could be based on local stories which she heard as she grew up in this area, or, quite likely, could be from her training. Whereas cow dung is considered "filth" in Black Sea villages, it is used as fuel and building material in the dry and de-forested central Anatolian plateau. In official Turkish discourse about folk practices, Anatolian practices are taken as standard. It is possible that Nurse Rahime heard about an Anatolian practice of using cow dung in a manner unfamiliar to the Black Sea, and considered it to be a perfect example of the "bad old days."

In a similar vein, a young girl in the room at the time of my interview with Nurse Rahime, asserted that a woman had died because of the old practice of having a woman crouch over a pan of boiling water to cause the afterbirth to come out quickly.[3] This story reminded Nurse Rahime that, in some other regions of Turkey, they have a woman crouch over a kind of herb, set alight, to cause fertility. Because of the dangers of these traditional practices, she said, and because people are fully aware of the dangers of childbirth in general, and the potential for mistakes, no one now wants a traditional midwife.

The traditional procedures after birth seem to be connected to the humoral system of hot and cold balancing. In particular, the use of cow dung to produce heat and the crouching over boiling water or lighted herbs seem similar to the "mother roasting, steaming, and smoking" observed by Lenore Manderson in Malay society (2003). Manderson summarizes the widespread humoral medical theory which is incorporated into popular medical systems in many places of the world, in a way which suits the Black Sea case: "In popular form and as observed today, the critical element of the tradition is the classification of the body and foods as hot and cold, with lesser emphasis also on the effect of wind or air." (p. 139) She discovers that "…near universally in cultures with a humoral medical tradition, parturition is believed to deplete the woman of heat and to place her in a state of especial vulnerability to cold. Postpartum practices aiming to protect the woman from cold and wind and to restore her to health bear remarkable similarity cross-culturally." (p. 141)

---

2. MacCormack (1982) cites World Health Organization statistics specifically linking deadly neonatal tetanus with proximity to cattle, particularly cattle dung. (p. 16)

3. See Ransel (2000) for a discussion of "steam-bath cabin" used in northern Russia and the use of pans of hot water and the practice of lying on the home oven to aid birth in southern regions. (in his fifth chapter "Giving Birth")

In Medreseönü, contemporary postpartum practices include abdominal massage and binding, special foods, and protection from heat and the evil eye. The use of cow dung and of burning herbs seems to have disappeared, if it in fact they were ever local practices on the Black Sea, perhaps around the time of the suppression of village midwifery and the introduction of the trained clinic midwife.

CONFINEMENT AFTER BIRTH

The *lohusa zamanı* is the period, often counted as forty days, after birth, in which the new mother and infant are confined to the home and kept carefully away from dangers. A special, bright red, fruit drink made locally from stewed plums, called *şerbet* or *komposto*, is considered particularly appropriate for this time. A glass is offered to each guest, and the new mother is enjoined to drink a glass with each visitor to make sure she gets a sufficient quantity. The symbolic number of forty days, which is used with great precision to count the days after death in which the soul is not settled, is not necessarily taken literally in the postpartum case. Many women reported that they could not stay confined that long, and got up and about their daily business as soon as they felt ready (or when told to by their mothers-in-law or husbands). In discussion with Nurse Rahime, she mentioned limitations placed on the new mother during *lohusa zamanı* which she considered crucial for the health of the mother and baby. She explained that village women must be protected from doing too much physical work too soon after giving birth. Although visitors can come to bring good wishes and small gold coins for the baby, the mother is not supposed to leave her house during this time. There are special foods for mother and guests, and other ritual practices done by women close to the new mother. Special care is taken to counteract the possibility of *nazar*, to which post-partum mothers as well as newborn infants are known to be particularly susceptible.

SYMBOLIC BURYING OF THE PLACENTA

Tradition calls for the placenta to be taken out of the house where the birth has occurred and buried. The new mother and her mother-in-law can decide where the placenta is to be buried. The choice of location for burial usually concerns hopes for the child's future. For example, burying the placenta near a school yard expresses hope that the child will advance through life by studying. Burying near a busy road will bring about a lifetime of travel. Burial by a strong and tall tree will help the child to be healthy and tall. Burying a placenta improperly can result in a troubled life. For more on worldwide cultural practices involving the placenta, see Jones and Kay (2003).

Home Birth with a Clinic Midwife

Our discussion about the traditional midwives led to talk about the current situation in Medreseönü. According to Nurse Rahime, the Health Clinic midwife goes to attend birth in the woman's home because it is more comfortable to give birth at home than at the clinic. The ambulance stands by in case an emergency requires a trip to one of the area hospitals. For Nurse Rahime and for most local women, the important difference between home birth and hospital birth is that you know the home bed is clean. In contrast, those women who make use of the expensive private birthing rooms in hospitals comment on the cleanliness, the comfort, and the *ilgi* of a trained specialist as reasons to prefer them to home births.

In response to an inquiry of mine, she claimed that it does not matter if the midwife is male. I have never heard of a male midwife, and even the males in the Health Clinic who are not doctors are not nurses, they are "health officers." There are a growing number of female doctors, especially in the big cities, but most doctors who deliver babies in hospitals are male.

Home birth is done on a floor mattress with pillows to prop up the woman, who leans back sideways across the bed. The midwife brings a bag that contains what she needs to assist the birth, such as sanitizing fluid and a tool to cut the cord. I was invited to attend a home birth, but I have never actually been contacted when one was occurring.

In the context of talk about traditional birth practices, Nurse Rahime and her mother-in-law related that some women go to a local hot spring for infertility problems (I did not hear this elsewhere). Then, since I was a new mother myself, and possibly ignorant about proper Muslim practice, the elderly mother-in-law felt a duty to instruct me about the dangers of touching a baby when ritually unclean. She explained that after being sexually active, and before performing the complete ritual ablutions, it is very dangerous to touch or even look at a baby. Even if the baby is crying at night, one should wash up before touching it or looking at it. The women were curious about differences between Turkish culture and American culture, and brought up the importance of virginity in Turkish culture. They may have been hoping for a scandalous revelation or at least an amusing discomfort on my part, as they joked about sending a bride back if she is found to be not a virgin. I provided them with no interesting information.

Hospital Birth

In the nearest hospital, in Fatsa, there is a very high cesarean rate (around 80%), in part because women who are at risk for some reason are likely to give birth in the hospital, and in part because women who like the status and security of having a private doctor often ask for a cesarean to avoid labor pains. Talking about giving birth in an *özel oda* (private room) is a way to show that no expense was spared for the birth and to make sure that no one gets the impression that the birth took place in a regular, inferior hospital setting. Getting to a hospital for check-ups and when labor has started is much easier now than it had been even ten or twenty years ago. Technologies such as ultrasound are available in the hospitals, and give mothers who value the most modern techniques a sense of security. As more women have babies in hospitals, more doctors become known through personal channels, making it easier for women to trust them.

A hospital birth, with its medical attention to the mother and its expense, may be preferred by a *gelin* as a way to improve her own status vis-à-vis her mother-in-law. In a hospital setting, the mother is the focus of the doctor's attention, the husband must provide payment, and the new mother is kept in bed for a few days, being instructed in the modern technologies of formula feeding and baby care. A traditional home birth involves a period of rest for the mother and various forms of ritual attention to the mother and baby, but the scene is dominated by the mother-in-law and the local female experts. A *gelin* who wishes to go to a hospital for her birth may be showing a preference for modernity and science in opposition to tradition. This would fit a pattern generally observed by ethnographers of childbirth in settings where clinical methods have been recently introduced, including the historical evidence about the introduction of clinical techniques in Europe and North America. In a comparative study done in England of immigrant women from South Asia and "British" women (Homans, 1982), research showed that; "Women in Britain therefore have come to depend on medical intervention in pregnancy and childbirth, often equating hospital confinements with reduced mortality rates." (251)

MacCormack (1982), in a survey of studies on the social context of birth, finds that:

> Where patrilineal descent and patrilocal residence following marriage prevail, a bride often goes to live among complete strangers, under

the authority of her mother-in-law. In these circumstances, a woman prefers to return to her mother's household to give birth…but is not always allowed to do so. (p. 14)

More research would determine if women giving birth in Turkish hospitals are more easily visited by their own mothers, but I suspect that this is the case. In the village home birth, a woman's mother may visit after the baby is born, but the birth itself is most commonly attended by the mother-in-law and the local midwife.

BELGIN'S HOSPITAL BIRTH

For a clear picture of why women dread the thought of having a baby in a regular, State-run, free hospital, I offer the following story told to me by Belgin, a woman in Istanbul. Although this example is from Istanbul, the critique of the lack of *ilgi* shown to patients in the State-run hospitals is similar to stories told on the Black Sea Coast. In the villages, women who favor private doctors and private rooms over home birth critique the state hospitals in a similar manner.

Belgin went to a *sigorta* hospital (a free State-run hospital), to have her son, who is now five and has no siblings yet. She was advised by friends and relatives to withstand as much of her contractions at home as she could before going in to the hospital. Her contractions started in the afternoon, and by 2 a.m. she was unable to stand them any more. Her husband took her to the hospital, where her labor continued through the night. At 10 a.m. some doctors came in with a big group of medical students and they gave every woman a shot. [presumably of something to induce or speed up labor] All of the women were in a row of beds and they all delivered exactly ten minutes after the shot, right at ten after ten. Belgin laughed as she explained that the women who had come in at 6 or 8 a.m. had been quite pleased, whereas she had suffered much longer while waiting for the shot. She complained that the nurses at the *sigorta* hospitals pay no attention to the laboring women, spending their time drinking tea and talking on the telephone instead.

Belgin criticizes the nurses for their lack of *ilgi* in terms which could be used by anyone to criticize female family members in other circumstances. The judging of clinical practitioners in terms of family obligations for care is examined in detail in the following chapter.

Delaney (1991) details the abusive attitude shown by government doctors toward village women in a hospital in Ankara and contrasts hospital births with a midwife-assisted birth at home. (61–64) She also devotes considerable attention to the period of *loğusalık (lohusa zamanı)*. (64–72)

Birth at the Fatsa Hospital

No one in the villages would go all the way to Istanbul for a State-run hospital. They would only feel the trip worth the time and expense if a private doctor is involved. A young mother told me that she had good care from a private doctor in the Fatsa Hospital, but that there was a woman in labor in the room with her who was terribly ignored. She was screaming for help from the nurses, who were sitting close by, drinking their inevitable glasses of tea. Only when the baby fell out onto the bed did the nurses rouse themselves to action. The woman telling me the story had suffered a previous miscarriage and had been under strict supervision with this pregnancy since a threatened miscarriage at one-and-a-half months. She was very pleased with her private doctor, who sent her home under strict orders to have complete bed rest until past three months (His exact words were, "Don't even stir soup!"). Her baby had been in breech position, which worried her mother-in-law, the same woman whose breech births had been assisted by Aunty Emine, but the baby turned to normal presentation just before birth. Her doctor had been prepared to do a cesarean, but expressed the hope that she, being young and likely to want more children in the future, could have a normal delivery, which is how it happened.

Yildiz's Cesareans

A neighbor of Aunty Emine, Yıldız, who is in her late twenties and has two children, told me about her hospital births during an interview in 1996. On the tape, she relates that her first pregnancy was twin girls, but she didn't know she had twins. Ten days before the birth, she fell flat on her back outside her house. She did not realize it, but the fall had harmed one of the fetuses. When she finally had contractions and went to the hospital in Ordu, the doctor discovered that it was a double pregnancy and that one fetus was dead. She had a cesarean by the Head Doctor at the Ordu Hospital, who performed as a private doctor with a fee. Her second child was also born by cesarean in the same hospital. She prefers the hospital, because it is safer. She tells me that the biggest danger of having a baby at home is bleeding, because some women bleed to death. She stayed in the hospital for eight days, and then had to get back to work at home when she arrived. After the second child, she stayed nine days in the hospital and then was able to stay in bed for twenty-four days at home. She says she thinks cesareans are better. The place where she gave birth was a section of the hospital reserved for birthing.

Yıldız's daughter, the twin who survived, was about seven years old when this interview took place, and she contributes details as her mother speaks. She says that the doctor had told her mother that, if she had come to him immediately after the fall, the other twin would have been saved. This child has heard the story of the pregnancy and tragedy all her life, absorbing the details from hearing the story told by her mother and others in the family (she would not have heard directly from the doctor). In this case, we can see that the mother is held responsible for the health of her unborn child, and blamed, if not for falling, then for delaying seeking help after the fall.

Esra's Private Room Birth

In 1997, I interviewed Esra, a woman younger than me by a few years. She was brought up in Perşembe, a town not far away, and now lives with her husband in the village of Gebeşli (1997). She was visiting her friend Nazmiye, daughter of Aunty Emine, her sisters-in-law and her two children, one four years old, the other four months old. I asked her about her birthing experiences.

Esra: I had normal deliveries in the Fatsa Government Hospital, in a private room. I was in the hospital for a week. The second pregnancy, I was sick all the time, throwing up, dizzy. I deliver in just half an hour! I go in for a check up when the time is near, and they tell me to come in the next day to deliver. I'm afraid of the contractions, so I go to the hospital. Because I deliver without contractions, I don't trust myself, I'm scared, so that why I go to the hospital. They say it's better at home, but I'm used to the hospital. I stay there a day and then rest at home for fifteen days.
Sylvia: What do they do for *lohusa zamanı* (the lying in period after birth)?
E: You lie down, you know, they come to see the baby. They don't let you go out in the cold. You're not supposed to get cold at all, you sweat a lot!

S: Are there special foods?

E: They make *komposto* [a fruit syrup drink] and soup for the mother.

S: And for the visitors?

E: If the baby's a boy, you give the visitors *pilav* [a rice dish], if it's a girl, you give *helva* [a sweet]. They put a red ribbon in your hair [the mother's].

In this interview we can see the concern for hot and cold, according to the idea that birth can deplete a woman of heat, and the use of a red ribbon, often used for happy occasions in protection against the evil eye.

INFANT FEEDING TRENDS IN MEDRESEÖNÜ

Rima D. Apple, in her *Mothers and Medicine: A Social History of Infant Feeding, 1890–1950* (1987), traces way infant feeding, once considered a purely domestic concern, was slowly taken up by the medical profession as a realm for intervention. She finds that:

During the second half of the century [19th century in the U.S.A.], concern for the high rate of infant mortality stimulated interest in the question of infant feeding, since a high proportion of infant deaths were blamed on inadequate nutrition, due either to deficient breast milk or to poor artificial food. Using the finding of contemporary science, research-oriented physicians fashioned theories of healthful infant feeding. Faced with breast-fed infants who did not thrive and mothers who could not or would not nurse their children, practitioners too wanted a satisfactory substitute for mother's milk. Commercial infant-food products, typically devised by chemists, appeared on the market, providing alternatives to maternal nursing. Furthermore, women who feared their milk was deficient wanted an artificial food that they could use safely." (p.4)

In the villages I studied, mothers of young infants seemed to follow a fairly regular pattern of exclusive nursing for a month or two, after which *Can Bebe* cookies mashed in warm cow's milk were introduced. Women would explain this introduction of foods as a necessity, saying *"Sütüm yetmedi."* (My milk was not sufficient.). Nursing at the breast then continued mainly as a method to put a baby to sleep, but the milk supply dwindled until the baby was weaned. Pacifiers are commonly used, including pacifiers with an evil eye protection motif or light blue color as a part of traditional baby accessorizing. *Can Bebe* cookies, a type of sweet white cookie enriched with vitamins and minerals, are almost exclusively preferred over baby formula because they are cheaper and available everywhere.

Aunty Emine related that her first child, a boy, suffered from insufficient mother's milk, so the family purchased a goat specifically to give him goat's milk. Her later children were less fortunate: as the family fell into a period of poverty which then stretched on, they were faced with periods of chronic hunger, parasitic infestations, malnutrition leading, in one child, to cravings for dirt, and the shame of being caught stealing food. The social network of the village meant that there were homes the children could visit for food, but a malnourished mother may not produce sufficient milk and a poor family cannot keep a milk animal. Store-bought infant cookies or formula were unheard of in the village at the time, but a poor family would not have been able to buy them in any case.

Esra on Breast-Feeding

Esra, who had her baby in a private room at the Fatsa hospital, relies on the doctor's advice about infant feeding. She never cited tradition or the advice of women in our conversation.

S: Are you nursing your baby?
E: My first, I [nursed and] gave formula once a day for the first five months, this one, I'm just nursing, no formula. The doctor says, "the best thing is mother's milk."
[She doesn't seem to worry that I will cause *nazar* to her milk supply, either because she knows I am nursing myself, or perhaps because she thinks of this interview in terms of a medical interview. We turn to other subjects, and later circle back to nursing]
E: Here the doctors say "Don't nurse your baby after one year, it's bad for the baby." Is it bad?
S: Oh no, not at all.
E: It's bad for the mother, if anything, not for the baby.
S: [Referring to Timur] Sometimes he bothers me, but it's good for his health.
E: Of course it's good for health. They grow up without getting sick all the time! This one [indicates four-year-old], was sick a lot. Babies get fever, bronchitis, we were always going to the doctor. At home,

we made tea, gave honey and milk, we would rub Vicks on his chest, but it doesn't go away without the doctor.
S: To be sure…
E: Yes, still it is better to go to the doctor.
S: I look at my friends, and the healthiest babies are nursing.
E: Yes, it's the best.

✶✶✶✶✶

The Fallen Stomach Revisited

One of my unmarried informants told me about a woman like Hatice who had had trouble conceiving. She had been taken up to her mother's village (Afırlı), where a woman had performed the stomach pulling technique. The effectiveness of the treatment had been immediately destroyed because of the bumpy ride down the road back to her home. A second try had failed for the same reason. Finally, the family asked the woman to visit them at home for the treatment. Subsequently, I was told, the patient became pregnant.

Although this woman was the *gelin* of Aunty Emine's next-door neighbor, although we had babies of similar ages and various family ties in common, and although I saw her frequently, we had never been alone together. One night, the two of us were alone in her room, swinging Timur in a blanket held like a hammock, trying to get him to sleep. When I asked her about how she had overcome her problems in conceiving, and asked her about the effectiveness of the stomach pulling technique, she pulled me close and whispered, 'Those things are empty/futile (*boş*). I got pregnant after going to a doctor.' Because her mother and mother-in-law both value the traditional practices and believe in their effectiveness, she dared not express such views in front of them. She is, however, absolutely certain (if secretive) in her attribution of success to the doctor's medicine (she had been given a fertility drug), and has a fine son to prove it. She may also have been reaching out to me, as a Western *gelin* in the home of a traditional midwife, expecting me to share both her secrecy and her faith in clinical medicine.

"Stomach-pulling" as a treatment for infertility is used in other parts of Turkey. An acquaintance from Adana told me that her own mother had been unable to conceive for six years after the birth of her first child. After being diagnosed and treated for a "fallen stomach" by a traditional expert in the local woman's bath house, she became pregnant. The woman relating this story is thus living proof of the efficacy of this traditional practice.

Other Problems with Reproductive Health

Lale, who was quoted in Chapter 5 on the subject of *nazar*, also told me about the biggest health problem in her life, ovarian cysts which interfered with her fertility:

Sylvia: I'm collecting information about health, so I'd appreciate it if you could give me examples from your lives. Have you had any illnesses?
Lale: I was sick, I had an operation. I had *kis.*
S: What's that? (I look it up and find it is fibroids or an ovarian cyst)
L: It happens in your ovaries.
S: What remedy did you use?
L: I had an operation in Istanbul. I got pains, I went to the hospital, had an operation. Then we had this girl [indicates her approximately ten-year-old daughter]. When she was 7 months old, I got it again, I had another operation. One of my ovaries was removed. When she was a year-and-a-half, it happened again, so they removed the other ovary.
S: Was it a private hospital?
L: Yes, a private one, we don't use insurance. We'd rather pay and get good care. I had two operations in one place, and then switched doctors. In case he had diagnosed wrong...But the second doctor said the same thing, so I got the operation. Now, Thank God, I'm fine, but I get headaches, nervousness, I get depressed.

Lale's story reflects the common distinction between the bad care provided for free through state insurance and the good care which must be obtained from a private doctor. The switch to another doctor seems to have been driven by the fact that Lale's fertility would be permanently terminated by the removal of the second ovary, leaving her with one child.

The Contemporary Mix of Options for Birth and Reproductive Health

I have tried to show the range of choices in birthing practices available for the women of Medreseönü. The traditional birthing was at home with the assistance of a village midwife. The current hospital birthing options include the technologies to monitor fetal development and heart rate during birth, I.V. medicines, a full range of pain reducing medications, the anesthetics and surgical equipment necessary for performing a cesarean, and the standard equipment such as forceps, umbilical cord-cutting tools, and incubators for care of babies. Hospitals also provide various surgical procedures and fertility medicines in case of problems in reproductive health. Each individual woman, in consultation with family members (usually including seriously considered input from her mother-in-law), negotiates a strategy for obtaining her preferred care during pregnancy and birth. Of course, the circumstances sometime dictate a change in plans, such as when an emergency occurs. All women state their appreciation for the expanded options available since the introduction and expansion of local clinics and hospitals, although they often complain about the cost of getting good care. The Turkish government has always expressed an obligation to provide free care to Turkish villagers and workers, but ordinary citizens are aware of a large gap between the political promises they hear and the reality they experience.

In the case of Hatice and Mehmet, the traditional practice of "stomach-pulling" was the first remedy tried for infertility. When it brought no results, they then turned to a series of doctors in ever more distant locations. The price of procedures in the hospitals became a deciding factor in their choice of action, although the success of the Istanbul doctor in helping Hatice's sister through her pregnancy increased their hopes in him. In the case of the "stomach-pulling" technique's failure to work, older women explained that Hatice must have spoiled the effects of the treatment by moving around too much or lifting something heavy. At the time, the couple worried that leaving the hospital too soon and undertaking a strenuous journey might cause the failure of the operation, a concept that is parallel to the model of ruining a "stomach-pulling" through over exertion.

Reproduction, family planning, and birth are health issues of great importance to women in this area. They are held responsible for success and failure. Young women are taught necessary information about these issues, which they are expected to apply to their own lives after marriage. Women past childbearing age are generally respected for their knowledge of reproductive health along with all types of health, and consulted in the normal settings of visiting and conversation. Clinical techniques, supported by the national media, local practitioners, and success stories in the local society, offer a new range of options for women with reproductive concerns. There are cultural benefits which may be associated with medical procedures such as cesarean birth, making them popular. A medical procedure may instill terror, as it did in the case of Hatice and Ahmet's traumatic trip to Istanbul, but the hope of positive results, and the stigma and sorrow of childlessness, lead people to them when local methods have been exhausted. The availability of clinical techniques to assist with reproduction, in combination with the cultural authority of doctors, has led some young women to doubt the wisdom of their elders. In general, however, women see reproductive health as a part of overall health, and mix available methods in a practical way to ensure the best results. The following chapter goes into greater detail about the variety of institutions of clinical medicine, the type of medicine promoted by the Turkish state, the provision of which, however, is often hampered by a lack of resources.

CHAPTER 8

INSTITUTIONS OF
CLINICAL MEDICINE

Beni Türk Hekimlerine Emanet Ediniz.
Entrust me to Turkish Doctors

—Mustafa Kemal Atatürk

İnandık doktorlara; Öyle böyle dediler
Ayrılık defterini elimize verdiler
Doktorlar da ne bilur ciğerun acisini
Cerrahpaşa'ya koydum canumun yarisini
We believed the doctors when they said "It's this, It's that…"
They gave us our walking papers
What do doctors know about the pain in your liver?
I left half of my life at Cerrahpaşa Hospital

—Anonymous, sung by Volkan Konak, Maranda, 2003

The Health Clinic occupies one floor of the municipal building on the shore road, in the small cluster of buildings which make up the center of Medreseönü. I am hurrying there because I am late for vaccination day, and I had expressly asked to be able to observe the workings of the clinic on this day. The staff is quite familiar with me by now, as I have come often to sit with them drinking tea and asking about the clinic's operations. I immediately cross through the waiting room, where several families with small children wait with the characteristically glum attitude that seems to come over Turkish people in line for government services. I pass through the doctor's examining room, where a baby is expressing dismay about the whole frightening procedure of vaccination. The doctor gives me a nod, I open the next door, and am met by the instant attention of the entire staff. All the nurses are having their cigarettes, in direct violation of all the advice of the anti-smoking posters up in the waiting room, and they are thus quite alert when someone enters their office, in case they need to quickly dispose of the evidence of their unhealthy

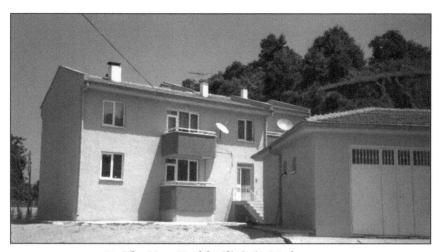

31. The New Health Clinic in Medreseönü

habit. They ask me why I am so late, and I tell them that I have spent the night in Ordu and had to wait for a ride back. It is around noon, and twenty-one of the infants to be vaccinated have been seen to, leaving thirty-seven yet to be done. The nurses joke that it is the pride of those who live near the shore road which has made them dally, in contrast to the villagers from farther away who have to get the vaccination over with in the morning and get on with the rest of their daily tasks.

True to the requirements of government regulations, the walls of the nurses' office display various enlarged tables of data they have collected, including data on population growth, mother and child health, immunizations, family planning, sanitation efforts, and other health-related statistics. Each room has, bolted to the wall, a signed, stamped, and framed list of all the contents of the room. Above everything, in each room, is a portrait of Atatürk, the modernizing leader and personification of the patriarchal Turkish state which has provided and regulates such Health Clinics.

The walls of the waiting room display posters meant for the patients and their families. Anti-smoking posters show children's drawings picked from a national search. One shows a boy crying huge spurting tears at the grave of his father, with a pack of cigarettes over-laid with the red circular symbol of negation. An old poster carries the title "You're Expecting a Baby." In three out of the six sections, pregnant women, who seem to have come out of an early 1970's fashion spread—complete with mini skirts and flipped hair—are shown brushing their teeth, taking a shower, lounging on a lawn chair, dancing with a partner, riding a horse, and taking a stroll on the arm of a suitably

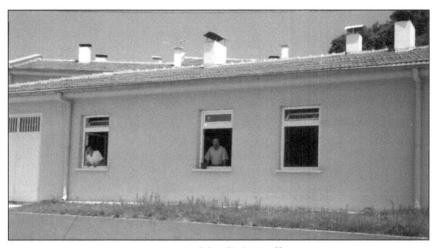

32. Health Clinic Staff

fashionable man. One section shows a variety of appropriate foods, and the remaining two sections show pregnant village women, wearing village-style head scarves, carrying a load of sticks, lifting a cauldron, washing laundry in a tub, and washing the floor. Each section has a written text which explains what should be done or not done ("Keep clean." "Don't do difficult sports." "Eat a variety of healthy foods." "Stroll in fresh air and relax." "Don't lift heavy loads." and "Don't do difficult and tiring work.") For an illiterate person, however, it is impossible to tell that some pictures show recommendations and others are admonishments. One could easily extrapolate a message that rich pregnant women dance, flirt with men, enjoy running hot water, and ride horses while pregnant village women carry on with their same round of chores—and although this was probably not the intended message of the poster, it is not far from the realities known well by those waiting in this room. An anti-cholera poster shows in graphic detail the types of filth encountered in village life which can harbor the disease: animal dung, swarming flies, exposed outdoor toilets, sewage running into drinking water supplies, and a thin old person in bed with a puddle forming underneath. As pictures of the desired healthy state, advertising from European drug companies are hung about—usually showing a fat, blue-eyed, blond baby with a dimpled smile. Local contributions fill a glass-fronted cabinet—embroideries made by young local women in stitching classes, and crocheted baby mittens and hats. In the corner, a poster of a blond, blue-eyed nurse in standard nursing uniform with her finger to her lips and a stern look disciplines the waiting room.

The nurses are here in full force today, and two midwives who live in their own villages rather than in Medreseönü have come in as well. This is the first time I am meeting the youngest midwife, and I am surprised by her attire. She is wearing the new style of Islamic dress, which includes an overcoat, a large polyester headscarf, a long-sleeved blouse, and a skirt which almost touches the ground over her fashionable platform shoes. Inside the clinic, she removes her overcoat, but the rest stays unchanged. When I get a chance to talk to her alone, I ask her about what she is wearing. I know that it is against the law for government employees to wear the clothes that mark them as Islamic traditionalists. This midwife's photograph on the clinic wall shows her in standard nursing uniform. In response to my query, she laughs, saying "And this is supposed to be a Muslim country!" She tells me that many of her patients are more comfortable with her because of her modest dress.

The staff spends the afternoon of the vaccination day calling around to try to bring in the children who had not shown up in the morning. The staff's knowledge of the familial and social relationships of the villagers is crucial to the success of contacting the parents. In many cases, a neighbor or relative is called in order to try to get a message to the parents who were not found by a direct telephone call. Since each staff member knows a particular network of people, everyone works together to try to close the net on the parents on the list. There is a lot of joking and light-hearted gossiping as the calls are placed (from the "back-stage" area of the nurse's office).

One family is reached and the man answering tells the midwife not to worry about calling another family of his relatives because he was going to see them anyway. The staff is working from a list provided by the downstairs post office (which is also the telephone center) and photocopied in the government office copier located one floor up from the clinic. The midwife from Büyükağız has only two families left, and wonders aloud if she should take the two shots and go home. A few more families come in, and I take my leave because the car that can give me a ride up the hill is waiting in the lot in front of the clinic.

✶✶✶✶✶

The Clinic as Representative
of the Turkish State

Many recent theorists have worked to expose the complex relationships between the individual and the state. Their theories, which are based mainly on print media, have tended to assume literacy, and a kind of "trickle-down" nationalism, focusing on intellectuals, politicians, and generals. They also tend to assume a "blank-slate" kind of citizen ready to be inscribed with national identity. This kind of study does not examine the role of "regular" individual citizens, who are often minimally exposed to literature, in the negotiation of national identity. Foucault has shown that the state can have a visceral impact on the individual's body and identity, through imprisonment, medication, and other forms of control.

In his history of the clinic as an institution, Foucault notices that:

> "For clinical experience to become possible as a form of knowledge, a reorganization of the hospital field, a new definition of the status of the patient in society, and the establishment of a certain relationship between public assistance and medical experience, between help and knowledge, became necessary; the patient had to be enveloped in a collective, homogeneous space." (196)

Post-colonial theory has shown that states have a great deal of power over their citizens, who thus occupy a subaltern position.[1] This power, however, is applied neither consistently nor constantly over time. Individuals both respond to and initiate relations with state power, in a complex process that includes both contestation and negotiation. Foucault (1963) has shown that a clinic is a particular kind of institution, with a vested interest in a certain world view and a specific set of technological tools. By looking at the interaction between the state and the individual, in the context of a health clinic, we can get an idea about how this kind of negotiation takes place.

With the creation of a modern nation-state, various state institutions are established which have an impact on the daily life of citizens. One of the institutions, which can have a very personal effect on individuals, is the institution of national health care. The modern Turkish state introduced a national program of medicine based on a western clinical model, which was spread throughout the countryside to promote a specific type of integration and modernization of the Turkish citizens. The implications of the fact that a western model was adopted are vast, but, as stated in Chapter 1, my concern in this research is with the difference between the clinical model and the local, traditional model, more than the historical origins and political impact of the origins of the clinical/biomedical model.

---

1. Post-colonial theorists whose works have informed this book's concept of the interdependencies between state and individual citizen include: Anderson 1991, Bhabha 1990, Clifford and Marcus 1986, Clifford 1988, Enloe 1989, Hertzfeld 1986, 1987, Hobsbawm and Ranger 1983, Jusdanis 1991, Minh-ha 1989, Said 1978, Spivak 1988, 1990, and Webber 1991.

After describing the ways in which the clinic's physical set up, its medical philosophy, its personnel, and its rules and regulations represent the state in a local setting, this chapter will examine the ways members of the health clinic staff shift their behaviors and loyalties in different situations because they both represent the state and have local identities. Individuals enter into power relations with the clinic, using various strategies of body language and rhetoric, in order to achieve their desired health-care goals. Interactions between the state and the individual will be illustrated using the example of vaccinations provided by the state to village children. It should again be stressed that focus on the "individual," simplifies the actual Turkish cultural situation in which at least one family member will accompany a patient to the clinic and participate in health-care decisions. This chapter then examines the regional hospital and describes a trip to a private doctor in Ordu in order to show the ways such a trip differs from a trip to the clinic.

Reading the Clinic

The clinic is a representative of the state because it is founded, funded, and furnished by the state. The most important and recognizable symbols of state affiliation are the flag outside and the portrait of Atatürk above the doctor's desk. In every room is a small framed list of the furnishings of the room, a reminder of the bureaucratic attention to detail typical of state institutions. In the waiting room, posters that seem to be mostly from the 1970's, show which health issues particularly concern the state—the improvement of pre-natal care, the prevention of cholera, and the reduction of smoking-related deaths. A poster of a nurse with her finger to her lips conveys a need for patients to respect and obey the rules of the clinic, and, by extension, the state.

Along with the physical furnishings of the clinic comes a crucial yet invisible component of the clinic's operations: the western medical model of sickness and health. In a philosophical universe in which illnesses are caused by drafts, by eating cold foods, by the evil eye, by walking barefoot on a tile floor, and so on, the microbiological model is not used to explain illnesses, and in fact can seem a bit silly. The state's promotion of the biological model has made some inroads into local awareness, however, through the institutions of the health clinic, schools, television, and newspapers, and through the exposure of locals to other cultures through travel and work.

The Staff

The state also determines the staff of the clinic, as all health clinic doctors, nurses, health officers, and midwives are trained in state institutions and assigned to their locations by the state. Turkish doctors are mostly trained in urban centers at the state's expense, and then sent to peripheral and rural areas to perform a four-to-six-year assignment that is seen as a national duty and a repayment for education. In the Medreseönü clinic, the doctor is not from the Black Sea area and may move on to another assignment when this one is completed. He has extended his stay once, and people report with pride that he likes the place. They also conspire to marry him to a local so that he will stay. The other staff members were trained in the small cities near their home villages, also at the state's expense, but with the expectation that they would return to their home town and serve the adjoining villages. Their uniforms are meant to mark them as state employees, and they are supposed to follow procedures according to state regulations.

The Work of the Clinic

The everyday work of the clinic includes examining patients, prescribing medications, administering vaccinations, discussing and dispensing birth-control, identifying and tracking pregnancies, and performing tasks such as giving injections, stitching wounds, or treating burns. The health clinic staff also goes on rounds of the villages, checking sanitation, visiting confined patients, and gathering census information. The clinic is sometimes the agency that refers a patient to a doctor or hospital for more extensive testing or treatment than available at the clinic. The rules and regulations for these tasks are spelled out in a handbook provided by the state to each clinic. Much of the staff's time is spent filling out reports and entering census data into charts provided by the state. In this direct way, the state meets and tracks its citizens through the health clinic. Campaigns to lower infant mortality include pregnancy monitoring, vaccination, birth-weight and weight gain recording.

As representatives of the state, the health clinic staff can charge fines for unsanitary toilets or stables. In this case, the health clinic staff represents the state right at the homes of its citizens, with the power to judge their cleanliness. Besides the fact that a lack of sanitation is linked to diseases such as cholera, the state's concern with the disposal of wastes is a part of the national goals of modernization and westernization and shows the extent of the state's wish for control over the populace. In practice, however, conditions deemed unsanitary by official standards are often overlooked if personal relations are good between the clinic staff and the homeowner, or, conversely, turned into a hotly contended issue if the relations are bad. The task of enforcing cleanliness is seen by both the government and the populace as a health-related one, as it fits both the germ model of illness and the local ideas about filth (*pislik*) as an agent of illness.

The Handbook of Clinic Regulations

A handbook is provided by the state to regulate and standardize the workings of all health clinics in the country. In this text (*Sağlık Ocağı Yönetimi,* 6th edition, 1993), we can find evidence of the state's official position and attitude about villagers and their health care system. In the discussion of special problems relating to women's reproductive health, the handbook states:

> For example, it is necessary to get to know and visit more often, even if it disrupts the routine, those mothers who are candidates for the danger of pregnancy toxemia, those children who are undernourished, and those families whose care and education is hampered by the grandmother's age and ignorance (*yaşlılık ve bilgisizlik*). (106)

This shows that the government considers "old wives' knowledge" to be a hindrance to the proper care of its citizens. The handbook also makes clear that the staff of the clinic is hierarchically ranked, with the doctor at the top and the midwives at the bottom. The midwives are asked to attend local social functions, such as weddings and female gatherings, in order to achieve comfortable social relations within their villages. Doctors are likewise instructed to attend male social functions. The doctors and midwives are not equals, however; the doctors are meant to supervise and correct the work of the nurses and midwives. The handbook tells the doctors:

> A point which should not be forgotten when participating in this kind of house visit with a midwife is that, if the midwife has a deficiency or if her procedure is not correct, it is important that you give the proper instruction after the visit, when you are alone with the midwife, in order not to harm the respect the midwife has in the eyes of the family. (111)

Midwives, then, should be integrated into village social life and earn the respect of villagers, but must still be under the direct supervision of the doctor.

Although, in theory, the state exerts almost total control over the furnishings, funding, staff, and procedures of the health clinic, in practice, there is still some room for local autonomy. One significant example of this autonomy is the fact that the clinic's ambulance was purchased by a local group of families who work in Germany and thus constitute a kind of local moneyed class. It stands outside the clinic as a sign that local charitable donations can provide something that the state was unable or unwilling to provide. The competition between the central government and local pious or charitable foundations to provide resources to the common people is a feature of Turkish culture that has been widely noted in Ottoman history.

Power Dynamics

To get an idea about the state-local power dynamics in the arena of health care, we can examine the complex social behavior of the health clinic staff: The doctor, for example, is the most powerful representative of the state. At the same time, however, he is an outsider who needs to act with care in order to be accepted and respected in the local setting. The others can move more fluidly between representing the state and claiming insider status as long-standing members of the local community. Two of the four midwives spend more of their working hours in their home villages than they do in the clinic. The doctor, the health manager, the two nurses, the secretary, and the remaining two midwives live close to the clinic and report to work there. There is no person who comes into the clinic who is not somehow connected to the social networks of the villages and the town. Even if a complete stranger should happen to need emergency care at the clinic, he or she will be asked questions about origins and family so that some familiarity can be established. For example, if an American tourist ever turns up in the area, he or she could be quickly integrated into the networks of familiarity by virtue of the fact that one local family now has contacts in America. Patients can be friends, relatives, classmates, enemies, neighbors, or guests, and their reception in the clinic in part depends on these relationships. There is no place for anonymous or impersonal treatment. Because staff members have all lived elsewhere, at least for their medical education, they have formed ideas about the differences between local life and life elsewhere. Health clinic staff members become something like "big fish in a small pond," acquiring status because of their education and their experience in the wider world. When talking with people with as much or more experience in the outside world, however, they are quick to show that they realize the limitations of their situation. This strategy comes from the awareness that outsiders or locals who have "made it" in the big cities or abroad can be derisive toward those who have returned to work in their hometown.

Discussions of traditional healing practices, when conducted within the clinic, are fraught with insider/outsider tension. When I asked what the health clinic policy was about religious amulets worn for healing or protection, the staff members were quick to explain that amulets are tolerated because people like them and because they do no harm. The assumption seemed to be that an outsider (especially a westerner) would consider them useless or even a cause of backwardness, and thus expect the clinics to work to stop their use. It also seems that the official rule book ignores traditional healing practices altogether, thus implying that they are not worthy of attention. Outside the clinic, staff members kept up an attitude of skepticism about many local practices and beliefs, although they also told me about instances in which the local practices met with success. It is possible for a staff member to be skeptical or even derisive about certain traditional healing practices and yet hold others to be efficacious. The practices that are regarded as valuable are taken as examples of the practical knowledge of the elders, while the ones regarded as harmful are spoken of as the fruit of ignorance. One nurse, who would probably attribute most illnesses to microbes rather than to the evil eye, still wears a protective blue bead on her necklace. The clinic staff, especially the midwives, consistently practices the traditional uttering of *"Maşallah"* when looking at a new baby in order to avert the evil eye. The midwives also play along with the tradition that food should be given to the midwife who delivers a baby so that the baby will never go hungry.

"On-Stage" and "Back-Stage" Behavior

Staff members at the health clinic have what could be called performative and "backstage" ways of behaving in the clinic. This contrast of performance and "backstage" behavior was introduced by Goffman in *The Presentation of Self in Everyday Life* (1959) and used by many scholars, including Makhlouf (1979) who found spaces of "on-stage" and "backstage" behavior to be important in the dynamics of social visiting among women in Yemen. Goffman's examination of the ways humans perform certain roles as they go about their normal daily activities is useful to ethnographers and others entering a new culture as they try to make sense of local behavior. As a foreign ethnographer and an incoming family member, I needed to understand social behavior and learn appropriate behavior. It was fairly easy for me to notice switches between clearly distinct registers of behavior, for example between formality and informality in an institutional setting such as the Health Clinic.

When they greet patients in the waiting room, staff members tend to be stern and business-like, speaking in short sentences and using the imperative case. They hold their bodies straight and faces serious. In contrast, in their own office, where they invited me to sit down, have some tea, and chat, they tell stories, laugh, and slump in their chairs. All of the female staff members smoked cigarettes "backstage," but when I tried to take a picture of a midwife with a cigarette, she strongly protested. Everyone laughed and joked about what Americans would think about Turkey's smoking nurses. Turkish women who smoke do not do so in all situations and often prefer that their habit not be known by everyone—thus it is usually a "backstage" activity, in the clinic or elsewhere. In public, the nurses support the state's anti-smoking campaign, but behind the scenes at the clinic they personally subvert it. Another interesting subversion of official rules is the Islamically-marked clothing and behavior of the youngest midwife. This woman even uses the nurses' office to do her prayers. This situation would have been unthinkable before the 1990's, but after the Islamically-minded Refah party gained considerable influence, more people have begun to mark themselves publicly as active Muslims.

Patient Tactics

The clinic employees alter their behavior according to whether they feel most like state representatives or like locals, whether they are "on stage" or "backstage." When I observed the behavior of people coming into the clinic because of various health problems, I could see that they also actively manipulate their social identities to obtain the maximum benefit from their visit. A patient is literally putting his or her body on the line when asking for state help in the intimate arena of physical health. The most common type of approach to health clinic staff is that of the humble petitioner, accompanied by a body language conveying apprehension, respect, embarrassment, and hope. This is a perfect complement to the stern and stiff behavior of the staff—and usually leads to a smooth transaction. The tendency of the staff to loiter "backstage" a bit before seeing patients heightens the patient's awareness of the power the clinic holds and increases the humility of the patient's self-presentation. Of course, this is a delicate negotiation with certain boundaries—if a staff member loiters too long or shows actual disrespect while "on stage," patients would have every right to grumble, complain, or spread stories later, depending on the situation.

Another patient tactic is one most often used by elderly women, in which the patient tries to place herself in a familial relationship with someone on the staff. Because this is a small town, there is usually some close familial tie, but I have seen this tactic used even in big city settings. An elderly woman patient might greet a nurse by saying "Hello, my girl," (*kızım*, which is also "my daughter") or, if she feels she has a better chance of getting the best treatment from another nurse, she might ask, "Is my aunt's daughter's girl here?" This would prompt the nurse she is addressing to ask about the family connections being referred to, leading to a shift of power to the elderly woman, who is the expert in knowing who is who. Even if it is quite a stretch, a patient could ask "Aren't you so-and-so's kid?" and still draw a staff member into a discussion of family relationships.

Another example of the use of familial patterns of relationship is the strategy used by a person bringing in a dependent to be seen by the staff. Because taking responsibility for a dependent is such an important act in Turkish culture, the responsible person can act in an assertive way toward state employees. While the dependent remains absolutely passive (often looking very ill), the responsible person stays on foot, actively pressing for quick service by staying near the door to the doctor's office or speaking with any nurse who passes through the waiting area. This is typically a male strategy, but women can use it if it seems a better strategy than the petitioner style of address or the appeal to the respect due elders.

Some patients fully expect to be welcomed "backstage," because of their previous relationships with staff members. In this case, they carry themselves upright and, moving quickly, stick their heads into the back office, smile, and wait to be welcomed in. This behavior elicits a welcome even if the staff does not immediately recognize the person—"if they act this way, then we must know them." These strategies of self-presentation are put to use, not only in state-run health clinics, but also in virtually any state-run office or in settings like banks where the power relationships are seen to favor the institution, not the individual.

Vaccination

State-subaltern power relationships manifest themselves in the behavior of state employees and of those who need to obtain services from them. For a concrete example of the ways in which state authority can make itself felt in the physical bodies and social lives of individuals, I have described the health clinic's vaccination campaign. It is important to point out that there is nothing "natural" about vaccinations. In the United States, we have been conditioned by decades of promotion and education to consider vaccinations an essential and beneficial practice (although there are some who oppose the practice on religious grounds). The theory behind vaccinations fits in with our understanding of viruses, microbes, the immune system, and illness in general. As a result, we subject our children to the temporary pain of shots and the discomfort of the reaction to vaccinations, firm in our convictions that it is best in the long-run. In contrast, many Turkish villagers seem to be highly ambivalent or downright mistrustful of vaccinations—taking their children for shots only because the law requires it rather than because they believe in the benefits of vaccinations. This often frustrates the staff members, who have been trained to take the benefits of vaccination for granted.

For the sake of a counter-example, in Turkey, parents have their sons circumcised with a firm belief in the long-term benefits of the practice. In the

U.S., we used to consider male circumcision to be so beneficial to health and hygiene that it was a near-universal practice. Now that the tide of national consensus seems to be shifting to the opinion that circumcision is not necessary for health, many experts are speaking against its universal application and some have taken up a campaign against it on the grounds that it causes unnecessary pain to infants and may cause long-term psychological damage. When discussing this issue with a Turkish man, I was told that he found vaccination to be a much greater source of anxiety and pain than circumcision had been. In other words, while pain may be a cross-cultural universal, there are significant cultural differences in the perception of pain based on cultural explanatory models of health and illness. (See Good, 1999)

I came across three examples of the ambivalence most villagers feel about vaccinations. The first is that parents often try to scare their children into good behavior by telling them that, if they are bad, one of the people in the group will stick them with a needle—give them a shot (*"Yenge sana iğne yapar!"*) A second example was the widespread alarm caused by a newspaper article that reported that two babies who had been given bad vaccinations had required amputations because of gangrene. The Health Minister was reported as saying that the government vaccinations were inferior and insufficient (*kalitesiz ve yetersiz*). The health clinic I observed received queries from concerned parents after this article was published. The third example I found of mistrust of vaccinations was a widespread rumor that powerful foreign countries, concerned about Turkey's rapid population growth, were sending a new type of vaccination that would render Turkish children sterile in later life. The woman who told me about it said it had been in the newspapers and that Turkish doctors had proved it. The rumor seems to have been connected with the introduction of the oral polio vaccine—administered by drops rather than by injection. This unfamiliar method of administration and the state's insistence that all children receive them, even if they had already been vaccinated, seems to have led to the scare. The scene was set for such a rumor because of the general mistrust of vaccinations and because it is common knowledge in Turkey that Europeans and Americans are alarmed by the Turkish population growth rate.

In short, the Turkish Health Bureau allocates significant resources for a national campaign of vaccination for all children, and the health clinic is responsible for carrying it out in the villages and neighborhoods across the nation. In the clinic I observed, the midwives are responsible for keeping track of all babies through the period of completing their vaccinations. Instead of having parents bring their babies in for shots individually according to their own specific age, the clinic has special vaccination days on which it administers shots to babies from the same age group. When the ambulance was first presented to the clinic, it was used to drive to all the villages to administer vaccinations door-to-door. That practice has been discontinued, to the displeasure of many villagers who find it difficult, because of the nature of their agricultural work, to bring their children into the clinic on any one set day. One nurse complained to me that the villagers are too demanding, especially when the vaccinations are a free service. In this case, we see a clear state directive to vaccinate all the children, taken up by the health clinic staff, who have to cajole a recalcitrant population into dropping everything and bringing in children for a shot which is known to be painful and not necessarily considered beneficial.

The local health clinic, then, is a setting in which power relationships between the state and its citizens are played out. These power relationships are shaped by the fact that the state intends to impose a western medical model on a population that has had a different working model of health and illness. The staff members of the clinic have to find a balance between their duties to the state and their local social obligations. People who choose to enter the health clinic know they are entering a government office and use strategies to obtain the care they are seeking and still retain a measure of autonomy. The state provides free or low-cost health care for everyone who is willing to use the clinic. In return it asks for its citizens to accept the western model of medicine and to comply with rules regarding such issues as sanitation and vaccination. In the interaction between the health clinic and its patients we can get an idea about the complex and critical contestations and negotiations between state and citizen.

Women's Social Interactions at Institutions of Clinical Medicine

In Yemen, Makhlouf (1979) observed that new institutions such as clinics were creating new types of social interactions for women:

> "…medical facilities provide new alternatives for knowledge and social interaction. They bring women into contact with a wide range of people. It is the Yemeni mother who takes the child to the clinic, and there she interacts with specialists (doctor and nurses) as well as with other women, some friends and some strangers, who have similar problems. They also acquire new knowledge about a sector of life which they share with others outside the home. All women attempt to understand medical treatments and tend to follow the innovations in this field. A number of times I observed women exchanging informa-

tion about new drugs and giving advice to one another, or trying to explain sickness in terms of their recently acquired knowledge." (66)

Makhlouf leaves room for the possibility that this new context for female interaction may be modeled on older forms of health-seeking behavior, like shrine visits or visits to a traditional healer, which may have provided the same type of interaction between unacquainted women. Along the Black Sea coast and throughout Turkey, women meet strangers as they pursue health-care benefits for themselves and their families. They try to establish familial-style relationships with health care providers in order to obtain good care. In a crowded waiting room, women seek information and referrals, taking care to behave properly with unfamiliar men. This behavior can be seen as an extension of the usual village forms of building social networks. If an illiterate, elderly villager arrives in a hospital to seek help, the first order of business is to find someone in the noisy, chaotic hustle and bustle to ask directions. With any luck, some advance connection has been established and the villager has a name of a doctor or a nurse in the hospital. If this person can be found, then the villager can feel assured that he or she will be taken care of. If there is no such advance connection, the villager will try to establish one, either by asking a likely person (such as the guard at the door) about his village of origin, with the hope of discovering some actual family relationship or at least an acquaintance in common, or by using terms such as *oğlum* or *kızım* ("My son," "My girl") to set up a fictitious kinship in the hope of getting respect and assistance.

THE RANGE OF HEALTH CARE PROVIDERS

The individual is not expected to take care of his or her own illnesses, and a person without female relatives to provide care is pitied. The closest female relatives are responsible for care in a time of illness: mother, wife, sister, daughter-in-law, daughter, and sister-in-law. Neighbors, relatives contacted by telephone, and local female traditional experts can be consulted as an extension of the female relatives' circle. Close male relatives are called in if the illness requires more than available home care: if a medicine or product must be purchased, if a specialist must be brought to the home or the patient taken to a specialist, if transportation to a clinic, doctor's office, or hospital is needed, or if cash payment is required. In the clinic, nurses and midwives function in a manner similar to female relatives, providing the basic care and advice, while the doctor is called in for consultation if his expertise is needed or if a referral is required. The options for families to consider when an individual needs medical treatment range from the home and neighbors to the city hospital, from local to distant, familiar to unknown, and from free-of-charge to expensive.

In choosing how to treat a health problem, families take into account what they have heard from others or had recommended by others, but acknowledge that sometimes people choose a treatment based mostly on what they are used to (from *alışmak*), what is traditional or personally preferred. Some use this phrase to make a kind of apology for what could be called "less than modern" behavior on their own part, or especially to explain older family members' old-fashioned ways. When I asked Esra, the woman who lives in Perşembe and had her babies delivered at the Fatsa state hospital, whether her mother-in-law likes to go to the doctor, she replied:

> Esra: No, she doesn't like it much. You would have to force her to go to the hospital. Unless she wants it, she won't go, she'll stand the pain.
> Sylvia: She likes the old ways, then?
> E: Yes, She's used to that. Before, they didn't have doctors, they did everything in the village. That's what they're used to. It's not that they're scared of doctors, they just don't like going. They like the village stuff.
> S: Also, stuff is expensive...
> E: Yes, it's really expensive here [she has heard about the system in Germany], the medicine is expensive. They take money from you.
> S: No insurance?
> E: No, nothing like that. It's really expensive, but for your health, you go.

Esra is distinguishing her own preferences from that of her mother-in-law, showing herself to be a town dweller with disposable income in distinction to her mother-in-law who is a traditionalist villager. Her approach also shows that, although the family is usually involved in decisions about health care, older women are able to decide for themselves that they will or will not go to a hospital. To understand how this decision is made, one must understand the workings of a Black Sea hospital.

THE HOSPITAL

A basic provincial hospital in Turkey is not set up to provide the patients with the comforts of home. A hospital stay, unless it is in an expensive, private room, means that family members feel obliged to bring food, sheets and towels, changes of clothing, and visit with the patient to pass the time. A patient who has no family in evidence in a hospital room is greatly pitied and often brought into the circle of a more fortunate patient with gifts of food and conversation. The most frequently heard criticisms of the local hospitals are that they are dirty and smelly, that the nurses are overworked and either neglect patients or treat them roughly, that they are depressing, and that they are a source of illness because sick people are all thrown in together. In contrast, home care is considered much more sanitary, comfortable, gentle, and healthy.

The doctors and nurses in the hospitals realize the benefits that family visits can bring to the patient. They do not deny the lack of resources such as food and bedding for patients, although they consider their conditions to be much more sanitary than home conditions, especially in villages. A compromise is continuously being worked out as the hospital staff tries to restrict the numbers and noise-levels of visitors, while each patient's family and friends try to maximize the benefits of the stay for the patient. As in all Turkish institutions, most official rules are flexible, according to the social connections of the patient and his or her family.

The Hospital as Family

In Turkish culture, the hospital is judged in direct relation to family care at home. The strongest critiques of hospital care are those which find it lacking the emotional support, wholesome food, cleanliness, and *ilgi* which can be found at home. When hospitals are praised, it is generally for their technologies and for the skills of specialists, not for their atmosphere or sympathetic care. If the family is the primary care unit, then all other health care is judged by the standards of the family. White (1994) has noticed parallels between the Turkish family and larger societal relations:

> Just as in the family the father assures the normative reproduction of traditional family relations, so the Turkish state manages the economy along lines laid down by the liberal economists, raising prices, adjusting interest rates, providing incentives and punishments. Meanwhile, just as the mother in the family reproduces relations moment by moment in practice, the Turkish people renegotiate their material reproduction day by day by acting out norms such as those of reciprocity, steering small amounts of money over and around the systematic channels imposed from above. (67)

In terms of the state-run hospitals, it is no wonder that the institutions of the *devlet* (state) are seen to lack the *ilgi* required to get well—the patriarch is meant to be aloof from day-to-day care—that is the business of women. The state builds physical structures, like hospitals and clinics, which are concrete examples of the patriarchal ability of the state to provide care for the "family" of citizens. What goes on in the daily routine inside the hospital is of less concern to the state, which is meant to maintain a dignified and elevated status.

The women within the state hospital, mostly the nurses who are meant to provide the daily care, are criticized by patients for their lack of *ilgi*, as if they were members of the family structure, bad *gelins* or ungrateful daughters. The irony is that they *have* no family obligation, and their rewards are small enough for the work they do. Like all state employees, they can consider themselves secure in their jobs but have no motivation to provide anything but the absolute minimum of service.

There is a growing literature on nursing which shows a wide-spread cross-cultural linkage between an ideal of female nurturing and the provision of compassionate medical care in a professional setting. In a close ethnographic study of a British ward staffed by female nurses caring for middle-aged men suffering from gastro-intestinal problems, Jan Savage (1999) shows that:

> Through a particular set of embodied practices, nurses were very often able to define the nature of the ward's symbolic space and whether it was taken to represent a public or private sphere. In doing so, they were able to suggest a quasi-kinship between themselves and patients.... these references to the domestic domain were surface representations of deeper, moral principles that informed nursing care, namely the principles of closeness, openness and sameness, which might be differently represented in other contexts. (182–183)

In a manner which seems similar to the Turkish case, British nursing is viewed as "women's work," with resulting expectations of morally informed care without adequate professional pay. (Savage, 185) Although researchers have found that many cultures link nursing knowledge and "motherhood knowledge," Savage found that the nurses in the ward she studied tried to downplay maternal symbols while reinforcing a type of family or domestic sphere that she characterizes as "closeness". (186) In the Turkish hospital, it seems that the nursing ideal is more closely linked to the *gelin* than the mother, with the benefit to the patient that this work is meant to be both fully caring and unpaid. If the nurses within the *devlet* hospital do not show enough *ilgi*, then the families must step in to take up the slack—bringing foods (even if they have been

forbidden in the restricted diet —*perhiz*— prescribed by the doctors), clothing, sheets and towels, and by spending time with the patients.

Outside of the relations between state and citizen, private hospitals and
clinics offer better services in return for cash. They put much stronger con-
trols on the visitors to patients—keeping strict hours, limiting the number of
visitors allowed, and regulating or prohibiting the items brought from home.
The understanding is that the patient will be well taken care of in exchange
for the high price of care. The extra-familial coldness of this kind of cash-
based transaction is mitigated by webs of social networks which make certain
specialists familiar (because they treated a family member or acquaintance),
or by the fact that the money needed for private care must be procured by tra-
ditionally-shaped negotiations within families.

Turks express surprise that the German state cares so well for Turkish workers, even illegal ones—and that free care is of a quality far superior to that
available in Turkey. Many take this as proof that the German state is either
foolish or so rich as not to care, an overindulgent patriarch who should be
taken advantage of as much as possible.

Nurses

Nurses who work in government hospitals (*Devlet Hastanesi* or *Sigorta Hastanesi*) are underpaid and overworked. Many of the nurses who have been
working the longest are graduates of a nursing middle school program. In this
type of program, girls from villages would be sent to boarding schools to be
trained as nurses. This was often done when families had several daughters
and little chance of marrying them all well. It was a way to have a daughter
enter the cash economy, save her from village labor, and widen her social circle so that she may marry well (perhaps even a doctor!). In other words, it
was a strategy for upward mobility, for one girl, and thus for her family as a
whole. Now, after years of overwork and a subsistence salary, the long-term
nurses are now seeing new nurses with better education (either high school or
college training) coming in with better salaries and fewer responsibilities. The
only way to make life at the job bearable is to make friends with the other
nurses, become immune to the suffering of patients, and find ways to maximize leisure (tea and cigarettes are the nearly universal pleasures of all government workers) and minimize work. With increased privatization, nurses
can supplement their work in government hospitals and clinics with work in
private ones. While the government jobs are very secure and poorly paid, the
higher wages of a private clinic come with the possibility of being fired for
poor performance. A nurse who is very comfortable and can get away with

showing little *ilgi* to the patients in a government hospital will change her attitude as she enters her private workplace, becoming serious, careful, respectful to patients, and hard-working.

Private Clinics

The state-run hospitals, although free, are not the preferred option in cases of serious illness. Even people who first try state clinics and doctors in order to save money will proceed to private practices if illness persists and money can be called in from some family member or acquaintance. Private clinics are located in nice neighborhoods, and are distinguishable from the state clinics and hospitals by their state-of-the-art equipment, new paint, new and stylish staff uniforms, and the pleasant demeanor (or *ilgi*) of those who greet and serve new patients.

Lale, whose operations for ovarian cysts were discussed in the previous chapter, compares the university hospital of Samsun (which has a better reputation than the state hospitals of Fatsa and Ordu) to private clinics in a conversation we had when she and her daughter were in the village from their home in Samsun, visiting the husband's relatives. (1997)

> Sylvia: Where are you from?
> Lale: Here, but we're in Samsun.
> S: Are the doctors good?
> L: Yes, the *Fakülte* [University Hospital] is pretty good. But you go to a private doctor—They look after you. If you go to the State Hospital, then they just look at you from across the room. They do check ups, they give you medicine, but it's up to chance. In the private one, they pay attention (*ilgi gösteriyorlar*).
> S: There are private rooms, too.
> L: Yes....
> S: Do you know any traditional medicine, have you heard about it?
> L: Yes, it happens around here. I hear they do it in the villages, but I don't know...
> S: Some go to doctors in the hospital and they're not happy and they say village stuff is better—especially bone-setting.
> L: Yes, there are a lot who get it [bone-setting] done, but because we never had it happen to us... [she can't say much about it]
> S: May God prevent it.
> L: Yes, May God prevent it.

S: There are teas…
L: There are many different teas, linden, we use linden when we have
flu. There's quince leaf, I put in carnation, I squeeze lemon.
S: Mixed?
L: Yes mixed, we drink it.
S: Is village food healthy?
L: According to me it is.
S: Do you bring it from the village [to the city]?
L: Yes, it's healthier, fresh.
S: Natural.
L: Yes, everything in the village is natural. We like it. We eat what we
like. All those vegetables, greens, the leaves, everything

So, while Lale is happy to bring the fresh produce of the village to her home
in the city, she finds little use for village medical practices. Her knowledge of
teas is easily transferred from a rural environment to the city, and the teas may
in fact be store-bought even if the knowledge may come from her village up-
bringing. Although she may ask her apartment neighbors for their opinions
about health and advice for home treatment, like villagers who ask for the advice of those nearby, Lale is more likely than her parents to consult a clinical
practitioner for simple problems, and to seek the best clinical treatment available. While the residents of the village studied here use urban institutions of
health care only in the most serious of circumstances, expressing pride in their
independence and stalwartness and preferring to try local and free-of-charge
methods, urban dwellers are more savvy and frequent consumers of clinical
medicine.

CHAPTER 9

DEPARTURES

This bleating eventually stops. The wolf appears.
We run off in different directions,
with always some thought of how lucky we are.
But nothing floats for long.
Death floods the mouth and the ear.
Every head goes under and away.

—Rumi, Open Secret, #65

Azrailin gelir kendi
Ne ağa der ne efendi
Sayılı günler tükendi
Yolun sonu görünüyor

Your own Azrael comes
He doesn't call you 'Lord' or 'Sir'
The numbered days are up
The end of the road comes into view

—words by Dursun Ali Akınet, sung by İbrahim Tatlıses

I could see now that my soul had left my body and that I was cupped in
Azrael's hand. My soul, the size of a bee, was bathed in light, and it shuddered
as it left my body and continued to tremble like mercury in Azrael's palm.
—Orhan Pamuk, 2001. My Name Is Red, 176

After so much suffering, a calm came over me. Death did not cause me the
pain I'd feared; on the contrary, I relaxed, quickly realizing that my present
situation was a permanent one, wheras the constraints I'd felt in life were only
temporary. This was how it would be from now on, for century upon century,
until the end of the universe. This neither upset nor gladdened me. Events I'd

once endured briskly and sequentially were now spread over infinite space and existed simultaneously. As in one of those large double-leaf paintings wherein a witty miniaturist has painted a number of unrelated things in each corner—many things were happening all at once.

—Orhan Pamuk, 2001. My Name Is Red, 176–177

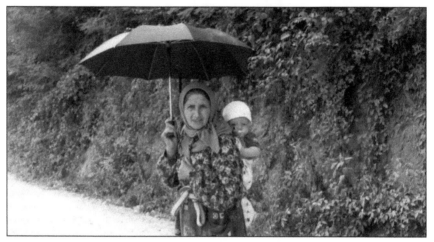

33. Aunty Emine and Timur

Care for the Elderly and Dying

In the traditional family setting, a man and his wife age and eventually die in their own home, cared for by their daughters-in-law and visited by their daughters. With fewer families organized in this manner, many elderly villagers travel to stay with their grown children in order to get access to the superior health care in bigger cities (or even to free care in Germany). During a severe and prolonged illness, or at the end of a person's life, a female family member usually takes charge of caring for a patient, including washing, feeding, and providing company. In the traditional family structure, it is the *gelin*, daughter-in-law, who cares for the ailing parents, and this is considered to be one of the most difficult tasks a *gelin* is bound by duty to perform. Daughters who happen to live nearby may also help with the care of their ailing parents. This task requires enormous effort and patience on the part of the woman who is providing care, and she receives the public accolades of her family and neighbors and is said to be preparing a place for herself in heaven. This personal social and spiritual reward for the *gelin* is in addition to her work as part of a debt the son (her husband) owes to his mother. Cynical observers note that those elders with significant wealth get better care from their family members than those who have nothing.

A serious illness in the family causes all of the traditional family dynamics to come into sharp focus. Traditionally, an older parents would be cared for by their daughters-in-law, who would be living in the same house or close by. Their sons would make sure the financial means are available to get care—to pay for specialists, medicines, and transportation. Married daughters would come when they could, but would be excused if their own family obligations were too pressing or the distance to their homes was great. The situation on the Black Sea Coast now has changed so that few sons live with or close to their parents because they have moved to work in Turkish or European cities. In some families, the daughter-in-law lives with the husband's family while he is away. This situation is considered unfavorable by most *gelins*, who will try to join the husband and escape the village rigors and the control and burden of their parents-in-law. Once the husband has saved up enough to support a family in the new place, and once the *gelin* has had a baby or two, she usually goes to join him. When a young woman and her family are considering marriage, they closely consider the possible burden of care for the parents of a prospective groom.

The parents, then, in this new arrangement, are left without the traditional source of health care for their old age. If there are several married sons, they will try to get at least one to settle in the village. If they have managed to marry a daughter within the village or nearby, they can usually expect some care from her. Cash money for clinic and hospital treatment become easier to obtain as the children move away for salaried jobs, but the traditional, at home attention and care (*ilgi*), is increasingly hard to secure.

Women's Roles at a Time of Death in the Family

Women, especially the *gelins*, are held most responsible for the care of the dying. This customary insistence that the *gelin* performs the difficult tasks associated with serious illness is not unquestioned by the women themselves. While most *gelins* will help in the care of their elderly in-laws, they also are known to resist through various means such as public complaints, private negotiations with their husbands, stalling or ignoring requests, attempts to separate households by moving away, and the extremely serious option of withholding forgiveness as a tyrannical parent-in-law is dying. Forgiveness is not considered a paramount virtue in the local belief system, and a *gelin* who has been abused by her in-laws can display her resistance in this locally acceptable way. She may say: "*Bana yaptıklarını af etmem.*" ("I will not forgive what you have done to me."), "*Hakımı helal etmem.*" ("I will never forgive what you owe to me."), or "*Öbür dünyada yakana yapışacağım.*" ("I will grab onto your collar in the next world."). This implies that the dying person will face punishment for her or his sins after death.

Functions to be performed by women at a time of death include sitting up with the body for one night, washing and performing the ritual ablutions for the body of a female relative in preparation for burial, lamenting at the home of the deceased, preparation of food for those visiting to pay respects to the family, and informal discussion of the life of the deceased, including attempts to gain forgiveness for any debts or slights. These duties are performed by all of the women in the family together, with the behaviors of daughters, *gelin*s, and other relatives carefully monitored for appropriateness of respect, grieving, and statements made during lamentation.[1] The bodies of male family members are usually washed by male relatives or ritual experts. When the body is taken from the home of the deceased, the women mourners stay within the yard of the household while the men accompany the coffin in a procession to the graveyard.

The integration of the area into the national and international cash economy means that people are increasingly turning to paid professionals to do the most difficult tasks, including care for the bed-ridden, the preparation of the corpse, and sometimes even ritual lamenting. Visiting the graves of relatives and performing at least the basic prayers is still considered family duty and is performed periodically even by those who practice few other Muslim rituals and prayers. Grave visiting is also an occasion which prompts even the

---

1. Distinctive semi-musical descending tones of women's laments, speaking eloquently, often in improvised rhyme, of both the good and bad aspects of the life and character if the deceased, have been observed in diverse Black Sea cultures, including Russian and Georgian. For an ethnomusicological examination of Russian laments, see Margarita Mazo, (1994) "Wedding Laments in North Russian Villages." in *Music Cultures in Contact.* edited by Margaret Kartomi and Stephen Blum. Basel: Gordon and Breach Science Publishers: 21–40. and Margarita Mazo, (1994) "Lament Made Visible: A Study of Paramusical Features in Russian Laments." in *Theme and Variations. Writings on Music in Honor of Rulan Chao Pian.* edited by Bell Yung and Joseph Lam. Harvard University and the University of Hong Kong: 164–212. Funeral lamenting is currently practiced in Medreseönü, but I observed that people critique the ability of contemporary mourners, remembering better practices in the past, and cast doubt on the motives of mourners. This type of critique is, of course, often a part of the preservation of culture, and may not reflect an actual degradation of the tradition. The general trends away from oral culture toward literate and mass media culture, however, may leave little room for such traditional forms of improvisation.

most avowedly secular women to make a gesture toward covering their heads in public.

DEATH IN GURBET

In Fakir Baykurt's novel of Turkish workers in Germany, the main protagonist, a middle-aged widow named Kezik Acar, needs to find a way to balance her obligations to her homeland and husband buried there with the growing reality that her children will not be leaving Germany for Turkey. She goes with her children and their partners and children to visit the overseer of a German graveyard:

> *Müdür Beyefendi, biz Duisburg'ta kalıcıyız. Birkaç yıl önce ev aldık. Çocuklarımın eşi, arkadaşı Alman. Okullarını bitirip burada iş alacaklar. Torunlarım burada büyüyecek. Gerçekte ben kendim dönmeyi düşünüyordum. Varıp kocamın yanına uzanacaktım. Çocuklar, torunlar burada kalınca, ben de kalmaya kara verdim. Artık buraya gömüleceğim. Kocamı bu yüzden getirmek istiyorum. Park gibi gömütlüklerinizin köşesinde yan yana yatarız ...*" (p. 45)

Mr. Manager, sir, we are here in Duisburg for good. A few years ago we bought a house. My children's wife and boyfriend are German. They are going to finish school and get jobs here. My grandchildren will grow up here. Actually, I was thinking about going back myself. I was going to go back and stretch out beside my husband (in the next grave). With the children and the grandchildren staying, I decided to stay. I'll be buried here instead. This is why I want to bring my husband. We will lie side by side in some corner of your park-like graveyard.

This scene shows the adjustments made necessary because of labor migration, and shows that, for this character, the familial duties of visiting the grave and the wish to be buried in proximity as a family are chosen in preference to any sense of attachment to a particular piece of land in Turkey. The sense of "homeland" seems to have shifted as the permanent location of the family shifted. The concept of "return" loses its strength for this woman because her priorities are with her children and grandchildren. It is possible to argue that this type of loyalty to family over land fits the traditional role of *gelin* particularly well, as if the move to Germany is just a typical move to the husband's residence. The body of the husband, then, seems to his widow to be misplaced. Further study of male discourse about the proper place for burial would be needed to understand if it differs from this story of female priorities in *gurbet*.

The most poignant songs about *gurbet* come when return is impossible. The following song reflects the agony of a fatally ill person in a foreign country. The presence of a doctor, even the head doctor of a hospital, brings no relief for the suffering heart of the patient.

> *Hastahane önünde incir ağcı*
> *Doktor bulamadı bana ilacı*
> *Baş talip geliyor yaramdan acı*
> *Hasta düştüm yüreğime dert oldu*
> *Ellerin vatanı bana yurt oldu*
> *Mezarımı kazın bayıra düze*
> *Yönünü çevirin sıladan yüze*
> *Benden selam söyleyin sevdiğinize*
> *Başına koysun karalar ağlasın*
> *Gurbet elde kaldım diye ağlasın*
> *Garip kaldım yüreğime dert oldu*
> *Ellerin vatanı bana yurt oldu*

A fig tree in front of the hospital
The doctor could find no medicine for me
The head doctor is coming, more painful than my wound
I fell ill, my heart is troubled
The foreigners' land has become my residence
Dig my grave anywhere, steep or flat
Just so it faces my homeland
Tell the one you love I send my greetings
Let her wear black and weep
Let her cry because I remained in gurbet
I stayed a stranger, my heart is troubled
The foreigners' land has become my residence

—Hastahane Önünde
Anonymous, sung by Volkan Konak, on *Maranda*, 2003

The refrain for each line of the song is *annam* (mother) with the last few syllables repeated, suggesting that the mother is being addressed as the one to hear the suffering of the patient. In typical poetic multivalence, the one who is to mourn the death of the singer could be the beloved, the mother, or anyone back at home.

*****

As her health declined, Aunty Emine went to a private doctor in Ordu. She had been feeling faint, tired and overworked. She had pains in her left side and in her leg. She was worried about her age and the constant worry of tending a milk cow. Because her son agreed to pay for her trip to a doctor, she made the full-day expedition and arranged to stay with her daughter for the night in Ordu. Dr. Deniz found high blood pressure, high cholesterol, and congestive heart failure. He prescribed dietary and lifestyle restrictions, three kinds of pills to be taken morning, noon, and night, and three injections. She bought the expensive medications in the pharmacy below the doctor's office. Aunty Emine had a woman in her daughter's apartment building give her the first shot before leaving Ordu. The second shot was given at the Medreseönü health clinic by a clinic nurse the following day, when Aunty Emine returned from Ordu. She had the third shot given by a woman in her home village of Gebeşli. The woman had to be persuaded because the previous shot she had given to someone else had caused a severe reaction necessitating a rushed trip to the Fatsa hospital. To understand the prescription medications, Aunty Emine had one of her granddaughters read the print on the pill bottles as she memorized the pills by their shape and color. As for the dietary restrictions and the admonishment by the doctor to sell her cow, they were slowly adapted into her life. She was canny about the value of her cow as a meat animal, and refused to sell it for almost a year, waiting for the price to go up. From the U.S., all we could do was ask her to take care and send money for medications.

Aunty Emine died in February of 2003, after a series of strokes, visits to doctors in Samsun and Ordu, and quadruple by-pass surgery in Ankara in August of 2002. Her family gathered around as each crisis unfolded, all trying to get the best care possible for her. The stress of the travel and inconvenience required to get recommended medical treatments compounded the hardships of heart disease for Aunty Emine. She had to endure long journeys by car and ambulance, prolonged hospital stays, and extended visits to various relatives, including her daughters. With her sons all in *gurbet*, Aunty Emine had lost the basic traditional source of comfort in her old age, the ministrations of a *gelin*. She herself had cared for her husband's parents in turn as they aged and passed on, but the new systems deprived her of the old *ilgi* while substituting a modern clinical *ilgi* which was expensive, physically torturous, carelessly administered, and difficult to obtain. After years of marriage and the raising of seven children to adulthood, she had become the central figure in the health care of her family and community. She knew she would be buried and remembered in her husband's village, but she wished to be buried on the side of the graveyard near the road which led back up the mountain to natal home. In this, she attained her desire.

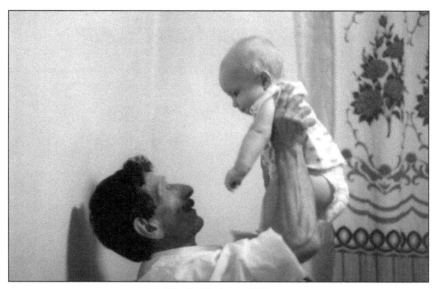

34. Uncle Ferit and Timur

Uncle Ferit passed on in late November of 2004, in his mid 80s, and is buried next to Aunty Emine. May they both rest in peace.

*****

CONCLUSIONS

It is my hope that this research will contribute to the recently expanding academic literature on health care systems. It can add to the ethnographic literature on Turkish culture, especially because Black Sea culture has been studied far less than Anatolian Turkish culture. As a case study on Turkish women, it will increase the number of specific and in-depth studies of women in modern Muslim culture, studies which are needed to counter popular stereotypes about Muslim women which have caused misunderstanding and hostility between Western countries and the Middle East. On another level, I believe that if the dynamics of the interactions between traditional and clinical medicine in one local setting can be understood, then the communication between patients and healers in a variety of settings may be improved for the benefit of all concerned. Folklorists in the United States have recently become involved in helping hospitals negotiate the treatment of patients from widely differing cultural backgrounds and individual life stories.

Hufford (1995b) advocates cultural training for medical students with the assumption that "the social, cultural and psychological aspects of human diversity can be as important to accurate diagnosis and effective care as are the biological facts of health and disease." As patients ourselves, it is important to realize that clinical medicine has its own culture, which varies in different local contexts and times, and this culture is always forced to interact with the medical cultures and expectations of patients. This book aims to contribute to a growing awareness of the complex relationships between traditional and clinical medicine by examining health care in one agricultural region of Turkey. I hope I have been able to show that both traditional and clinical medicine provide culturally-mediated explanations and treatments for illness, and that the cultures of all individuals and groups involved are important in providing the best care for patients. As in any cross-cultural encounter, the potential for misunderstanding exists alongside the potential for new understanding. My goal was to describe the interactions between traditional and clinical healing practices in such a way as to facilitate understanding on personal, inter-personal, and academic levels.

Often, as I went around the villages, I would be looked over by an elderly woman trying to see whom I resembled. I would feel included and accepted if she exclaimed that I looked just like so-and-so, because I knew that she was finding a way to make me part of the family, part of the "web of mutual support" described by White (1994). Likewise, I hope that this work will be examined by those older and wiser than I and be found to have a family resemblance to the work of the scholars and the thoughts of the people I like to consider as my relations. As Hufford (1995a) puts it:

> Life experience must coexist and share authority with technical expertise in order for a society to develop and maintain a rich and human view of itself and the world in which it lives. Folk belief traditions are an enormous and invaluable resource for this process. With the wisdom that they offer, we have the capacity to enrich our lives without rejecting the benefits that have come with scientific and technical progress....the problem of the modern world is not too much intellectual activity and reasoning, and science and rational analysis do not contradict basic spiritual beliefs. The problem is a too-narrow view of what intellectual activity is and who has the capacity to reason soundly. Folklore as a field has the capacity to help our society find more democratic ways of sharing cultural authority. (40)

✳✳✳✳✳

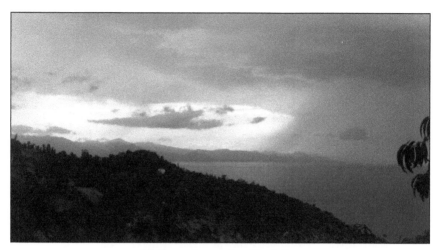

35. Sunset over the Black Sea

Having approached Medreseönü by bus at dawn, I'd like to conclude my description of the place by sitting under the pine trees, overlooking the sea at sunset. The little hill-crest with pine trees, called Çamlık (pine-treed), is one of the few places around not actually cultivated. There are corn stalks, beans climbing up their poles, and fruit trees coming right up to the grassy crest, of course, but this place has its value without being cultivated. The girls have boisterous picnics here, the boys run away from their chores to flop down on their bellies and wonder what lies over the sea. Even the grownups sometimes take a stroll up here, maybe to check the sky for signs of tomorrow's weather, to remember their childhood, or to send unspoken messages to family far away. The grass is full of wildflowers because the cows are not brought here to graze. The pine trees have a special pungent smell, and give off a strange whistling moan, even in a slight breeze.

As the sun drops lower, the lights of Fatsa come on across the bay. Some small twinkling fishing boats head for harbor, while others head out for night fishing. The corn stalks rustle and mothers call to their children in the distance. The sun turns orange and swells, staining the sea.

I am here in the dusk with two of Nazmiye's daughters. They have been asking me about America and my family. I have been soliciting their help to match name and stories with faces and families. They are patient with me and amused because my mind gets twisted up in the threads of extended family relationships and the local terms for these most important ties. They learn standard Turkish grammar and pronunciation in the local school, and can "translate" local terms for me. They are well-versed in national culture, especially the music and lives of pop stars, because their hilltop house gets good reception and they have at least five channels of TV. Their father also brings home a daily newspaper with national circulation, and they have cut out various articles about health care for me.

One of the girls asks me why I am writing a book about this place, when it will be finished, and what job I will get when I'm done. I tell her that, in America, people are curious about other cultures. That, although we have doctors and clinics and fine hospitals and all sorts of medicines, we wonder about the old ways, when people used to take care of themselves and each other. That I am looking for a kind of meaning, a closeness found in the way an elderly village woman wants to sit up with a sick person, touching her hand, bringing her special tea, discussing what went wrong and how to remedy the problem. I want to describe the difference between the old faith that all health and all illness had a reason, that they were part of God's plan for all people who must live and die, that they fit into a system of shared meaning—and the more recent feeling that doctors don't really know their patients, don't really listen to them or explain carefully to them, that they are experts in taking money, using machines, and giving medicine, but can't explain the flame inside an old woman's chest.

The girls agree that doctors can be expensive, but they know many people who have been helped by them. They worry that I am being too conservative, not giving enough credit to modern advances. The younger sister points out that I like visiting the village, but that I wouldn't want to be stuck here. She reminds me that all the young people talk about is how they are going to get away from the mind-numbing routine of constant chores, lifting, carrying, taking the cows to graze, washing, scrubbing, harvesting, mending, with almost no cash income to show for all that work. They can't even study for school properly, with all the work there is to do—and school or marriage are the only tickets out for the girls—the boys can run away to work in the cities, find a job on a fishing boat, or buy a minibus and start a route along the coast road.

They're glad to help their American *yenge* with her project, they'd love to see a book about their little spot on the Black Sea Coast, but even more, they'd like to know if their *yenge* might find a way to bring them away from the village, even to America. To them, young and optimistic, the promise of modernization is a golden one. The local clinic may have some faults, but that is just because it lacks resources. If one doctor's recommendations are not helpful, there must be a better doctor, in a bigger city, whose treatments would be. The old ways are nice, comforting, more spiritual, and sometimes better, but they are fading, becoming objects of nostalgia, dying as the older generation passes away, as it must be in this age of progress.

Sitting under the pine trees on a grassy hill scattered with wildflowers, it is easy to romanticize the village. I love the fresh milk, the fruits, the vegetables, the clean air. I want my son to know his family, his language, his culture, and his place here. I haven't been poor, I haven't worked hard to produce my own crops, I haven't lost family members to childbirth, accidents at sea, infection, war, or hunger. I come for the weddings, make a show of helping out, spend some dollars, and leave before the first frost. My family and friends in Medreseönü are praying for the success of my work, they send me home with mulberry syrup, hand-knit sweaters, and advice on how to cool a feverish baby. We speak by telephone on the holidays, and they know they can call on us if some emergency arises.

With this work, I have hoped to show a vibrant and active culture and community, in which Muslim women of all ages are actively creating, molding, changing, and improving their own health care system, so that it will continue to work for their community as it changes and grows. I have tried to depict village life on the Black Sea Coast of Turkey at the end of the twentieth and beginning of the twenty-first century, showing real people with real concerns. I have tried to show how I learned what I never would have known without becoming a part of this family, of this world; and I hope my descriptions reflect my respect for those who taught me.

This talk is like stamping new coins. They pile up,
While the real work is done outside
By someone digging in the ground.

—Rumi #617, from Open Secret

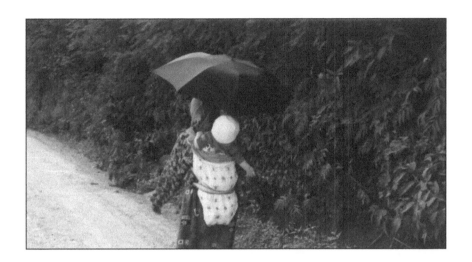

Glossary of Turkish Terms

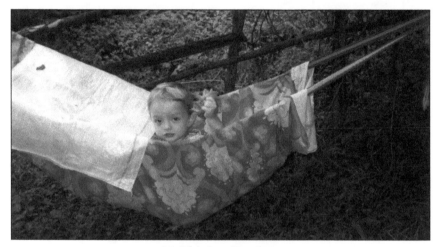

36. This is a Hazelnut

Words for People

Açık
uncovered, a woman not wearing a headscarf, literally "open"

Ağabey
older brother, can be used as a term of respect for a non-relative

Almancı
this word combines the word for German: Alman with the professional ending, with the literal result being something like "Germanist" but which means one who migrated to Germany or Europe for work

Amca
uncle, can be used as a term of respect for an older non-relative

Anne/Anna
mother

Annem/Annam	my mother, used when addressing one's own mother or mother-in-law
Aşık	folk poet or minstrel
Bey	title for a man, used with a given name or professional title
Buralı değil	"not from here" or someone who comes from elsewhere, perhaps now living locally
Damat	son-in-law, groom
Delikanlı	a young man (sometimes a young woman), literally "crazy-blooded"
Doktor	clinical doctor
Dul kadın	widow or divorced woman
Ebe	midwife
Evliya	saint
Gelin	(from gelmek: to come): the one who comes, the bride
Hacı	a person, male or female, who has performed the hac to Mecca
Hekim	medical doctor, now replaced by "doktor"
Hemşire	nurse, based on a word for sister
Hoca	religious expert of a village. In the villages I studied, this was a man assigned by the state, who came from another region, and who administered the activities at the local mosque, taught Koran school for children, and performed the call to prayer five times each day.
Kapalı	head-scarf wearer, literally "closed," "covered"
Kız	girl, daughter, virgin
Kocakarı	old woman
Köy ebesi	village midwife, not trained in a school
Lokman hekim	herbalist
Nine	(pronounced Nee-neh) a diminutive used for a grandmother

Oğlan	boy, youth
Oğul	son
Tanıdık	aquaintance
Teyze	aunt, can be used as a term of respect for an older non-relative
Yabancı	foreigner, could be from another town or from another country
Yar	sweetheart, used in poetry and song
Yenge	a woman married into the family who is older than oneself

PLACE NAMES

Gecekondu	shanty town on city outskirts
Köy	village
Mahalle	neighborhood
Merkez	city center
Varoş	suburb
Yayla	the upland summer pastures used by animal herders

CULTURAL CONCEPTS

Aman	mercy
Aptes	ritual ablution
Arabesk	a style of music associated with rural migrants and their problems of longing
Ayaz	frost, a time when Granny processes herbal remedies
Ayrılık	separation, a cause of suffering
Bakmak	to look at, to look after someone
Bismillahirrah-manirrahim	The Arabic prayer 'In the name of God, the Compassionate, the Merciful,' used as a prayer for beginning any project, journey, meal, prayer, healing technique, etc.

Cin	pronounced jin, a "genie" or supernatural being that lives on earth
Devlet	the State
Devlet Baba	"Father State"
Divan şiiri	Ottoman classical poetry
Ecinni	Arabic plural of cin, in Turkish it is an entirely negative type of being
Ezan	the call to prayer, heard five times per day, also the first thing whispered into a baby's ear at birth
Garip	strange, lonely, forlorn, living in a foreign land
Gunah	sin
Gurbet	exile, wandering, separation, loneliness, migration to work far from home
Hac	(pronounced "haj") the pilgrimage to Mecca, required of any Muslim who can afford it once in a lifetime
Hava	weather or air, often used by Granny to describe the sense of relief from pain
Helal etmek	to renounce claims or forgive wrongs, particularly at a funeral
Himaye	patriarchal patronage, protection or support
Hortlak	a horrible, tormented, unhappy soul that can wander the earth
İdare etmek	to manage, get by in life, to survive on minimum effort
İlgi	care, concern, interest
İlgi göstermek	to show interest, concern
İmam-Hatip Okulu	A state religious school
İyi niyetli	well intentioned (said about a person)
İzin	patriarchal permission

Karabasma	a night-mare, "old hag" that causes night paralysis, literally "black pressing"
Maşallah	"Wonder of God" said to ward off nazar
Melek	angel
Muska	protective amulet, often containing a written prayer and worn on the person
Nazar	the 'evil eye'
Nazar duası	prayer against the 'evil eye'
Niyet	intention
Peri	fairy
Peştemal	traditional waist wrap, usually striped and showing regional distinction
Ruh	spirit, ghost, but literally "soul"
Sevap	a good deed, merit towards the afterlife
Sini	round table top tray traditionally used to eat while seated on the floor
Temiz kalplı	clean hearted (said about a person)
Tesettür	Islamically-marked modest dress as worn by urban women
Torpil	pull, influence, social connections
Uğraşmak	to struggle, to work hard, to strive
Yalnızlık	lonliness, a cause of suffering
Yayla	summer highland pastures

Words about Traditional Medicine

Batıl inançlar	superstitions
Boş	empty, futile
Eski işler	old stuff, old ways
Geleneksel tedavileri	traditional remedies
Geri kafalı	retarded, backward

Kocakarı ilaçları	old woman's medicine
Kocakarı inançları	old woman's beliefs
Köy işleri	village stuff, village ways
Ottan, yandan ilaç	herbal, local medicines
Saçma sapan	ridiculous
Uyduruk	made-up, false

Words about Clinical Medicine

Devlet Hastanesi	State-run hospital
Doktor işi	doctor stuff, doctor business
Doktor Moktor	as in the Yiddish 'Doctor Schmoctor' a sign of disparagement
Hastane işi	hospital stuff, hospital business
Özel oda	private room in a hospital or clinic
Sağlık Ocağı	Health Clinic
Sigorta Hastanesi	Welfare hospital, State hospital
Tıp Fakültesi	Medical School

Ritual Celebrations and Social Events

Altın günü	women's credit rotation party
Düğün	wedding
Gelin Gezdirmek	"to take the bride around" the way a mother-in-law introduces her new daughter-in-law to the female society of the village
Gelin Görmeye Gitmek	"to go to see the bride" semi-formal visits to the home of a new gelin

İmece (sometimes meci) communal work, most commonly a group of
women performing agricultural tasks or a group of
men undertaking the construction of a building or
road.

Kabul günü women's credit rotation party

Kına Gecesi henna night, the female send-off party for the bride

Lohusa Zamanı the forty days after giving birth, in which the new
mother and baby must be careful

Mevlûd a reading of Süleyman Çelebi's Mevlidi Şerif, a four-
teenth-century Turkish poem on the birth of the
Prophet Muhammed. A mevlûd is generally held in a
home, as a family commemorates the fortieth day
after a death of a loved one, or gives thanks for the
granting of a prayer, also Mevlit, the contemporary
spelling for the poem and the night of the birth
(Redhouse Dictionary) or Mawlid (from the Arabic)

Nikâh marriage ceremony, often refers to the religious ceremony which is not recognised by civil law

Sünnet Düğünü circumcision celebration (lit.: circumcision wedding)

Zikir/Zikr Sufi ritual of remembrance of God

MEDICAL TERMS

Acı pain

Afiyet health, eating or drinking with pleasure

Aşı vaccination, vaccine

Ateş fire, fever

Bunalmak to feel smothered, oppressed, depressed

Çare cure, remedy, antidote

Çekmek to suffer, endure, to pull

Çıkık displaced joint tendon or muscle

Çıldırmak to lose one's mind, go mad

Deli	insane, crazy
Derman	cure, medicine, energy
Dert	problem, trouble, sickness, complaint, worry, disease
Divane	mad, crazy with love
Düşük	miscarriage, abortion
Grip	flu, influenza
Güneş çarpması	sunstroke
Hal	condition, state
Hasta	the word means "ill" and also the "person who is ill" i.e. the patient
Hastalık	illness
Hava çalması	catching a cold
Isıtma	heating, warming, sometimes fever
İçi yanmak	to be very thirsty, deeply grieved
İğne	needle, shot, syringe
İlaç	medicine
Kalp	heart problems
Kırık	fracture
Kırıkçıkıkçı	specialist in treating breaks, fractures, and displacements
Kis	cyst
Kolonya	cologne, often lemon-scented, used to sterilize
Kurşun dökmek	to pour lead, a diagnostic procedure and treatment for nazar
Kurt	parasitic worm
Kurt dökmek	to pass a worm, literally 'to drop a worm'
Mecnun	crazed by love, insane
Merhamet	mercy, compassion, pity
Mide bulantısı	nausea
Mide çekmek	pulling the stomach, the remedy for a fallen stomach

Mide düşmesi	the falling of the stomach
Mide düşüklüğü	ailment caused by a fallen stomach
Mide üşümesi	stomach flu
Mikrop	microbe or annoying pest
Mum dökmek	to pour wax, a diagnostic procedure and treatment for nazar
Özel oda	private room in a hospital or clinic
Perhiz	restricted diet prescribed by a doctor
Perişan	wretched, miserable, regretful
Pislik	filth, can be a cause of illness
Ruh hastası	person suffering from mental illness, literally 'soul sickness'
Ruh hastalığı	mental illness, literally 'soul sickness'
Sancı	cramp, gripping pain
Sızı	ache
Sigorta	insurance
Sigorta Hastanesi	free State-run hospital
Solucan	parasitic worm
Şeker	diabetes, literally 'sugar'
Şifa	recovery of health
Tansiyon	hypertension
Tenya	parasitic worm
Teselli	consolation, comfort, solace
Tıp Fakültesi	medical school
Tutmak	lit: "to hold" for the bones to knit back together
Üşümek	to feel cold
Üşütmek	to catch a chill
Yağ	cholesterol, literally 'fat' or 'oil'
Yara	wound
Yaramaz	naughty, (a food that is) bad for one
Zayıf	weak, thin, puny

BODY LANGUAGE

Bağır	bosom, breast, heart, bowels
Bağırsak	intestine
Can	soul, life, vitality
Ciğer	liver, the classical seat of the emotions
Et	flesh
Gerdan	upper chest, breast (an important place to keep covered to avoid catching a cold)
Göğüs	breast
İç	insides, innards (often "bleeding" or "constricted" in poetry and song)
Kalp/gönül/yürek	heart
Kemik	bone
Mide	stomach
Rahim	womb
Yumurta	egg, ovum

FOOD USED FOR HEALTH

Acı bakla suyu	broth of tonka bean
Ayran	yogurt with water and salt
Ayva	quince
Ayva Yaprağı	quince leaf
Bal	honey
Can Bebe	brand name of a sweet white cookie enriched with vitamins and minerals, used mixed with cow's milk to feed babies
Defne	laurel
Fırın ekmeği	bakery bread, made with bleached wheat flour
Gıda	nourishment, nutrition

Helva	sweet confection made with sesame oil and various grains
Ihlamur	linden (the flowers of the tree are used as tea)
Isırgan otu	stinging nettle
Karanfil	carnation, sometimes clove
Keşkek	a dish made of pounded wheat and broth, served at weddings and mevlûds
Komposto	beverage made from stewed fruit, often plum
Lahana tohumu	in standard Turkish, collard green seeds
Limon	lemon
Mısır ekmeği	corn bread
Nar kabuğu	pommegranate skin
Pancar	(in standard Turkish) sugar beet, (in the Black Sea Region) collard greens
Pancar tohumu	(in Black Sea Turkish) collard green seeds
Pekmez	molasses made from mulberry (most common in the Black Sea region) or grape
Pelin otu	wormwood, absinthe
Pilav	cooked rice dish
Süt	milk
Şerbet	a sweet drink, often of stewed fruit and sugar
Taflan	cherry laurel

Appendix on Local History and Ethnicity

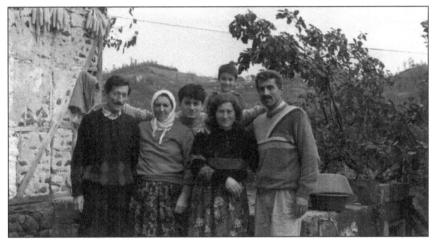

37. The Bearers of Local History

History

The history of the area includes early mention of the Hittites, Thracians, Phrygians, and the colony of Miletus. Coveted by the Seljuk and Ottoman Turks in turn, the region was the last stronghold of the Byzantine Empire, under the Pontic Greeks, after the fall of Constantinople. It was under brief Mongol and Timurid rule until finally coming under Ottoman rule in 1461. Ordu, the capital of the province called Ordu which includes the villages described in this book, is flanked by Sinop and Samsun to the west and Giresun and Trabzon to the east. It grew from a small castle with a surrounding village to a city only in the 19th century. After a big fire in 1883, the city was rebuilt with a new plan which, more or less, remains the basic outline of the city today. Archaeological evidence, including recent underwater exploration off of Sinop, shows that the Black Sea coastal region of Asia Minor was often better connected by water to other parts of the coastline than across the mountains into the Anatolian interior.

The geography of the Black Sea coast of Turkey has determined its economic relations with other lands. Meeker (2002) explains the links between land, water, and the human occupations of the region:

> As homelands, the valleys were not what they first appeared to be, motley groups of people living in isolated hamlets dispersed across the landscape. The valleys were instead transit systems whose inhabitants had a large stake in the security of the people, animals, and goods moving through them....each valley system comprised an integrated social network....the peoples of the coastal region, densely settled and agriculturally impoverished, were also oriented toward outside markets of all kinds, for labor, skills, services, and goods. And given the existence of networks of relationships and lines of communication inside their homelands, they were in a position to make their way in the world abroad beyond their coastal valleys. As a consequence, the rural areas of the coastal valleys have been inhabited for many, many centuries by cash-croppers, soldiers, miners, carpenters, sailors, metal-workers, weavers, rope-makers, dyers, masons, cooks, laborers, and traders, as well as a small minority of extortionists, counterfeiters, smugglers, gunrunners, kidnappers, bandits, pirates, and assassins. The residents of the rural areas have plied all these legitimate and illegitimate activities in their homelands since ancient times, but they have also left their homelands to go abroad as migrants when there was an opportunity to do so. Similarly, just as these rural societies have been oriented to external market conditions, so, too, outsiders were always in a position to become insiders among them. Certain kinds of "specialists" have always infiltrated the coastal region when they had something to offer its resident peoples. (note 27) Among them we find animal transporters, religious teachers, military officers, stone-layers, wood-carvers, metalworkers, shipwrights, and so on. In this respect, the coastal region, which is otherwise completely rural in character, bears a resemblance to an urban center. (96)

Magnarella (1998) also connects geography with economic choices available to Black Sea coastal residents:

> Historically the rugged topography had limited agriculture, and alternative land based industries have been virtually absent. Hence many

Black Sea men have had to search abroad for work. Owing to their legendary reputations for seaworthiness and bravery, they were eagerly recruited into the Roman, Byzantine, and Ottoman armies and navies. They are still actively sought out by the Turkish navy and merchant marine. Black Sea men have also emigrated to major cities in the Ottoman Empire, Persia, Russia and Poland to work as cooks, bakers, restauranteurs, and pastry chefs. After earning their "fortunes," many have returned to their Black Sea villages to retire. Others have stayed in their newly found homes, establishing families and passing business on to their sons. Today every Turkish city and many European ones have at least one bakery, pastry shop or restaurant run by Black Sea men from Turkey. (178)

Neal Ascherson (1995) describes, in the accessible style of a scholar-journalist, the history of the peoples all around the Black Sea, and outlines the effects of twentieth-century nationalism on the Pontic Greeks, the Lazi, and other Black Sea peoples. Charles King's history of the Black Sea (2004) gives a succinct summary of the history of names in the region (including the various theories for the choice of "black" to name the sea). This book is an extensive yet readable history of the region from the mythical times of Hercules and Jason with his Argonauts, through the history of Herodotus and memoirs of Ovid, the impact of Scythians, Persians, Khazars, Arabs, and Slavs, the economic colonies of Genoese and Venetians, the Empires of the Byzantines, Seljuks, Mongols, Comneni, Ilkhanids, and Ottomans—all the way through the upheavals of the twentieth century and the contemporary political, environmental, and economic challenges of the present day. King notes that, at the turn of the twentieth century, travelers to the region, expecting to find examples of various "races," "…instead found individuals and communities for who plural identities and mixed cultures were the norm." As the century progressed, however, "it was the idea of the timelessly pure nation that eventually won out, often with tragic results." (191) King's account of Russian, Bulgarian, and Romanian writings of the period clearly shows that Turkey was not the only nation of the Black Sea in which "the theories of ethnic purity and religious piety being expounded by poets and historians were… sorely at odds with the multifarious reality of the coast." (204) His section "The Unpeopling" addresses the tragic consequences of the ideologies of national, religious, and racial purity as played out upon the Black Sea peoples.

War with Russia and the nationalist struggles in the Caucasus had a strong impact on the Black Sea Coast. Elders in the area I studied remembered the difficult times at the turn of the twentieth century. For example, Aunty Emine's father spent seven years as a prisoner of the Russians before walking home to join the nationalist army of Mustafa Kemal. An gripping and thorough history of the struggles between Russia and the Turks during this period can be found in Bülent Gökay's *A Clash of Empires: Turkey between Russian Bolshevism and British Imperialism, 1918–1923* (1997).

In the First World War, Pontic Greeks in the area agitated for a restoration of an independent Greek state, aided in turn by the Russians, Armenians, and British who had various interests in the area. An army sent from Ankara in 1921 put an end to these efforts. Greek presence in the area of my research survives mainly in the local good-natured admission that Greek blood (as well as Circassian, Georgian, Armenian, Laz, and various other types) runs in the veins of many.

In terms of primary sources from the difficult war years, Sonyel (1993) cites a report on the condition of the Muslim population of the Black Sea coast that Ameer Ali of the British Red Crescent Society forwarded in 1916 to Lord Robert Cecil and the Russian press. The report was made by M. Philips Price, who had seen the area before the war and had at that point been in the region for eight months. His report claimed that the eighteen months of warfare had left the Turkish and Laz peasantry in a "lamentable state." (416)

It was difficult for me to solicit historical information about the area, in part because of the sensitivity of issues of ethnicity and nationalism, but mainly because I did not have the occasion to spend time with the older men who tell historical stories, usually while sitting in the all-male environment of the coffeehouse. Fortunately, Michael Meeker (2002) has published the results of more than forty years of ethnographic research done in this type of male setting on the Black Sea Coast. Although the local history he solicited is centered to the East of my research area, many of the social constructs he describes are similar in basic outline to those common in the villages in Ordu province. In fact, the male informant I was closest to, Uncle Ferit, comes from a family that moved to their current location from Sürmene, which falls within Meeker's region of study, during the war with Russia at the turn of the twentieth-century.

The Cold War division of the Black Sea nations into opposing camps violated the historical connectivity of that body of water. Family histories prove the not-so-distant interactions across and around the sea. For instance, Aunty Emine's family background is at least partly Circassian (*Çerkez*). Meeker's inclusion of gunrunning and smuggling in the list of centuries-old activities in the coastal regions fits with local lore about the weapons smuggled from the Soviet Union and used in the communist insurrection and defense of Fatsa in 1979. The "Fatsa incidents" were a serious affront to the ideology of national unity and to the Cold War anti-Communist, pro-NATO rhetoric of the Turkish government. The severe military reaction from Ankara to these events naturally tempers the local telling of history, and yet the "Fatsa incidents" validate Meeker and Magnarella's claims for long-standing trade and communications across the water. With the end of the Cold War era, the older connections reasserted themselves, bringing a rush of enterprising shuttle traders and opening the doors for new types of interpersonal relations (such as unregulated prostitution and modern forms of banditry) which paid no heed to purity of morals or ethnicity. Slowly these informal relations have been settling into more formal types of regional economic cooperation. In the villages examined in this book, several families in the area "remembered" their Georgian heritage as soon as the Soviet Union collapsed, some even turned out to have language skills which allowed them to communicate with Georgians coming across the border to trade.

ETHNICITY

Ethnic identification has been a tricky issue on the Black Sea Coast (as well as in the rest of Turkey) since the end of the heterogeneous Ottoman Empire and the start of the Turkish nation state, which was conceived as a nation of Turks. Many top-down efforts to homogenize the population were implemented, from the severity of massacres and forced migrations, to attempts to re-write the history of Kurds so that they would be seen as "mountain Turks" rather than as a separate ethnic group. On the Black Sea Coast, historically a mixed area where many ethnic groups have lived side-by-side for centuries, most people today automatically call themselves Turks, although they accept the humorous (and incorrect) stereotypical reference to all Black Sea dwellers as "Laz" and make light of their own mixed blood. In other words, ethnic identity is only fore grounded when it is rhetorically important to emphasize difference from Europeans, Arabs, Greeks, or others, usually in a political discussion. Recently, the distinction between Kurds and Turks has been very much in public debate, both in the Turkish media and in local places of political talk, such as the coffeehouses. In terms of local identity, however, ethnicity is usually taken for granted.

Despite recent interest and public discussion of ethnic diversity within Turkey, research into ethnohistory yields no simple answers. As Meeker finds:

> The role of non-Turkic peoples in the social history of the Muslim
> population in the eastern Black Sea region was undisputed. The problem was that none of these non-Turkic groups could be considered
> to have been a preponderant influence throughout the coastal dis-

tricts. The Muslim population in this part of Turkey was formed relatively recently out of many different ethnic groups, including peoples of Turkic, Lazi, Kurdish, Greek, and Armenian background. The influence of each of these ethnic groups varied in different parts of the region, from valley to valley as well as from the lower to the upper parts of a single valley." (30)

Diversity in ethnic or religious identity was "smoothed out" as the Turkish nation coalesced at the beginning of the century—non-Muslims, especially Orthodox Christians, were at times exiled or killed, and at times migrated voluntarily or made conscious efforts to blend in. National efforts were required to integrate the many incoming Muslims from the Balkans and the Russian empire, efforts which were never wholly successful. In general terms, however, citizenship in Turkey is spoken of in simple terms conflating Turkish ethnicity and language with Muslim religion. The varieties of Muslim legal schools, differences between Sunni and Alevi sects, as well as tarikat or "dervish lodge" affiliations, which had been so important to public identity in Ottoman times, have recently taken a place in public discussions because of the increase in religious political discourse. For a long period of Republican history, these forms of identity were downplayed in secular education and the national media.

As a part of this simplification of identity, personal names and place names were Turkified to suit the ideology of a singular national ethnicity. For example, just to the east of Fatsa, the town called by the Greek name of Vona (and known as Porta Voon by the Genoese, see Freely, 1996, p. 99), was given the uninspiring name Perşembe, meaning "Thursday," because of its weekly market day.

Magnarella (1974, 1979, 1982 and 1998) has examined various aspects of Turkish Republican cultural change, including an examination of the Hemshin (Hemşin, Hemşinli) and Laz (also Lazuri) of northeastern Turkey and of identity maintenance and assimilation among Georgian communities in Turkey.

Beller-Hann and Hann (2001) have participated in a recent effort to describe the ethnic and linguistic mix present on the Black Sea Coast which has been downplayed during the Republican period under the homogenizing emphasis on Turkish citizenship. New publications have shown that the linguistically and ethnically complex Caucasian region extends quite far into Turkey. Recent ethnographic research by Hovann H. Simonian in the eastern Black Sea Region has turned up fascinating information on the Hemşin, a distinct group of Muslims who speak an Armenian language yet disassociate themselves from Armenian ancestry. (*ISIM Newsletter*, volume 14, June, 2004, pp. 24–25)

Howard Eissenstat, in a chapter "Metaphors of Race and Discourse of Nation," (2005) cites among materials from across Turkey two reports from the Black Sea coast—the 1940 report of a Turkish parliamentarian, which puts the Armenian population of Ordu at 500, and a letter from the Giresun CHP party chief mentioning several Jewish families who had migrated from Thrace and Istanbul, taking "Turkish and Muslim" family names. Eissenstat's chapter shows that the ideologies of race and nation were variously applied in an effort to re-configure the diverse population which had resulted from the break-up of a multi-ethnic empire, a series of regional and international wars, and waves of migration, both voluntary and forced. Discussions of ethnicity in Turkey are always held in a discursive field shaped on the one hand by family and local history and on the other by state ideologies of race and nation. This field is often so fraught with tension that discussion becomes impossible.

Focusing on contemporary village life, my research never aimed to reach certainties about ethnic identity or local history. With the complex local history of national, political, and ethnic battles in this century, most people seem to prefer to skirt historical re-tellings and debates. In contrast to Meeker's study of the male and public discourse which includes local history and is also based on relationships he has forged over decades, this study evolved from a contemporary, female, private, family-at-home social setting.

For those determined to delve into the ethnic mosaic underlying the current map of nations, several sources contain fascinating data. The 1989 volume *Ethnic Groups in the Republic of Turkey*, edited by Peter Alford Andrews with the assistance of Rüdiger Benninghaus contains a wealth of information about forty-seven major ethnic and religious designations. The sections on the Hemşinli, Pontic Greek-speaking Muslims (particularly concentrated in Trabzon), Circassians, Georgians, and Laz contain the most information relevant to the Black Sea region of Turkey. Gypsies are mentioned in Samsun city and Çarşamba town, in the cities of Giresun, Rize, and Zonguldak, as well as scattered villages in Artvin Province. R. Benninghaus is the major source cited in Andrews (1989) on the Hemşinli, Laz, and Pontic Greek-speaking Muslims. His twenty-two page article on the Hemşinli is in German, while his five-page article on the Laz is in English. In the same volume, P. A. Andrews and İ. Aydemir (1974–75) are the major sources listed on the Black Sea Circassians (particularly in Samsun and Sinop), and Batıray Özbek provides a nine-page article in German about them. The scant ethnic information on the towns of Ünye, Fatsa, and Perşembe of Ordu Province seems to indicate that more research is needed in the area. (See Andrews, 1989)

Salahi R. Sonyel's *Minorities and the Destruction of the Ottoman Empire* (1993), put out by the Turkish Historical Society Printing House in Ankara, brings together diverse and often differing sources on the populations in conflict in the period around the First World War. Some sources included are reports to the Paris Peace Conference in 1919, reports by the the Archbishop of Trabzon, and Ottoman Turkish government statistics of the time.

For information on the exchanges of populations, forced migrations, and mortality in Anatolia in the period around the First World War, a useful summary can be found in Erik J. Zürcher's *Turkey: A Modern History* (1993). Zürcher provides the following figures on the exchange of populations between the nations of Greece and Turkey, as mandated by the Treaty of Lausanne in 1923:

Greek Orthodox population sent to Greece: about 900,000 people

Muslims of Greece sent to Turkey: about 400,000 people

He writes that in the ten years between 1913 and 1923, with Anatolia becoming a theater of war in 1915, followed by the Great War and the Turkish War of Independence, "some 2.5 million Anatolian Muslims lost their lives, as well as between 600,000 and 800,000 Armenians and up to 300,000 Greeks. All in all, the population of Anatolia declined by 20 per cent through mortality, a percentage 20 times as high as that of France, which had been the hardest-hit country among the European belligerents in the World War." (Zürcher, 171) Although the Balkan War of 1912–13 had brought hundreds of thousands of Muslim refugees into Anatolia, the larger emigration of Armenians (several hundred thousand) and Greeks meant that the total net loss of Anatolian population by migration alone was about 10 per cent. (Ibid.)

Discussions of ethnicity along the Black Sea coast of Turkey held on the list-serve H-TURK have brought up some interesting resources, including the works of a Pontic Greek writer from Salonika, Yorgo Andreadis, who has four books published about the Pontic experiences of population exchange, in Turkish, through Belge Press in the 1990's (see: www.h-net.org: letter by Michael Meeker, 6 Sept. 2000).

A sampling of recent publications in Turkish includes Mehmet Bilgin's *Doğu Karadeniz: Tarih, Kültür, İnsan/The Eastern Black Sea: History, Culture, Peoples* (Trabzon: Serander Yayınları, 2000), an ethnohistory covering the broad recorded history of the Black Sea coast of Asia Minor, with an emphasis on Trabzon. *Türkiye'nin Etnik Yapısı: Halkımızın Kökenleri ve Gerçekleri/ Turkey's Ethnic Composition: Our People's Roots and Realities*, by Ali Tayyar Önder (İstanbul: Pozitif, 4th printing, 2002), includes short sections about the Çerkez (Circassian), Laz, and Gürcü (Georgian) ethnicities, although most of the book evaluates the identities of various Kurdish and Alevi forms of identification. İbrahim Tellioğlu's *Osmanlı Hakimiyetine Kadar Doğu Karadeniz'de*

Türkler/ Turks in the Eastern Black Sea until the Ottman Rule (Trabzon: Serander Yayıncılık, 2004) is a scholarly work bringing together Turkish, Ottoman, Byzantine, Georgian, Armenian, French, English, and other sources on the pre-Ottoman Turkish period. Using sociological research techniques such as questionaires in two areas of the Eastern Black Sea coast, Ethem Yıldız and Muammer Ak attempt to address globalization and cultral identity in their book *Doğu Karadeniz'de Kültürel Kimlik/ Cultural Identity in the Eastern Black Sea* (İstanbul: Çatı Kitapları, 2002). On the Hemşin, see Ali Gündüz (2002), who includes notes on the Georgians and Laz.

We can expect that stories of identity and belonging will continue to be written and re-written by and about the peoples of the Black Sea littoral as new configurations and political exigencies emerge.

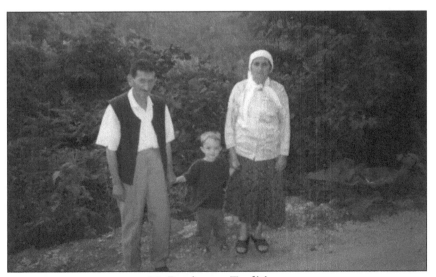

38. Passing on Traditions

BIBLIOGRAPHY

Abadan-Unat, Nermin.
1982. "The Effect of International Labor Migration on Women's Roles: the Turkish Case," in Kağıtçıbaşı, Çiğdem, ed. (with the assistance of Diane Sunar) *Sex Roles, Family, & Community in Turkey*. Bloomington: Indiana University Turkish Studies.
1993. "Impact of External Migration on Rural Turkey," in Stirling, Paul, ed. 1993. *Culture and Economy: Changes in Turkish Villages*. Huntingdon: The Eothen Press.

Abadan-Unat, Nermin, ed.
1982. *Women in Turkish Society*. Leiden: E.J. Brill.

Abou-El-Haj, Rifa'at Ali
1991. *Formation of the Modern State: The Ottoman Empire, Sixteenth to Eighteenth Centuries*. Albany: State University of New York Press.

Abrahams, Roger D.
1976. "The Complex Relations of Simple Forms" in Dan Ben-Amos, ed. *Folklore Genres*. Austin: University of Texas Press, pp. 193–214.

Abu-Lughod, Lila
1986. *Veiled Sentiments: Honor and Society in a Bedouin Society*. Berkeley: University of California Press.
1995. "A Tale of Two Pregnancies" in Ruth Behar and Deborah A. Gordon, eds. *Women Writing Culture*. Berkeley: University of California Press, pp. 339–349.

Acar, Feride
1991. "Women in the Ideology of Islamic Revivalism in Turkey: Three Islamic Women's Journals," in Richard Tapper, ed. *Islam in Modern Turkey: Religion, Politics and Literature in a Secular State*. London: I.B. Tauris & Co. Ltd.

Akşit, Bahattin
1991. "Islamic Education in Turkey: Medrese Reform in Late Ottoman Times and Imam-Hatip Schools in the Republic," in Richard Tapper, *Islam*

in Modern Turkey: Religion, Politics and Literature in a Secular State. London: I.B. Tauris & Co. Ltd.
1993. "Studies in Rural Transformation in Turkey: 1950–1990," in Stirling, Paul, ed. 1993. *Culture and Economy: Changes in Turkish Villages.* Huntingdon: The Eothen Press.

Akşit, Belma
1993. "Rural Health Seeking: Under Fives in Sivas, Van and Ankara," in Stirling, Paul, ed. 1993. *Culture and Economy: Changes in Turkish Villages.* Huntingdon: The Eothen Press.

Althusser, Louis
1970. "Ideology and Ideological State Apparatuses (Notes towards an Investigation)" from *Lenin and Philosophy and Other Essays.* translated by Ben Brewster, New York: Monthly Review Press, 1971.

Anderson, Benedict
1991. *Imagined Communities: Reflections on the Origin and Spread of Nationalism.* revised ed. London: Verso.

Andrews, Peter Alford, compiler and editor
1989. with the assistance of Rüdiger Benninghaus. *Ethnic Groups in the Republic of Turkey.* Wiesbaden: Dr. Ludwig Reichert Verlag.

Andrews, Walter G.
1985. *Poetry's Voice, Society's Song: Ottoman Lyric Poetry.* Seattle: University of Washington Press.
1997. "Ottoman Lyrics: Introductory Essay" in Walter G. Andrews, Najaat Black, and Mehmet Kalpaklı, editors and translators. *Ottoman Lyric Poetry: An Anthology.* Austin: University of Texas Press, pp. 3–23.
2001. "Other Selves, Other Poets and the Other Literary History: An Essay in Three Movements" in Walter Andrews ed., *Intersections in Turkish Literature: Essays in Honor of James Stewart-Robinson,* Ann Arbor: University of Michigan Press.

Andrews, Walter G., Najaat Black, and Mehmet Kalpaklı, editors and translators
1997. *Ottoman Lyric Poetry: An Anthology.* Austin: University of Texas Press.

Andrews, Walter G. and Mehmet Kalpaklı
2005. *The Age of Beloveds: Love and the Beloved in Early-Modern Ottoman and European Culture and Society* Durham North Carolina: Duke University Press

Appadurai, Arjun, Frank J. Korom, and Margaret A. Mills, eds.
1991. *Gender, Genre, and Power in South Asian Expressive Traditions.* Philadelphia: University of Pennsylvania Press.

Apple, Rima D.
1987. *Mothers and Medicine: A Social History of Infant Feeding, 1890–1950*. Madison: University of Wisconsin Press.

Ardener, Shirley and Sandra Burman, eds.
1995 *Money-Go-Rounds: The Importance of Rotating Savings and Credit Associations for Women* Oxford: Berg Publishers.

Ascherson, Neal
1995. *The Black Sea*. New York: Hill and Wang.

Atkinson, Paul
1990. *The Ethnographic Imagination: Textual Constructions of Reality*. London: Routledge.

Başgöz, İlhan
1978. "Folklore Studies and Nationalism in Turkey," in Felix J. Oinas, ed. *Folklore, Nationalism and Politics*. Slavica Publishers, Inc. pp. 123–137.

Bauman, Richard
1984. *Verbal Art as Performance*. Prospect Heights, Illinois: Waveland Press. [1977]

Beeman, William O.
1986. *Language, Status, and Power in Iran*. Bloomington: Indiana University Press.

Bellér-Hann, Ildikó and Chris Hann
2001. *Turkish Region: State, Market and Social Identities on the East Black Sea Coast*. Santa Fe: School of American Research Press.

Bennett, Gillian
1987. *Traditions of Belief: Women, Folklore and the Supernatural Today*. London: Penguin Books.

Benninghaus, Rüdiger
1989. "The Laz: An Example of Multiple Identification" in Peter Alford Andrews, compiler and editor, with the assistance of Rüdiger Benninghaus. *Ethnic Groups in the Republic of Turkey*. Wiesbaden: Dr. Ludwig Reichert Verlag.

Bhabha, Homi K, ed.
1990. *Nation and Narration*. London: Routledge.

Blum, Richard H. and Eva Blum
1965. *Health and Healing in Rural Greece*. Stanford, CA: Stanford University Press.

Boddy, Janice
1989. *Wombs and Alien Spirits: Women, Men, and the Zār Cult in Northern Sudan*. Madison: The University of Wisconsin Press.

Bowen, John R.
1993. *Muslims through Discourse: Religion and Ritual in Gayo Society.* Princeton: Princeton University Press.

Brettell, Caroline B.
1993. *When They Read What We Write: The Politics of Ethnography.* London: Bergin & Garvey.

Briggs, Charles L.
1986. *Learning How to Ask: A Sociolinguistic Appraisal of the Role of the Interview in Social Science Research.* Cambridge: Cambridge U. Press.

Bruner, Edward
1986. "Ethnography as Narrative," in Victor Turner and Edward Bruner, eds. *The Anthropology of Experience.* Urbana: University of Illinois Press, pp. 139–155.

Bourguinon, Erika
1991. *Possession.* Prospect Heights, Illinois: Waveland Press. [1976]

Chittick, William C. and Peter Wilson
1982. Fakhruddin 'Iraqi: *Divine Flashes* (Classics of Western Spirituality with preface by Seyyed Hossein Nasr. Paulist Press Series: Classics of Western Spirituality.

Chock, Phyllis Pease
1986. "The Outsider Wife and the Divided Self: The Genesis of Ethnic Identities," in Phyllis Pease Chock and June R. Wyman, eds. *Discourse and the Social Life of Meaning.* Washington D.C.: Smithsonian Institution Press.

Clifford, James
1988. *The Predicament of Culture: Twentieth-Century Ethnography, Literature, and Art.* Cambridge, MA: Harvard University Press.

Clifford, James and George E. Marcus, eds.
1986. *Writing Culture: The Poetics and Politics of Ethnography.* Berkeley: University of California Press.

Creyghton, Marie-Louise
1992. "Breast-Feeding and *Baraka* in Northern Tunisia," in V. Maher, ed. *The Anthropology of Breast-Feeding: Natural Law or Social Construct?* Oxford: Berg.

Dankoff, Robert
1991. *The Intimate Life of an Ottoman Statesman: Melek Ahmed Pasha (1588–1662) As Portrayed in Evliya Celebi's Book of Travels.* Translated with commentary; Historical Introduction by Rhoads Murphey. Albany: State University of New York Press.

Davis-Floyd, Robbie E.
1993. "The Technocratic Model of Birth" in Susan Tower Hollis, Linda Pershing, and M. Jane Young, eds. *Feminist Theory and the Study of Folklore.*
Urbana: University of Illinois Press.

Delaney, Carol
1991. *The Seed and the Soil: Gender and Cosmology in Turkish Village
Society.* Berkeley: University of California Press.
1993. "Traditional Modes of Authority and Co-Operation," in Stirling,
Paul, ed. 1993. *Culture and Economy: Changes in Turkish Villages.*
Huntingdon: The Eothen Press.

del Valle, Teresa, ed.
1993. *Gendered Anthropology.* London: Routledge.

Dorson, Richard M., ed.
1978. *Folklore in the Modern World.* The Hague: Mouton Publ.

Donaldson, Bess Allen
1938. *The Wild Rue: A Study of Mohammadan Magic and Folklore in Iran*
pp. 13–23 on the evil eye reprinted in Allan Dundes, ed. *The Evil Eye: A
Casebook.* 1992, pp. 66–77.

Doubleday, Veronica
1990. *Three Women of Herat.* Austin: University of Texas Press.

Doumato, Eleanor Abdella
2000. *Getting God's Ear: Women, Islam, and Healing in Saudi Arabia and the
Gulf.* New York: Columbia University Press.

Dube, Leela
1986. "Seed and Earth: The Symbolism of Biological Reproduction and
Sexual Relations of Production," in Leela Dube, Eleanor Leacock, and
Shirley Ardener, eds. *Visibility and Power: Essays on Women in Society and
Development.* Delhi: Oxford University Press.

Dube, Leela, Eleanor Leacock, and Shirley Ardener, eds.
1986. *Visibility and Power: Essays on Women in Society and Development.*
Delhi: Oxford University Press.

Duben, Alan
1982. "The Significance of Family and Kinship in Urban Turkey," in
Kağıtçıbaşı, Çiğdem, ed. (with the assistance of Diane Sunar) *Sex Roles,
Family, & Community in Turkey.* Bloomington: Indiana University Turkish
Studies, pp. 73–99.

Dundes, Alan
1977. "Who Are the Folk?" in William R. Bascom, ed. *Frontiers of Folklore.* Boulder: Westview Press.
1980. "Texture, Text, and Context," in Alan Dundes, ed. *Interpreting Folklore.* Bloomington: Indiana University Press, pp. 20–32.
1992. *The Evil Eye: A Casebook.* Madison: University of Wisconsin Press. [1981]

Dundes, Lauren, ed.
2003. *The Manner Born: Birth Rites in Cross-Cultural Perspective.* Walnut Creek, CA: AltaMira Press.

Early, Evelyn A.
1993. *Baladi Women of Cairo: Playing with an Egg and a Stone.* Lynne Rienner Publ: Boulder & London.

Enloe, Cynthia
1989. *Bananas, Beaches and Bases: Making Feminist Sense of International Politics.* London: Pandora.

Ewing, Katherine
1984. "The Sufi as Saint, Curer, and Exorcist in Modern Pakistan," in E. Valentine Daniel and Judy F. Pugh, eds. *South Asian Systems of Healing.* Contributions to Asian Studies, vol. 17. Leiden: E. J. Brill, pp. 106–114.

Farrer, Claire R., ed.
1986. *Women and Folklore: Images and Genres.* Prospect Heights, Illinois: Waveland Press. (originally published as JAF special issue, 1975)

Feld, Steven
1982. *Sound and Sentiment: Birds, Weeping, Poetics, and Song in Kaluli Expression.* Philadelphia: University of Pennsylvania Press.

Fernea, Elizabeth Warnock
1969. *Guests of the Sheik: An Ethnography of an Iraqi Village.* Garden City, N.Y.: Anchor Books.
1992. "Research on Middle Eastern Women: State of the Art." in Marilyn Robinson Waldman, Müge Galin, and Artemis Leontis, eds. Understanding Women: The Challenge of Cross-Cultural Perspectives. Papers in Comparative Studies, vol. 7, (1991–1992), Columbus: The Ohio State University. pp. 55–79.

Field, Mark G.
1975. "Comparative Sociological Perspectives on Health Systems: Notes on a Conceptual Approach," in Arthur Kleinman, Peter Kunstadter, E. Russell Alexander, and James L. Gale, eds. *Medicine in Chinese Cultures: Compar-*

ative Studies of Health Care in Chinese and Other Societies. Washington D.C.: U.S. Department of Health, pp. 567–587.

Foucault, Michel
1961. *Madness and Civilization: A History of Insanity in the Age of Reason.* trans. by Richard Howard. New York: Vintage Books, 1988.
1963. *The Birth of the Clinic: An Archaeology of Medical Perception.* trans. By A.M. Sheridan Smith. New York: Vintage Books, 1973, 1994.
1966. *The Order of Things: An Archaeology of the Human Sciences.* translator not cited. New York: Vintage Books, 1973.
1969. *The Archaeology of Knowledge and The Discourse on Language.* trans. by A. M. Sheridan Smith and Rupert Sawyer. New York: Pantheon Books, 1972.

Freely, John
1996. *The Black Sea Coast of Turkey.* Istanbul: Redhouse Press.

Geertz, Clifford
1973. *The Interpretation of Cultures.* New York: Basic Books, Inc.
1976. "From the Native's Point of View: On the Nature of Anthropological Understanding," in Keith Basso and Henry Selby, eds., *Meaning in Anthropology,* pp. 221–238. Albuquerque: University of New Mexico Press.
1983. *Local Knowledge: Further Essays in Interpretive Anthropology.* New York: Basic Books.
1984. "Anti Anti-Relativism," *American Anthropologist* 86: 263–278.

Gerson, Elihu
1976. "The Social Character of Illness: Deviance or Politics?" *Social Science and Medicine* 10, pp. 219–224.

Gevitz, Norman, ed.
1988. *Other Healers: Unorthodox Medicine in America.* Baltimore: Johns Hopkins University Press.

Gilmore, David D.
1982. "Anthropology of the Mediterranean Area," *Annual Review of Anthropology* 11, pp. 175–205.

Glassie, Henry H.
1993. *Traditional Turkish Art Today.* Bloomington: Indiana University Press.

Goffman, Erving.
1959. *The Presentation of Self in Everyday Life.* New York: Anchor Books.

Good, Byron J.
1977. "The Heart of What's the Matter: The Semantics of Illness in Iran." *Culture, Medicine and Psychiatry* 1, 25–58.
1994. *Medicine, Rationality, and Experience: An Anthropological Perspective.* Cambridge: Cambridge University Press.

Good, Byron J. and Mary-Jo DelVecchio Good
1989. "Toward a Meaning-Centered Analysis of Popular Illness Categories: "Fright Illness" and "Heart Distress" in Iran" in Anthony J. Marsella and Geoffrey M. White, eds. *Cultural Conceptions of Mental Health and Therapy*. Dordrecht: D. Reidel Publishing Co.
1992. "The Comparative Study of Greco-Islamic Medicine: The Integration of Medical Knowledge into Local Symbolic Contexts," in Charles Leslie and Allan Young, eds. *Paths to Asian Medical Knowledge*. Berkeley: University of California Press. pp. 257–271.

Grima, Benedicte
1992. *The Performance of Emotion Among Paxtun Women: "The Misfortunes Which Have Befallen Me."* Austin: University of Texas Press.Gürsoy-Tezcan, Akile
1991. "Mosque or Health Centre?: A Dispute in a *Gecekondu*," in Richard Tapper, *Islam in Modern Turkey: Religion, Politics and Literature in a Secular State*. London: I.B. Tauris & Co. Ltd.

Hahn, Robert A.
1984. "Rethinking 'Illness' and 'Disease' " in E. Valentine Daniel and Judy F. Pugh, eds. *South Asian Systems of Healing*. Contributions to Asian Studies, Vol. 17. Leiden: E.J. Brill, pp. 1–23.

Hahn, Robert A.
1995. *Sickness and Healing: An Anthropological Perspective*. New Haven: Yale University Press.

Handler, Richard and Jocelyn Linnekin
1984. "Tradition, Genuine or Spurious," *Journal of American Folklore* 97: 273–90.

Hann, C[hris] M.
1990. *Tea and the Domestication of the Turkish State*. Huntingdon, England: Eothen Press.
1993. "The Sexual Division of Labour in Lazistan," in Stirling, Paul, ed. 1993. *Culture and Economy: Changes in Turkish Villages*. Huntingdon: The Eothen Press.

Hann, C[hris]. and I. [Beller]-Hann
1992. "Samovars and sex on Turkey's Russian markets," *Anthropology Today* 8 (4)" 3–6.
1998. "Markets, morality and modernity in north-east Turkey," in T. Wilson and H. Donnan, eds. *Border Identities: Nation and State at International Frontiers*. Cambridge: Cambridge University Press, pp. 237–62.

Heper, Metin
1982. "The Plight of Urban Migrants: Dynamics of Service Procurement in a Squatter Area," Kağıtçıbaşı, Çiğdem, ed. (with the assistance of Diane Sunar) *Sex Roles, Family, & Community in Turkey.* Bloomington: Indiana University Turkish Studies.

Herzfeld, Michael
1986. *Ours Once More: Folklore, Ideology, and the Making of Modern Greece.* New York, NY: Pella Publishing Co.
1987. *Anthropology through the Looking-Glass: Critical Ethnography in the Margins of Europe.* Cambridge: Cambridge University Press..

Hinojosa, Servando Z.
2001. "'The Hands Know': Bodily Engagement and Medical Impasse in Highland Mayan Bonesetting." *Medical Anthropology Quarterly* 16 (1): 1–19.

Hobsbawm, Eric and Terrence Ranger, eds.
1983. *The Invention of Tradition.* New York: Cambridge University Press.

Holbrook, Victoria Rowe
1994. *The Unreadable Shores of Love: Turkish Modernity and Mystic Romance.* Austin: University of Texas Press.

Holden, Pat, ed.
1983. *Women's Religious Experience.* London: Croom Helm.

Hollis, Susan Tower, Linda Pershing, and M. Jane Young, eds.
1993. *Feminist Theory and the Study of Folklore.* Urbana: University of Illinois Press.

Holquist, Michael
1990. *Dialogism: Bakhtin and His World.* London: Routledge.

Homans, H.
1982. "Pregnancy and Birth as Rites of Passage for two groups of Women in Britain," in Carol P. MacCormack, ed. *Ethnography of Fertility and Birth.* London: Academic Press. pp. 231–268.

Hoskins, Janet
1996. "From Diagnosis to Performance: Medical Practice and the Politics of Exchange in Kodi, West Sumba," in C. Laderman and M. Roseman, eds. *The Performance of Healing.* New York: Routledge.

Hufford, David J.
1976. "Ambiguity and the Rhetoric of Belief," *Keystone Folklore* vol. 21, no. 1, pp. 11–24.
1982. *The Terror That Comes in the Night: An Experience-Centered Study of Supernatural Assault Traditions.* Philadelphia: University of Pennsylvania Press.

1983. "Traditions of Disbelief," *New York Folklore Quarterly* 8, Nos. 3–4 (Winter, 1983): 21–30.

1988. "Inclusionism vs. Reductionism in the Study of the Culture-Bound Syndromes," (manuscript, in press, 1988, *for Culture, Medicine, and Psychiatry*) review of Simons and Hughs, *The Culture-Bound Syndromes* (1985).

1995a. "Beings Without Bodies: An Experience-Centered Theory of the Belief in Spirits," in Barbara Walker, ed. *Out of the Ordinary: Folklore and the Supernatural*, pp.10–45.

1995b. Project Description for the "Diversity in Medicine Project," at the Penn State College of Medicine, Hershey, Pennsylvania.

1995c. "The Scholarly Voice and the Personal Voice: Reflexivity in Belief Studies," *Western Folklore* 54, (January, 1995), pp. 57–76.

1995d. "Whose Culture? Whose Body?" *Perspectives from the Humanities*, vol. 7, no. 4, Department of Humanities, Hershey, PA: Penn State College of Medicine.

Hughes, Donna M.
2000. "The 'Natasha' Trade—The Transnational Shadow Market of Trafficking in Women: In the Shadows: Promoting Prosperity or Undermining Stability?" *Journal of International Affairs*, Spring, pp. 1–23.

'Iraqi, Fakhruddin
1982. *Divine Flashes* (Classics of Western Spirituality) written and translated by William C. Chittick and Peter Wilson, with preface by Seyyed Hossein Nasr. Paulist Press Series: Classics of Western Spirituality.

İncirlioğlu, Emine Onaran
1993. "Marriage, Gender Relations and Rural Transformation in Central Anatolia," in Stirling, Paul, ed. 1993. *Culture and Economy: Changes in Turkish Villages*. Huntingdon: The Eothen Press.

Jordan, Rosan A. and Susan Kalcik, eds.
1985. *Women's Folklore, Women's Culture*. Philadelphia: University of Pennsylvania Press.

Jusdanis, Gregory
1991. *Belated Modernity and Aesthetic Culture: Inventing National Literature*. Minneapolis: University of Minnesota Press.

Kağıtçıbaşı, Çiğdem, ed. (with the assistance of Diane Sunar)
1982. *Sex Roles, Family, & Community in Turkey*. Bloomington: Indiana University Turkish Studies.

Kağıtçıbaşı, Çiğdem
1982. "Sex Roles, Value of Children and Fertility in Turkey," in Kağıtçıbaşı, Çiğdem, ed. (with the assistance of Diane Sunar) *Sex Roles,*

Family, & Community in Turkey. Bloomington: Indiana University Turkish Studies.

Kamppinen, Matti
1989. *Cognitive Systems and Cultural Models of Illness: A Study of Two Mestizo Peasant Communities of the Peruvian Amazon*. Helsinki: Academia Scientiarum Fennica.

Kandiyoti, Deniz
1982. "Urban Change and Women's Roles in Turkey: an Overview and Evaluation," in Kağıtçıbaşı, Çiğdem, ed. (with the assistance of Diane Sunar) *Sex Roles, Family, & Community in Turkey*. Bloomington: Indiana University Turkish Studies, pp. 101–120.

Kandiyoti, Deniz and Ay_e Saktanber, eds.
2002. Fragments of Culture: The Everyday of Modern Turkey. Rutgers University Press.

Katz, Richard
1982. *Boiling Energy: Community Healing Among the Kalahari Kung*. Cambridge: Harvard University Press.

Kazancigil, A. and E. Özbudun, eds.
1981. *Atatürk: Founder of a Modern State*. London: C. Hurst & Co.

Kemal, Yashar
1981. *Seagull*. London: William Collins Sons & Co. Ltd. (originally published in Turkey in 1976 as *Al Gözüm Seyrele Salih*. İstanbul: Cem Yayınevi)

Keyder, Çağlar
1993. "The Genesis of Petty Commodity Production in Agriculture." in Stirling, Paul, ed. 1993. *Culture and Economy: Changes in Turkish Villages*. Huntingdon: The Eothen Press.

Khatib-Chalidi, Jane
1992. "Milk Kinship in Shi'ite Islamic Iran." in V. Maher, ed. *The Anthropology of Breast-Feeding: Natural Law or Social Construct?* Oxford: Berg. pp. 109–132.
1995. "Gold Coins and Coffee ROSCAs: Coping with Inflation the Turkish Way in Northern Cyprus" pp. 241–261 in Ardener, Shirley and Sandra Burman, eds. *Money-Go-Rounds: The Importance of Rotating Savings and Credit Associations for Women*. Oxford: Berg Publishers.

King, Charles.
2004. *The Black Sea: A History*. Oxford: Oxford University Press

Kıray, Mübeccel
1982. "Changing Patterns of Patronage: A Study in Structural Change," in Kağıtçıbaşı, Çiğdem, ed. (with the assistance of Diane Sunar) *Sex Roles, Family, & Community in Turkey.* Bloomington: Indiana University Turkish Studies.

Kirshenblatt-Gimblett, Barbara
1988. "Mistaken Dichotomies," *Journal of American Folklo*re 101, pp. 140–155.

Kleinman, Arthur
1975. "Social, Cultural and Historical Themes in the Study of Medicine in Chinese Societies: Problems and Prospects for the Comparative Study of Medicine and Psychiatry," in Arthur Kleinman, Peter Kunstadter, E. Russell Alexander, and James L. Gale, eds. *Medicine in Chinese Cultures: Comparative Studies of Health Care in Chinese and Other Societies.* Washington D.C.: U.S. Department of Health, pp. 589–658.
1980. *Patients and Healers in the Context of Culture: An Exploration of the Borderland between Anthropology, Medicine, and Psychiatry.* Berkeley: University of California Press.

Kohn, Tamara and Rosemary McKechnie, eds.
1999. *Extending the Boundaries of Care: Medical Ethics and Caring Practices.* Oxford: Berg.

Koskoff, Ellen, ed.
1989. *Women and Music in Cross-Cultural Perspective.* Urbana: University of Illinios Press.

Kunstadter, Peter
1975. "The Comparative Anthropological Study of Medical Systems in Society," In Arthur Kleinman, Peter Kunstadter, E. Russell Alexander, and James L. Gale, eds. *Medicine in Chinese Cultures: Comparative Studies of Health Care in Chinese and Other Societies.* Washington D.C.: U.S. Department of Health, pp. 683–695.
1975. "Do Cultural Differences Make Any Difference? Choice Points in Medical Systems Available in Northwestern Thailand," in Arthur Kleinman, Peter Kunstadter, E. Russell Alexander, and James L. Gale, eds. *Medicine in Chinese Cultures: Comparative Studies of Health Care in Chinese and Other Societies.* Washington D.C.: U.S. Department of Health, pp. 351–383.

Laderman, Carol
1983. *Wives and Midwives: Childbirth and Nutrition in Rural Malaysia.* Berkeley: University of California Press.

1987. "The Ambiguity of Symbols in the Structure of Healing," *Social Science and Medicine* vol. 24, no. 4, pp. 293–301.

1988. "Wayward Winds: Malay Archetypes, and Theory of Personality in the Context of Shamanism," *Social Science and Medicine* vol. 27, no. 8, pp. 799–810.

1992. "A Welcoming Soil: Islamic Humoralism on the Malay Peninsula," in Charles Leslie and Allan Young, eds. *Paths to Asian Medical Knowledge.* Berkeley: University of California Press. pp. 257–271.

1996. "The Poetics of Healing in Malay Shamanistic Performances," in C. Laderman and M. Roseman, eds. *The Performance of Healing.* New York: Routledge.

Laderman, Carol and Marina Roseman, eds.
1996. *The Performance of Healing.* New York: Routledge.

Lloyd, Timothy C.
1995. "Folklore, Foodways, and the Supernatural," in Barbara Walker, ed. *Out of the Ordinary: Folklore and the Supernatural.* Logan: Utah State University Press.

MacCallum, F. L.
1943. *The Mevlidi Sherif by Suleyman Chelebi.* London: John Murray.

MacCormack, Carol P., ed.
1982. *Ethnography of Fertility and Birth.* London: Academic Press.

Magnarella, Paul J.
1974. *Tradition and Change in a Turkish Town.* Cambridge, MA: Schenkmann Publ. Co. Inc.

1982. "Civil Violence in Turkey: Its Infrastructural, Social and Cultural Foundations," in Kağıtçıbaşı, Çiğdem, ed. (with the assistance of Diane Sunar) *Sex Roles, Family, & Community in Turkey.* Bloomington: Indiana University Turkish Studies.

1998. *Anatolia's Loom: Studies in Turkish Culture, Society, Politics and Law.* Istanbul: The Isis Press.

Maher, Vanessa, ed.
1992. *The Anthropology of Breast-Feeding: Natural Law or Social Construct?* Oxford: Berg.

Makhlouf, Carla
1979. *Changing Veils: Women and Modernisation in North Yemen.* Austin: University of Texas Press.

Malarek, Victor
2004. *The Natashas: Inside the New Global Sex Trade.* New York: Arcade Publishing.

Maloney, Clarence, ed.
1976. *The Evil Eye.* New York: Columbia University Press.

Manderson, Lenore
2003. "Roasting, Smoking, and Dieting in Response to Birth: Malay Confinement in Cross-Cultural Perspective," in Lauren Dundes, ed. *The Manner Born: Birth Rites in Cross-Cultural Perspective.* Walnut Creek, CA: AltaMira Press, pp. 137-159.

Marcus, George E. and Dick Cushman, eds.
1982. "Ethnographies as Texts," *Annual Review of Anthropology* 11, pp. 25–69.

Marcus, Julie
1992. *A World of Difference: Islam and Gender Hierarchy in Turkey.* London: Zed.

Mardin, Şerif
1962. *The Genesis of Young Ottoman Thought: A Study in the Modernization of Turkish Political Ideas.* Princeton, NJ: Princeton U. Press.
1989. *Religion and Social Change in Modern Turkey: The Case of Bediüzzaman Said Nursi.* Albany: State University of New York Press.

Marsella, Anthony J. and Geoffrey M. White, eds.
1989, reprinted with corrections from 1982. *Cultural Conceptions of Mental Health and Therapy.* Dordrecht: D. Reidel Publishing Co.

Martin, Emily
1992. [1987] *The Woman in the Body: A Cultural Analysis of Reproduction.* second ed. Boston: Beacon Press.

Mazo, Margarita
1994a. "Lament Made Visible: A Study of Paramusical Features in Russian Laments," in *Theme and Variations. Writings on Music in Honor of Rulan Chao Pian.* edited by Bell Yung and Joseph Lam. Harvard University and the University of Hong Kong: 164–212.
1994b. "Wedding Laments in North Russian Villages," in *Music Cultures in Contact.* edited by Margaret Kartomi and Stephen Blum. Basel: Gordon and Breach Science Publishers: 21–40.

Mburu, F. M.
1977. "The Duality of Traditional and Western medicine in Africa: Mystics, Myths and Reality," in Philip Singer, ed. *Traditional Healing: New Science or New Colonialism?* New York: Conch Magazine Ltd. Publishers, pp. 158–185.

McGilvray, D.B.
1982. "Sexual Power and Fertility in Sri Lanka: Batticaloa Tamils and Moors," in Carol P. MacCormack, ed. *Ethnography of Fertility and Birth.* London: Academic Press, pp. 25–73.

Meeker, Michael E.
1971. "The Black Sea Turks: Some Aspects of Their Ethnic and Cultural Background," *International Journal of Middle Eastern Studies*, 2, pp. 318–345.
1976. "Meaning and Society in the Near East: Examples from the Black Sea Turks and the Levantine Arabs (II)," International Journal of Middle East Studies, 7, pp. 383–422.
1996. "Concepts of Person, Family, and State in the District of Of," in Gabriele Rasuly-Paleczek, ed. *Turkish Families in Transition*. Frankfurt am Main: Lang.
2002. *A Nation of Empire: The Ottoman Legacy of Turkish Modernity*. Berkeley: University of California Press.

Mills, Margaret
1985. "Sex Role Reversals, Sex Changes, and Transvestite Disguise in the Oral Tradition of a Conservative Muslim Community in Afghanistan," in Rosan A. Jordan and Susan Kalcik, eds. *Women's Folklore, Women's Culture*. Philadelphia: University of Pennsylvania Press, pp. 187–213.
1990. *Oral Narrative in Afghanistan: The Individual in Tradition*. New York: Garland.
1991. *Rhetorics and Politics in Afghan Traditional Storytelling*. Philadelphia: University of Pennsylvania Press.
1993. "Feminist Theory and the Study of Folklore: A Twenty-Year Trajectory toward Theory," *Western Folklore*, 52, (April, 1993) pp. 173–192.

Minh-ha, Trinh T.
1989. *Woman, Native, Other: Writing Postcoloniality and Feminism*. Bloomington: Indiana University Press.

Minkowski, William L.
1994. "Physician Motives in Banning Medieval Traditional Healers," *Women and Health*, vol. 21 (1), pp. 83–96.

Mitford, Jessica
1992. *The American Way of Birth*. N.Y.: Penguin Group (Dutton).

Morley, Peter and Roy Wallis, eds.
1978. *Culture and Curing: Anthropological Perspectives on Traditional Medical Beliefs and Practices*. London: Peter Owen.

Mulcahy, Joanne B.
1993. " 'How They Knew': Women's Talk about Healing on Kodiak Island, Alaska," in Joan Newlon Radner, ed. *Feminist Messages: Coding in Women's Folk Culture*. Urbana: University of Illinois Press.

Mullen, Patrick B.
1992. *Listening to Old Voices: Folklore, Life Stories, and the Elderly*. Urbana, Illinois: University of Illinois Press.

The National Geographic Magazine
2001. "Deep Black Sea" or "Black Sea Discoveries: Startling Evidence of an Ancient Flood" May Pages: 52–69 Contributor(s): Ballard, Robert D. Author and Olson, Randy Photographer
2002. "Crucible of the Gods" vol 202, no. 3 September, pp. 74–101 Zwingle, Erla, Author and Olson, Randy Photographer.
2004. "Ancient Wrecks Await: Ballard Expedition 2003" May, Volume: v. 205, no. 5 Pages: 112–129 Contributor(s): de Jonge, Peter Author McLain, David Photographer.

Nichter, Mark and Margaret Lock, eds.
2002. *New Horizons in Medical Anthropology: Essays in Honour of Charles Leslie.* London: Routledge.

O'Connor, Bonnie Blair
1995. *Healing Traditions: Alternative Medicine and the Health Professions.* Philadelphia: University of Pennsylvania Press.

Olson, Emelie A.
1982. "Duofocal Family Structure and an Alternative Model of husband-Wife Relationship," in Kağıtçıbaşı, Çiğdem, ed. (with the assistance of Diane Sunar) *Sex Roles, Family, & Community in Turkey.* Bloomington: Indiana University Turkish Studies, pp. 33–72.

Önder, Sylvia Wing
1994. "Dynamic interactions Between Traditional Folk Healing and Clinical Practices on the Black Sea Coast of Turkey." paper presented at the Joint Annual Meeting of the American Folklore Society and the Society for Ethnomusicology, October 19–23, Milwaukee, Wisconsin.
1995. "Negotiating the Turkish National Body: Health Care on the Black Sea Coast," paper presented at the 30th Annual Meeting of the Middle East Studies Association, November 21–24, Providence, Rhode Island.
1996. "Going Home for a Wedding: The Maintenance of local Identity by Black Sea Turks Who Work in Germany," paper presented at the Annual Meeting of the American Folklore Society, October 30 – November 2, Austin, Texas.
2000. "Indigenous Evaluations of Health Care in Turkey," International Institute for the Study of Islam in the Modern World, *ISIM Newsletter*, number 5, Spring, available on-line at (http://isim.leidenuniv.nl/newsletter/5/index.html).

Özbay, Ferhunde
1982. "Women's Education in Rural Turkey," in Kağıtçıbaşı, Çiğdem, ed. (with the assistance of Diane Sunar) *Sex Roles, Family, & Community in Turkey.* Bloomington: Indiana University Turkish Studies.

Özdemir, Adil and Kenneth Frank
2000. *Visible Islam in Modern Turkey.* foreword by Annemarie Schimmel. London: MacMillan Press Ltd.

Pamuk, Orhan
1998. *Benim Adım Kırmızı.* İstanbul: İletişim Yayınları (17. Baskı Eylül, 2001)
2001. *My Name Is Red.* New York: Alfred Knopf.

Paredes, Americo and Richard Bauman, eds.
1972. *Toward New Perspectives in Folklore.* Austin: University of Texas Press.

Peristiany, J.G., ed.
1976. *Mediterranean Family Structures.* Cambridge: Cambridge University Press.

Pierce, Joe
1964. *Life in a Turkish Village.* New York: Holt, Rinehart and Winston.

Radner, Joan Newlon, ed.
1993. *Feminist Messages: Coding in Women's Folk Culture.* Urbana: University of Illinois Press.

Radner, Joan N. and Susan S. Lanser
1993. "Strategies of Coding in Women's Cultures," in Joan Newlon Radner, ed. *Feminist Messages: Coding in Women's Folk Culture.* Urbana: University of Illinois Press.

Ransel, David L.
2000. *Village Mothers: Three Generations of Change in Russia and Tataria.* Bloomington: Indiana University Press.

Rasuly-Paleczek, Gabriele, ed.
1996. *Turkish Families in Transition.* Frankfurt am Main: Lang.

Ridington, Robin
1978. "Metaphor and Meaning: Healing in Dunne-Za," (manuscript) *The Western Canadian Journal of Anthropology* vol. 7, nos. 2,3,4.

Ritchie, Susan
1993. "Ventriloquist Folklore: Who Speaks for Representation?" *Western Folklore* 52 (April, 1993), pp. 365–378.

Robinson, Carol E.
1989. "Coming to Grips with Songs of Power," (manuscript) paper given at S.E.M. Annual Meeting, Nov., 1989.

Romanucci-Ross, Lola, Daniel E. Moerman, and Laurence R. Tancredi, eds.
1997. " 'Medical Anthropology': Convergence of Mind and Experience in the Anthropological Imagination," in Lola Romanucci-Ross, Daniel E. Mo-

erman, and Laurence R. Tancredi, eds. *The Anthropology of Medicine*. Westport, CT: Bergin & Garvey.

Rosaldo, Renato
1989. *Culture and Truth: The Remaking of Social Analysis*. Boston: Beacon Press.

Roseman, Marina
1991. *Healing Sounds from the Malasian Rainforest: Temiar Music and Medicine*. Berkeley: U. of California Press.
1996. "'Pure Products Go Crazy': Rainforest Healing in a Nation-State," in C. Laderman and M. Roseman, eds. *The Performance of Healing*. New York: Routledge.
2002. "Making Sense out of Modernity," in Mark Nichter and Margaret Lock, eds. *New Horizons in Medical Anthropology: Essays in Honour of Charles Leslie*. London: Routledge.

Rumi, Jelaluddin.
1984. *Open Secret: Versions of Rumi* translated by John Moyne and Coleman Barks. Putney, Vermont: Threshold Books. (Rumi lived between 1207–1273)

Rushton, Lucy
1983. "Doves and Magpies: Village Women in the Greek Orthodox Church," in Pat Holden, ed. *Women's Religious Experience*. London: Croom Helm, pp. 57–70.

Said, Edward W.
1978. *Orientalism*. New York: Vintage Books.

Savage, Jan
1999. "Relative Strangers: Caring for Patients as the Expression of Nurses' Moral/Political Voice," in Tamara Kohn and Rosemary McKechnie, eds. *Extending the Boundaries of Care: Medical Ethics and Caring Practices*. Oxford: Berg.

Scheper-Hughes, Nancy
1992 (paperback, 1993). *Death Without Weeping: The Violence of Everyday Life in Brazil*. Berkeley: University of California Press.

Schick, Irvin Cemil and Ertu_rul Ahmet Tonak, eds.
1987. *Turkey in Transition: New Perspectives*. Oxford: Oxford University Press.

Schiffauer, Werner
1993. "Peasants Without Pride: Migration, Domestic Cycle and Perception of Time," in Stirling, Paul, ed. 1993. *Culture and Economy: Changes in Turkish Villages*. Huntingdon: The Eothen Press.

Schubel, Vernon James
1993. *Religious Performance in Contemporary Islam: Shi'i Devotional Rituals in South Asia*. Columbia: University of South Carolina Press.

Sered, Susan Starr
1992. *Women as Ritual Experts: The Religious Lives of Elderly Jewish Women in Jerusalem*. N.Y.: Oxford U. Press.

Shahshahani, Soheila
1986. "Women Whisper, Men Kill: A Case Study of the Mamasani Pastoral Nomads of Iran," in Leela Dube, Eleanor Leacock, and Shirley Ardener, eds. *Visibility and Power: Essays on Women in Society and Development*. Delhi: Oxford University Press.

Shankland, David
1999. *Islam and Society in Turkey*. Huntingdon: The Eothen Press.

Shuman, Amy
1986. *Storytelling Rights: The Uses of Oral and Written Texts by Urban Adolescents*. Cambridge: Cambridge University Press.
1993. "Gender and Genre" in Susan Tower Hollis, Linda Pershing, and M. Jane Young, eds. *Feminist Theory and the Study of Folklore*. Urbana: University of Illinois Press.

Simonian, Hovann H.
2004. "History and Identity among the Hemshin," *ISIM Newsletter*, volume 14, June, 2004, Leiden: International Institute for the Study of Islam in the Modern World, pp. 24–25.

Simons, Ronald C. and Charles C. Hughes, eds.
1985. *The Culture-Bound Syndromes*. Hingham, MA: Kluwer Academis Publishers.

Snow, Loudell F.
1974. "Folk Medical Beliefs and Their Implications for Care of Patients," *Annals of Internal Medicine* 81, pp. 82–96.
1975. "The Religious Component in Southern Folk Medicine," in Philip Singer, ed. *Traditional Healing: New Science or New Colonialism?* New York: Conch Magazine Ltd. Publishers, pp. 26–51.
1998. *Walkin' over Medicine*. Detroit: Wayne State University Press. [1993]

Sonyel, Salahi R.
1993. *Minorities and the Destruction of the Ottoman Empire*. Ankara: Turkish Historical Society Printing House.

Spivak, Gayatri Chakravorty
1988. "Can the Subaltern Speak?" in Nelson and Grossburg, eds. *Marxism and the Interpretation of Culture*. Springfield: University of Illinois Press.
1990. *The Post-Colonial Critic: Interviews, Strategies, Dialogues*. edited by Sarah Harasym. N.Y.: Routledge.

Spooner, Brian
1975. "Arabs and Iran: The Evil Eye in the Middle East," in Charles Maloney, ed. *The Evil Eye*. New York: Columbia University Press.

Stewart, Kathleen
1996. *A Space on the Side of the Road: Cultural Poetics in an "Other" America*. Princeton: Princeton University Press.

Stirling, Paul
1965. *Turkish Village*. London: Weidenfeld and Nicolson.
1993. "Growth and Changes: Speed, Scale, Complexity," in his, ed. *Culture and Economy: Changes in Turkish Villages*. Huntingdon: The Eothen Press.

Stirling, Paul, ed.
1993a. *Culture and Economy: Changes in Turkish Villages*. Huntingdon: The Eothen Press.

Stirling, Paul and Emine Onaran İncirlioğlu
1996. "Choosing Spouses: Villagers, Migrants, Kinship and Time," in Gabriele Rasuly-Paleczek, ed. *Turkish Families in Transition*. Frankfurt am Main: Lang.

Stokes, Martin
1992. *The Arabesk Debate: Music and Musicians in Modern Turkey*. Oxford: Clarendon Press.
1993. "Hazelnuts and Lutes: Perceptions of Change in a Black Sea Valley," in Paul Stirling, ed. *Culture and Economy: Changes in Turkish Villages*. Huntingdon: The Eothen Press.

Stoller, Paul
1989. *The Taste of Ethnographic Things: The Senses in Anthropology*. Philadelphia: University of Pennsylvania Press.
1996. "Sounds and Things: Pulsations of Power in Songhay," in C. Laderman and M. Roseman, eds. *The Performance of Healing*. New York: Routledge.

Stone, Frank A.
1973. *The Rub of Cultures in Modern Turkey: Literary Views of Education*. Bloomington: Indiana University Press.

Strasser, Sabine and Ruth Kronsteiner
1993. "Impure or Fertile? Two Essays on the Crossing of Frontiers through Anthropology and Feminism: 'Women in the Field—Reflections on a

Never-Ending Journey,' and 'The Impurity of Research and Female Fertility' " (Translated by Michael Gingrich) in Teresa del Valle, ed. *Gendered Anthropology*. London: Routledge, pp. 162–177.

Tapper, Nancy
1983. "Gender and Religion in a Turkish Town: A Comparison of Two Types of Formal Women's Gatherings," in Pat Holden, ed. *Women's Religious Experience*. London: Croom Helm, pp. 71–88.
1991. *Bartered Brides: Politics, Gender, and Marriage in an Afghan Tribal Society*. Cambridge: Cambridge U. Press.

Tapper, Richard, ed.
1991. *Islam in Modern Turkey: Religion, Politics and Literature in a Secular State*. London: I.B. Tauris & Co. Ltd.

Tapper, Nancy and Richard Tapper
1987. "The Birth of the Prophet: Ritual and Gender in Turkish Islam." *Man: The Journal of the Royal Anthropological Institute*, New Series, Vol. 22, No. 1, March, pp. 69–92.

Tapper, Richard and Nancy Tapper
1991. "Religion, Education and Continuity in a Provincial Town," in Richard Tapper, *Islam in Modern Turkey: Religion, Politics and Literature in a Secular State*. London: I.B. Tauris & Co. Ltd.

Tekeli, Şirin, ed.
1995. *Women in Modern Turkish Society*. London: Zed Books.

Tual, Anny
1986. "Speech and Silence: Women in Iran," in Leela Dube, Eleanor Leacock, and Shirley Ardener, eds. *Visibility and Power: Essays on Women in Society and Development*. Delhi: Oxford University Press.

Turner, Kay and Suzanne Seriff
1993. " 'Giving an Altar to St. Joseph': A Feminist Perpective on a Patronal Feast" in Susan Tower Hollis, Linda Pershing, and M. Jane Young, eds. *Feminist Theory and the Study of Folklore*. Urbana: University of Illinois Press.

Turner, Victor
1986. *The Anthropology of Performance*. New York: PAJ Publications.

Van Maanen, John
1986. *Tales of the Field: On Writing Ethnography*. Chicago: University of Chicago Press.

Waldman, Marilyn Robinson, Artemis Leontis, and Müge Galin, eds.
1992. *Understanding Women: The Challenge of Cross-Cultural Perspectives*. Columbus, OH: Papers in Comparative Studies, no. 7.

Walker, Barbara, ed.
1995. *Out of the Ordinary: Folklore and the Supernatural*. Logan: Utah State University Press.

Webber, Sabra J.
1991. *Romancing the Real: Folklore and Ethnographic Representation in North Africa*. Philadelphia: University of Pennsylvania Press.

White, Evelyn C., ed.
1990. *The Blackwomen's Health Book: Speaking for Ourselves*. Seattle, Washington: Seal Press.

White, Jenny B.
1994. *Money Makes Us Relatives: Women's Labor in Urban Turkey*. Austin: University of Texas Press.
2002. *Islamist Mobilization in Turkey: A Study in Vernacular Politics*. Seattle: University of Washington Press.

Whitehead, Tony Larry and Mary Ellen Conaway, eds.
1986. *Self, Sex, and Gender in Cross-Cultural Fieldwork*. Urbana: University of Illinois Press.

Wilson, William A.
1973. "Herder, Folklore, and Romantic Nationalism," *Journal of Popular Culture*, 6, pp. 819–835.

Wolbert, Barbara
1996. "The Reception Day—A Key to Migrant's Reintegration," in Gabriel Rasuly-Paleczek, *Turkish Families in Transition*. Frankfurt am Main: Lang, pp. 186–215.

Wolf, Margery
1992. *A Thrice-Told Tale: Feminism, Postmodernism, and Ethnographic Responsibility*. Stanford, CA: Stanford U. Press.

Yalçın-Heckmann, Lale
1993. "Sheep and Money: Pastoral Production at the Frontiers," in Stirling, Paul, ed. *Culture and Economy: Changes in Turkish Villages*. Huntingdon: The Eothen Press.

Yenal, Hatice Deniz
2000. "Weaving a market: The informal economy and gender in a transnational trade network between Turkey and the former Soviet Union." Ph.D. Thesis, State University of New York: Binghamton.

Yoder, Don.
1965. "Official Religion versus Folk Religion," *Pennsylvania Folklore*, pp. 36–52.

1972. "Folk Medicine." in Richard Dorson, ed. *Folklore and Folklife: An Introduction.* Chicago: U. of Chicago Press, pp. 191–215.

1974. "Toward a Definition of Folk Religion," *Western Folklore* 33, pp. 2–15.

Young, Katherine and Barbara A. Babcock, guest eds.
1993. "Bodylore." *Journal of American Folklore* 107, no. 423.

Young, M. Jane and Kay Turner
1993. "Challenging the Canon: Folklore Theory Reconsidered from Feminist Perspectives," in Susan Tower Hollis, Linda Pershing, and M. Jane Young, eds. *Feminist Theory and the Study of Folklore.* Urbana: University of Illinois Press.

Zurcher, Erik J.
1993. *Turkey: A Modern History.* London: I.B. Tauris & Co. Ltd.

Books in Turkish

Mehmet Bilgin's *Doğu Karadeniz: Tarih, Kültür, İnsan, The Eastern Black Sea: History, Culture, Peoples* (Trabzon: Serander Yayınları, 2000), an ethnohistory covering the broad recorded history of the Black Sea coast of Asia Minor, with an emphasis on Trabzon. *Türkiye'nin Etnik Yapısı: Halkımızın Kökenleri ve Gerçekleri/ Turkey's Ethnic Composition: Our People's Roots and Realities*, by Ali Tayyar Önder (İstanbul: Pozitif, 4th printing, 2002), includes short sections about the Çerkez (Circassian), Laz, and Gürcü (Georgian) ethnicities, although most of the book evaluates the identities of various Kurdish and Alevi forms of identification. İbrahim Tellioğlu's *Osmanlı Hakimiyetine Kadar Doğu Karadeniz'de Türkler/ Turks in the Eastern Black Sea until the Ottman Rule* (Trabzon: Serander Yayıncılık, 2004)

Abadan-Unat, Nermin, Deniz Kandiyoti and Mübeccel B. Kiray, eds.
1979. *Türk Toplumunda Kadın.* Ankara: Turkish Social Science Association.

Arısan, Kâzım
1992. "Geçen Yüzyılda İstanbul'da Ebeler ve Doğum," *Türk Tıp Tarihi Kongresi: Kongreye Sunulan Bildiriler.* Ankara: Türk Tarih Kurumu Basımevi, pp. 253–259.

Baykurt, Fakir
2002. (fourth edition, first edition 1997) *Yarım Ekmek.* İstanbul: Adam Yayınları. (a novel "Half a Loaf" about rural Turkish workers settling in Germany)

Belge, Murat
1983. *Tarihten Güncelliğe.* İstanbul: Alan Yayıncılık 3.

Çakır, Ruşen
1991. *Ayet ve Slogan: Türkiye'de İslami Oluşumlar*. third printing. İstanbul: Metis Yayınları.

Çavdar, C. Ayşenur
1992. "Günümüz Türk Halk Hekimliğinde İslam Öncesi Türk Tıbbının İzleri," *Türk Tıp Tarihi Kongresi: Kongreye Sunulan Bildiriler*. Ankara: Türk Tarih Kurumu Basımevi, pp. 253–259.

Çavuşoğlu, Mehmed
1978. "16. Yüzyılda Yaşamış bir Kadın Şair Nisayi." *Tarih Enstitüsü Dergisi* IX: 405–416, translation by Walter Andrews.

Eren, Nevzat and Zafer Öztek, eds.
1993. *Sağlık Ocağı Yönetimi*. 6th ed. Ankara: Palme Yayınları.

Gündüz, Ali
2002. *Hemşinliler: Dil - Tarih - Kültür*. Ankara: Yeni Gözde Matbaası. (A Study of the Hemşin, with chapters on language, history, and culture; includes notes on the Georgians and Laz of the Eastern Black Sea region)

Gürbilek, Nurdan
1991. *Vitrinde Yaşamak: 1980'lerin Kültürel İklimi*, second edition. Istanbul: Metis Yayınları.

Kalafat, Yaşar
1995. *Doğu Anadolu'da Eski Türk İnançlarının İzleri*. Ankara: Atatürk Kültür Merkezi Yayınları, Sayı No: 112.

Mihri Hatun. *Divan / Mikhri-Khatun* ; kriticheskii tekst i vstupitelnaia statia E.I. Mashtakovoi, Moskva: Izd-vo "Nauka", 1967 #23, p. 105–106, provided by Walter Andrews.

Seyman, Yaşar
2002. *Fındık Çiçek Açınca*. İstanbul: Sel Yayıncılık. (an account of the strike and march on Ankara by women hazelnut factory workers from fourteen towns along the Black Sea Coast in February of 1993)

Sosyalizm ve Toplumsal Mücadeleler Ansiklopedisi
1988. Volumes 6 and 7. İstanbul: İletişim Yayınları. Article on Fatsa Olayları

Terzioğlu, Arslan and Erwin Lucius, eds.
1993. *Türk Tıbbının Batılaşması*. İstanbul: Arkeoloji ve Sanat Yayınları, Kanaat Matbaası.

List of Illustrations

INDEX

fig. refers to illustrations, n refers to footnotes, informants and authors are listed in Name Index.

Name Index

Quotation marks indicate the pseudonym of an ethnographic informant.

301